AIDS: Facts and Issues

AIDS

Facts and Issues

Victor Gong, M.D. and
Norman Rudnick, Editors

Foreword by Congressman Ted Weiss

Rutgers University Press
New Brunswick and London

Second Printing, 1987

Library of Congress Cataloging-in-Publication Data

AIDS, facts and issues.

  Bibliography: p.
  Includes index.
  1. AIDS (Disease) I. Gong, Victor, 1956–
II. Rudnick, Norman. [DNLM: 1. Acquired Immunodeficiency
Syndrome. WD 308 A28824]
RC607.A26A3464   1986   616.97'92   86-20415
ISBN 0-8135-1201-8
ISBN 0-8135-1201-6 (pbk.)

British Cataloging-in-Publication Information Available.

First published by Rutgers University Press in 1985 as *Understanding Aids*. This
edition is a completely revised, expanded, and updated version of the original
publication.

To my parents,
Alfred Kar Gong and Shun Yee Gong,
for without their love and support
this book could not have been written,
and to the memory of Dr. Peter Ho.

Victor Gong

With love to my wife Selma
and my sons Evan and Paul.

Norman Rudnick

Names of the AIDS Virus

American discoverers called it human T-lymphotropic virus type III (HTLV-III). It was third in a series originally called human T-cell leukemia viruses. French discoverers called it lymphadenopathy-associated virus (LAV). Other American researchers named the virus they isolated AIDS-associated retrovirus (ARV). This book uses the most common designation, HTLV-III/LAV. However, a name likely to come into favor is human immune deficiency virus (HIV), recommended by the International Committee on Nomenclature of Viruses.

Contents

x   Contents

Foreword

Since the recognition of AIDS in 1981, the Public Health Service (PHS) has reported over 25,000 cases in the United States and estimates another 100,000 cases of ARC (AIDS-related complex). More than 12,000 men, women, and children have already died from the disease, and current projections indicate this number could climb to between 140,000 and 200,000 in the next five years. While these statistics are staggering, they cannot begin to convey the overwhelming human tragedy surrounding this killer. What they do demonstrate is that the AIDS epidemic is a national crisis that demands federal leadership.

The House Intergovernmental Relations and Human Resources Subcommittee has been investigating the federal response to the AIDS epidemic for over three years. What has become all too clear from this review is the continued reluctance of the current administration to deal adequately with this crisis on a number of levels. Although the Reagan administration has called AIDS this nation's "number one health priority," the agencies and programs that must lead the fight against the disease have been continuously underfunded, making budgetary constraints the major problem at the federal level. Each year since 1981, Congress has had not only to overcome the unwillingness of the Administration to request the level of funds that PHS scientists require but actually to battle proposed cutbacks.

In past health crises, it was public health officials who exerted leadership in the fight for action and funds. This has not been the case with AIDS. The Department of Health and Human Services (HHS) did not request additional AIDS funds until two years into the epidemic. Instead, the agency opted to transfer funds from other valuable health programs. Whether due to stigmatization of the groups chiefly at risk for AIDS—gay men and intravenous (IV)-drug abusers—or to the Administration's policy of overall reduction of the federal role in health matters, it has become clear that the consistently expressed judgment of PHS scientists of the need for additional AIDS money has been replaced by the judment of the Office of Management and Budget. This is no way for the federal government to handle its "number one health priority."

Until recently, the PHS had spent very little on public education and risk reduction for AIDS. These efforts had been left almost exclusively to local organizations, which did a remarkably good job. Had the federal government launched early public education and prevention efforts, much of the current panic surrounding AIDS could have been avoided. To achieve this end, somewhat belatedly, in June 1986 the PHS issued a report from a conference held to develop a plan for the prevention and control of AIDS. The report stated grim projections for AIDS incidence in the next five years and discussed long overdue programs for developing therapeutics and vaccines, public health control measures, education and risk reduction, preventing transmission by sexual practices and IV-drug abuse, and eliminating the contamination of blood and blood products. This is exactly the sort of coordination needed to fight AIDS. The report, however, failed to indicate how these programs will be funded and implemented. In view of the ominous forecast for this epidemic, it is critical that such programs be put into effect as expeditiously as humanly possible.

In addition, research in AIDS treatment has not been given a high priority. For years private researchers have been requesting grants to fund clinical trials to test drugs. The grant review process has been tragically slow, and, until recently, even the National Institutes of Health (NIH) had tested drugs on only a very small number of patients. In June of this year, HHS announced the development of fourteen federally funded Drug Treatment Evaluation Units. This program will receive $20 million a year for the next five years, a total of $100 million. While these long overdue Units will be centers of important research and testing of AIDS drugs that have shown some promise, they have been described by one noted private researcher as only a "drop in the bucket."

The burden of providing care and services to people who now have AIDS has been left entirely to state and local governments and community organizations. However, this country's health-care system is simply not equipped to handle the enormous drain that caring for AIDS patients places on funding, staff, and facilities. Individuals and local health-care delivery systems are already facing catastrophic costs. As case loads continue to grow, which they are doing at a staggering rate, local health-care organizations will demand federal intervention.

The problems with our health-care delivery system are not limited to AIDS and certainly have no simple solutions. I have introduced several bills designed to alleviate some of the burden imposed on individuals and health-care providers: one to set up a $60-million emergency fund for health care and services, another to waive the two-year Medicare waiting period for those receiving Social Security disability income checks, and a third, with Congressman Henry Waxman, an important leader in the fight against AIDS, to allow for home health care for persons with AIDS. As we progress further into the AIDS epidemic, the Administration will have to face head on the issue of health costs.

A recent development at the Justice Department will seriously hamper efforts by the PHS to halt the spread of AIDS. In response to an inquiry from HHS about the application of federal antidiscrimination laws to persons with AIDS, the Justice Department issued an opinion ruling that such people would not have the discrimination protections afforded other disabled persons. The decision, in effect, downplayed the medical opinion repeatedly endorsed by the PHS that AIDS is not transmitted by casual contact and allowed the irrational fear of getting AIDS in the workplace to be used as the legal basis for discriminating against persons with AIDS or ARC. The Justice Department's ruling, in a sense, pits one federal agency against another. It represents a major setback in the public health education efforts that the federal government is just beginning to fund, efforts designed to ensure that persons with AIDS are not subject to unfair discrimination. It could also undermine voluntary AIDS testing, now under way across the country, which can alert infected individuals and help reduce transmission.

These problems within the federal government have been compounded by actions of some members of Congress and others. Their proposals of laws that would, for example, prohibit students with AIDS from attending public schools or forbid persons with AIDS from holding certain jobs, seem to reflect social and political prejudices rather than a genuine understanding of the disease. Such proposals divert attention from the real issues of research, treatment, public education, health-care costs, and civil rights. They distort the medical and scientific evidence and PHS guidelines, frighten and mislead the public, and make it harder to implement programs to provide accurate information about AIDS.

Despite the poor federal response to this tragic epidemic, through congressional insistence AIDS funding *has* increased from $5.5 million in 1982 to $244 million for 1986. Also, although the president proposed cutting the budget for AIDS to $213 million for fiscal year 1987, the PHS requested much higher amounts—$351 million for fiscal year 1987 and $471 million for fiscal year 1988. (As of July 1986 the secretary of HHS had not yet agreed to this request.) Among other things, this money would be used for health education and risk reduction programs, development of a vaccine, drug development and testing, studies of the prevalence of AIDS in heterosexuals, AIDS in children, the effect of AIDS on the central nervous system, and the possible link between alcohol and drugs and susceptibility to AIDS. This PHS request may reflect a growing awareness among federal officials of the urgent need for a well-coordinated, efficient, and sufficiently funded program to fight this deadly disease.

The PHS has issued ominous projections of an increased incidence of AIDS, ARC, and infection with the AIDS virus. The cumulative total of AIDS cases is expected to rise to more than 270,000 in the next five years, and the number of deaths by 1991 to more than 140,000. According to PHS statistics, between 1986 and 1991 heterosexual cases will rise from 1,100 to about 7,000, with a dramatic increase in the number of cases outside New York City and

San Francisco, the current areas of highest AIDS incidence. If these projections are at all accurate, the pressures on the federal government to deal effectively with the crisis are going to be enormous. Through the efforts of Congress, the Administration has become better prepared, in terms of funding, organization, and communication, to fight the battle against AIDS. But a truly effective battle can be fought only if every available resource is mobilized and every possible effort made to develop and improve programs for education, risk reduction, drug research, and treatment.

AIDS: Facts and Issues is a comprehensive guide to the numerous problems surrounding this killer. It offers a broad outlook by examining a range of topics raised by AIDS and by providing focused studies by recognized experts of many complicated issues. It is a significant contribution to the public education efforts that must be pursued at every level of our government, schools, and health-care system.

It is my hope that this book will promote an understanding of these issues and an appreciation of the seriousness of the human devastation brought on by the AIDS epidemic. Armed with such understanding and appreciation, we can truly begin to treat AIDS as "our number one health priority" and take the necessary steps to assemble our resources and win this battle.

CONGRESSMAN TED WEISS, 17th District, New York,
Chairman, Subcommittee on Intergovernmental Relations and
Human Resources,
U.S. House of Representatives

Acknowledgments

We would like to express deep appreciation to the many friends and colleagues who provided invaluable assistance during the preparation of this book. Thanks go to Ms. Ginna Briggs, Lillian Gong, Joseph Lee, Evelyn Gong, Tina Green, Kathy Johnson, Joan-Cecelia Williams, Rose Mary Ryan, Mary Beth Thompson, Janet Netzke, Linda Masterson, Rose Marie Latronica, and Dr. Melvin Weinstein. Special thanks to Rutgers University Press, Karen Reeds, Kenneth Arnold, Barbara Tanz, and Lucille Engel.

One The Twentieth-Century Enigma

1   Facts and Fallacies: An AIDS Overview

VICTOR GONG

AIDS was first reported in 1981 as a unique and newly recognized syndrome characterized by a breakdown of the body's immune system and consequent vulnerability to infections healthy people ordinarily are able to fight off. Since its initial description AIDS has become a major public health problem in the United States and appears to forebode an equally challenging dilemma abroad. AIDS undoubtedly ranks as one of the most serious epidemics to confront modern medicine and is now a commonly encountered clinical problem, especially in large cities.

AIDS has received vast media coverage. Everyday we either read or hear something about the dreaded disease. However, the information conveyed is often incomplete, taken out of context, tainted by social prejudice, or premature in inciting optimism (for example, about a new drug that is merely being tested). It is clear that, as AIDS has received greater media and public attention, the need to understand the disease has only increased. Everyone "knows" something about AIDS, but many essential facts are not yet common knowledge. While there is still much to be learned about AIDS, the enormous amount of information amassed during the past five years has helped physicians, researchers, politicians, and others in battling this major public health dilemma. However, the public continues to fear AIDS out of proportion to the facts, which emphasizes the need for reliable information. This chapter will highlight the known facts and distinguish them from fears and fallacies.

DEFINING THE SYNDROME

AIDS, an acronym for acquired immune deficiency syndrome, is an impairment of the body's ability to fight disease. It leaves the affected individual vulnerable to illnesses that a healthy immune system might overcome. The name appropriately defines the condition. It is acquired, that is, not inherited but associated with the environment. Immune refers to the body's natural system of defense against disease, while deficiency indicates that the system is not functioning normally. Syndrome means a group of particular signs and symptoms that occur together and characterize a disorder.

AIDS patients are susceptible to diseases called opportunistic infections. These are illnesses due to organisms commonly found in the environment and harmful only to individuals with a weakened immune system. At first, AIDS patients feel as though they may have a cold, the flu, or some other viral illness. Early symptoms are usually benign and inconspicuous but may include fatigue, loss of appetite, fever, night sweats, swollen glands (enlarged lymph nodes) in the neck, armpits, or groin, unexplained weight loss, diarrhea, persistent cough, and various skin lesions. However, the symptoms may persist for months or worsen as opportunistic diseases exploit the body's collapsed defenses. Many (52 percent) develop an unusual pneumonia caused by the protozoan *Pneumocystis carinii*. Another third exhibit a rare cancer of the skin, Kaposi's sarcoma (KS), or contract one of many opportunistic diseases caused by fungi (yeasts), viruses, bacteria, and protozoans.

ETIOLOGY (CAUSE)

AIDS is believed to be caused by a virus belonging to the retrovirus family, viruses composed of genetic material called RNA (ribonucleic acid) instead of the more common DNA (deoxyribonucleic acid) found in most living things. Different investigators have given different names to the virus, but all appear to be the same or close members of the same family. In the United States it is termed human T-lymphotrhopic virus type III (HTLV-III) or AIDS-associated retrovirus (ARV), and in Europe it is called lymphadenopathy-associated virus (LAV). The common name is now HTLV-III/LAV. The virus has been isolated from body fluids (table 1). Infection with

TABLE 1. SOURCES OF THE AIDS VIRUS, HTLV-III/LAV

Blood	Breast milk
Semen	Vaginal/cervical secretions
Saliva	Spinal fluid
Urine	Lymph nodes
Tears	Bone marrow

this virus does not necessarily mean the inevitable development of full-blown AIDS. In fact, most infected persons remain in good health, while others experience a wide range of clinical diseases of varying severity.

AIDS TRANSMISSION

AIDS is spread by sexual contact, intravenous-drug use with contaminated needles or syringes, and, less commonly, through transfused infected blood or blood products, and from an infected mother to her baby in the womb or during birth. The virus is most commonly transmitted by an activity that exposes mucous membranes or the blood stream to infected blood or semen. Nevertheless, HTLV-III/LAV is a fragile virus outside the human body and is easily killed with soap, alcohol, hydrogen peroxide, or Clorox bleach solution.

AIDS is not an easy disease to contract. Unfounded fear that it can be acquired by casual contact has created unnecessary public hysteria. You cannot get AIDS by touching, hugging, shaking hands, or breathing the air near someone who is infected. Despite the presence of HTLV-III/LAV in the saliva and tears of AIDS patients, these are unlikely vehicles of transmission, and no such cases have ever been documented. However, deep kissing and prolonged swallowing of an infected partner's saliva may be risky and should be discouraged.

Even among health-care workers who have accidentally stuck themselves with needles and instruments contaminated with body fluids from AIDS patients, fewer than 1 percent have shown evidence of infection. None has developed AIDS to date. Studies of 619 household contacts of AIDS patients revealed no evidence of HTLV-III/LAV infection.

RISK GROUPS

The number of reported cases of AIDS in the United States now exceeds 22,000, and another 1–2 million are estimated to be infected with the AIDS virus. Most AIDS patients have been homosexual or bisexual men (73 percent) or intravenous-drug abusers (17 percent). Hemophiliacs requiring Factor VIII (a blood product that helps clotting) and blood transfusion recipients (prior to 1985) account for 1 percent and 2 percent, respectively. The advent of new techniques in preparing Factor VIII have eliminated the AIDS virus from this source. The screening of all blood products for antibodies to HTLV-III/LAV has virtually ensured an untainted American blood supply. Infants born to mothers with AIDS or known to have antibodies to the AIDS virus account for another 1 percent. Although exposure is usually before or during birth, some of the babies were infected by blood transfusions.

AIDS presents special problems for pregnant women. A newborn of an infected mother has about a 50 percent chance of contracting the disease, and each successive pregnancy increases the likelihood of transmitting the disease. The stress of pregnancy can also convert an asymptomatic infection in the mother into full-blown AIDS.

Sexual partners of members of a high-risk group are also at great risk. Although a small number of cases (about 5 percent) have been reported with no apparent relation to known risk factors, researchers believe that they probably were infected by sexual contact or had the virus introduced into their bloodstream.

DIAGNOSING AIDS

When should one suspect AIDS? AIDS should be suspected in patients under the age of 60 who develop recurrent or unusual infections under the circumstances summarized in table 2. Such patients usually appear emaciated and have a history of prolonged (3 months or more) fevers, night sweats, diarrhea, skin rash, and generalized swollen glands. Their personal histories may include homosexuality or bisexuality, intravenous-drug abuse, hemophilia, blood products transfusion, or sexual contact with another AIDS patient. (A child of a risk-group parent is also susceptible.) They are also free of other known causes of immunodeficiency, such as

TABLE 2. CLINICAL PROFILE OF AIDS PATIENTS

Age

Under 60

Personal Description

Homosexual and bisexual males
Intravenous-drug abusers
Hemophiliacs
Recipients of blood product transfusions
Sexual partners of patients with AIDS
Children of parent(s) with AIDS

Medical History

No previous diseases or drugs (cancers, chemotherapy, steroids, malnutrition, recent viral illnesses) that might weaken immunity

Symptoms

Night sweats
Prolonged fevers
Severe weight loss
Persistent diarrhea
Skin rash
Persistent cough
Shortness of breath

Signs

Generalized swollen glands
Emaciation
Blue or purple-brown spots on the body, especially legs and arms
Prolonged pneumonia
Oral thrush

Infections and Cancers (See Tables 3 and 4)

Laboratory Data

Tissue biopsy, sputum, blood, urine, etc., confirming opportunistic infection or cancer
Low (less than 1) helper/suppressor T-cell ratio

TABLE 2 (continued)

Abnormal results in immunologic skin tests
Unexplained anemia (low blood count)
Subnormal white blood count
Subnormal platelet count
Increased immunoglobulins
Positive HTLV-III/LAV antibody test result

cancers, malnutrition, and treatments with steroids, radiation, or anticancer drugs, and have not had a recent viral illness such as measles or mumps.

The Centers for Disease Control (CDC) in Atlanta, Georgia, has proposed strict surveillance guidelines for physicians for the diagnosis of AIDS. Such guidelines allow the CDC to obtain accurate data to detect disease patterns and monitor trends. The guidelines include characteristic infections (table 3) and/or cancers like Kaposi's sarcoma (table 4). These are considered "markers" of AIDS, indicative of and specific for an underlying immune defect. The symptoms of these otherwise rare diseases are often the first signals of the development of AIDS. Laboratory tests may also show evidence of a weakened immune state.

In June 1985 the CDC revised its original surveillance definition of AIDS to include cases that test positive for HTLV-III/LAV antibody or the virus itself, and the following additional criteria: (1) widespread histoplasmosis (a fungal infection), (2) isoporiasis causing chronic diarrhea, (3) candidiasis involving the lung, (4) non-Hodgkin's lymphoma, (5) Kaposi's sarcoma in patients no more than 60 years old. All patients diagnosed with AIDS must have detectable antibodies to HTLV-III/LAV and either a low number of helper T cells or a low ratio of helper-to-suppressor T cells. The CDC also issued a special surveillance definition for pediatric cases.

HTLV-III/LAV ANTIBODY TEST

A test for antibodies against HTLV-III/LAV (called ELISA, an acronym for enzyme-linked immunosorbent assay) is now widely used to screen blood for transfusions. It is also being used, with more controversy, to see who has been exposed to AIDS. It is important to

TABLE 3.   INFECTIONS INDICATIVE OF AIDS

Clinical Presentation	Causative Organism
Pneumonia (PCP)	*Pneumocystis carinii*
Enterocolitis	*Cryptosporidium*
Mucosal and skin lesions	Herpes simplex
Esophagitis	*Candida albicans*
	Herpes simplex
	Cytomegalovirus
Other pneumonias, meningitis,	*Toxoplasma gondii*
encephalitis (brain infection)	*Aspergillus*
	Cryptococcus neoformans
	Candida albicans
	Cytomegalovirus
	Nocardia
	Strongyloides
	Atypical *Mycobacterium*
Progressive multifocal	Papovavirus (J-C virus)
leukoencephalopathy (brain	
infection)	

TABLE 4.   CANCERS ASSOCIATED WITH AIDS

Kaposi's sarcoma	Cancer of the oropharynx (mouth)
Non-Hodgkin's lymphomas	Hepatocellular (liver) cancer
Hodgkin's disease	Chronic lymphocytic leukemia
Burkitt's lymphoma	Lung cancer (adenosquamous type)

realize that a positive test result is not an automatic indication of disease. The ELISA test does detect antibodies to the AIDS virus, produced by white blood cells one to two months after exposure. These antibodies are ineffective in destroying the AIDS virus, but their presence in the blood does not necessarily mean that a person has AIDS, will eventually come down with AIDS, or still carries the AIDS virus.

The ELISA test has been proven to be reproducible, specific, and sensitive, but no test is perfect. Therefore, any blood that tests positive on the ELISA test is tested again. If the result is still positive, the blood is subjected to an additional, complex test called the Western blot. If all three results are positive, they are taken as confirmation of exposure to the AIDS virus. A negative result, unfortunately, does not guarantee freedom from the virus. Antibodies may not yet have developed if exposure to the virus was recent.

The test has other inherent limitations. A small number of blood donors, usually people who have received blood transfusions or women who have had several pregnancies, may have a false-positive reaction to the ELISA test (that is, a flaw in the test makes it indicate antibodies to the AIDS virus that are not really present). However, these donors do test negative on the Western blot test. Even more serious are false negatives, indications that antibodies are absent when an individual is actually harboring the AIDS virus.

Despite these limitations, the HTLV-III/LAV antibody test is providing important information to medical investigators. AIDS appears to be considerably more widespread than was thought. Large numbers of asymptomatic homosexuals, intravenous-drug abusers, and hemophiliacs have antibodies to the AIDS virus in their blood but show no symptoms of AIDS. This means that many people have been infected without having the classic symptoms.

Extrapolating from confirmed test results, investigators estimate that possibly 2 million Americans may have antibodies to the AIDS virus in their blood. To repeat, a positive blood test result generally indicates exposure to the virus. It does not tell whether a person still has the virus or will definitely develop AIDS. In fact, most will not develop overt AIDS. At present, researchers cannot say which are immune to the disease, which are "carriers," and which will eventually develop AIDS.

SPECTRUM OF HTLV-III/LAV DISEASES

Only recently have researchers appreciated the responsibility of HTLV-III/LAV for multiple diseases and stages of infection. The term AIDS has been misapplied to represent the entire spectrum of HTLV-III/LAV diseases. AIDS is the end stage, the most devastating part of a wide range of HTLV-III/LAV infections.

This broad range of disease states is not unique to HTLV-III/LAV. For example, when any susceptible host is exposed to an infectious source, the response may vary widely. At one extreme is infection that results in death; at the other extreme is hidden or asymptomatic infection; in between are severe-to-mild illnesses from which the patients recover. The virus hepatitis B is a good example. Each year in the United States about 200,000 people, mostly young adults, acquire hepatitis-B infections. The majority of cases are undetected (asymptomatic) or exhibit nonspecific symptoms such as fatigue and nausea (often misdiagnosed as flu-like). About 50,000 have symptomatic illness with nausea, vomiting, abdominal pain, and jaundice (yellow skin and eyes), but eventually recover, and up to 20,000 (10 percent) then become carriers. Some 2,500 (1–2 percent) die from liver failure and/or liver cancer.

The incidence of AIDS is similarly deceptive. Thus, HTLV-III/ LAV disorders can be depicted as an iceberg: full-blown AIDS, above the water line, represents only a small proportion of the epidemic, while the majority of cases, below the water line, represent inapparent infections. The rigid CDC guidelines, however, do not cover the wide clinical spectrum of HTLV-III/LAV disease and might result in an underestimate of the extent and severity of the problem. The guidelines portray only one end of the spectrum and ignore milder forms of AIDS-related illnesses that have less clearly defined clinical courses but greater prevalence in the general population. The entire spectrum of HTLV-III/LAV-related conditions at present is thought to include asymptomatic HTLV-III/LAV infections, as well as symptomatic forms such as the lymphadenopathy syndrome, the wasting syndrome, AIDS-related complex (ARC), a variety of autoimmune diseases (caused by an overactive immune system), and full-blown AIDS.

What happens when an individual becomes infected with the HTLV-III/LAV virus? The majority, perhaps greater than 90 percent, will not develop either AIDS or ARC. While over 25,000 cases of AIDS have been reported in the United States, 1 to 2 million are estimated to be infected. Some will fortunately eliminate the virus from their bodies without any consequences. Others will develop a mononucleosis-like illness, with fever, rash, swollen glands, and joint aches, from which they will recover. A greater number will be asymptomatic. In some (about 60 percent) the AIDS virus will remain dormant and cause no signs or symptoms of disease. Others (about 25 percent) will develop ARC or the lymphadenopathy syndrome. The majority (80–95 percent) of asymptomatic infected patients will not develop overt AIDS. As many as 20 percent of ARC patients will develop full-blown AIDS within 5 years of onset of infection.

Why some patients infected with HTLV-III/LAV do not develop immune deficiency is not known. Various hypotheses have been proposed but none substantiated. Theories abound about the effects of the quantity of virus, the number of exposures, coincidental infections with other pathogens, immunosuppression by drugs and semen, and a natural variability in responses to infections.

Lymphadenopathy Syndrome

Some researchers believe that a condition characterized by swollen glands and other nonspecific signs and symptoms may be a preliminary stage of AIDS. Many patients with AIDS recall having had generalized swollen glands (lymphadenopathy) for many months prior to their diagnosis.

In May 1982 the CDC published reports of an increasing number of homosexual men with persistent, generalized swollen glands associated with fevers, malaise, night sweats, weight loss, and diarrhea. This was first called the "gay lymphadenopathy syndrome" but, since it has also been observed in others at increased risk for AIDS, it is now more appropriately renamed the "lymphadenopathy syndrome."

A patient is given this diagnosis if lymph nodes are enlarged in at least two separate areas of the body (excluding the groin) and show nonspecific inflammation. Many diseases can cause lymphadenopathy, for example, infections, especially viral such as mononucleosis, hepatitis, and cytomegalovirus, but also bacterial such as tuberculosis and syphilis. Drugs, cancers, and autoimmune disorders may also cause lymph node swelling. These causes must be excluded by appropriate laboratory and other tests before a diagnosis of lymphadenopathy syndrome is determined.

The lymphadenopathy syndrome appears to be related to AIDS in high-risk groups (homosexuals and drug users) who share many risk factors, for example, sexual promiscuity and frequent use of recreational drugs. They also have immunologic defects, such as a low white blood cell count and inversion of the T-cell ratio, but not as severe as their AIDS counterparts. Their blood usually tests positive for HTLV-III/LAV antibodies. The chance of progression from lymphadenopathy syndrome to overt AIDS is uncertain, but probably is as high as 10 percent.

AIDS-Related Complex

AIDS-related complex (ARC) is a term used since 1983 to describe HTLV-III/LAV-infected patients who develop prolonged symptoms of fatigue, fevers, night sweats, weight loss, and unexplained diarrhea. Almost all show evidence of T-cell disorders and chronic swollen glands. (Although there is no official CDC recognition of ARC, most clinicians accept as criteria at least two of the symptoms and at least two of the laboratory findings listed in table 2.)

Other terms used in reference to ARC include the lymphadenopathy syndrome and wasting syndrome. These syndromes both include general debilitation, persistent weight loss (as much as 40 percent) over several months, profound fatigue, diarrhea, and sometimes fever and swollen glands. Immunity is depressed, but not as severely as in AIDS, and one or more opportunistic infections may be present. Both meet the criteria for classification as ARC, but the wasting syndrome is more likely to progress to full-blown AIDS.

Autoimmune Diseases

The normal human immune system is able to discern the body's own cells and tissues (self) from alien cells and organisms. When it malfunctions, it may attack the body's own tissue by manufacturing antibodies directed against self misperceived as alien. The resulting destruction of tissue is called autoimmunity. In AIDS, a similar disorder, idiopathic thrombocytopenic purpura (ITP), directs antibodies against platelets, blood cells intimately involved in the clotting process. ITP may produce no overt symptoms, but the consequences of a reduced platelet count may be an increased susceptibility to bruising or frank bleeding.

AIDS

AIDS is the end point of the spectrum of HTLV-III/LAV infections. Its severe damage to the immune system makes patients easy prey for a variety of viruses, bacteria, protozoans, and fungi that can cause single or multiple recurrent infections, collectively categorized as opportunistic. We all have pathogens (disease-causing agents) in our body, for example, herpes virus, chicken pox virus, candidal fungi (yeast), and occasionally even cancer cells, but our immune surveillance system normally prevents them from harming us. If our immunity is impaired or nonfunctioning, these pathogens seize the opportunity to spread destruction, so that the localized infection becomes widely disseminated, or the single cancer cell multiplies and becomes a tumor. The immunodeficiency of AIDS does not directly cause sickness or death; rather, it lowers barriers and enables opportunistic pathogens to do harm.

SUMMARY

The acronym AIDS suggests the mystery of a syndrome that has become a major public health problem in the United States and abroad. The syndrome is seen primarily in groups of individuals at high risk and includes a variety of opportunistic infections and malignancies. Since the discovery of the AIDS virus, HTLV-III/ LAV, it has become apparent that AIDS is only the extreme end of a spectrum of infections with a common cause. A more accurate term is HTLV-III/LAV-related diseases, which encompasses a variety of illnesses including asymptomatic infections, lymphadenopathy syndrome, wasting syndrome, AIDS-related complex (ARC), autoimmune diseases, and full-blown AIDS. Since a diagnosis of AIDS places a stigmatizing label on a patient, it should conform with strict criteria. However, knowledge about the spread, distribution, and natural course of the disease is still evolving so that diagnostic criteria must continually be reevaluated as new information becomes available.

2   Assembling the AIDS Puzzle: Epidemiology

Keewhan Choi

In the late spring of 1981, Dr. Michael S. Gottlieb, four of his colleagues at the UCLA School of Medicine, and Dr. I. Pozalski at Cedars Mt. Sinai Hospital in Los Angeles came upon a remarkable medical mystery. Between October 1980 and May 1981 they treated 5 young male homosexuals hospitalized with *Pneumocystis carinii* pneumonia (PCP), a rare infection. All also had other "opportunistic" infections, normally seen only in organ transplant patients whose immune systems have been broken down intentionally to assist in acceptance of the new organ, and two of the men died during treatment. The sudden appearance of these diseases in so many otherwise healthy men was alarming. The doctors reported the cases in the June 5, 1981 issue of the Morbidity and Mortality Weekly Report (MMWR), published by the Centers for Disease Control (CDC) in Atlanta, Georgia, a periodical in which current public health problems and statistics are discussed.

At about the same time, Dr. Alvin Friedman of New York University called the CDC about an unusual number of cases of Kaposi's sarcoma (KS) he had found at New York University Hospital that past winter. Dr. Friedman and his colleagues reported in the July 3 issue of MMWR that 20 cases of KS had been discovered in New York and 6 in California in the 30 months from January 1979 to July 1981. All 26 were homosexual, their ages ranging from 26 to 51; 4 also had PCP. Within 2 years after diagnosis of KS, 8 were dead.

While this information was being digested, word came from California that 10 new cases of PCP had been identified. Again all involved homosexual men, and 2 also had KS. Concerned about these startling developments, the CDC, the federal agency responsible for controlling and preventing disease in the United States, formed a task force headed by Dr. James Curran that started a systematic search for cases of this as yet unnamed syndrome. They began looking for laboratory-proven cases of KS or opportunistic infections such as PCP in previously healthy people of either sex between the ages of 15 and 60. The target areas were chosen to include cities with varying proportions of homosexual men. The task force first contacted physicians, major hospitals, and tumor registries in New York State, California, and Georgia. The investigators also reviewed physicians' requests for pentamidine, a drug available only from the CDC and used to treat PCP. Later, the task force solicited detailed reports from physicians and health departments.

This early investigation went back to what the task force decided was probably the first case of the strange syndrome, one involving KS in New York City in 1978, and led to the conclusion that they were probably hunting down a totally new phenomenon. The next step was interviews with as many patients as possible to try to find out what was happening to homosexual men that was apparently not happening to anyone else. Dr. Harold Jaffe and other members of the task force went to San Francisco and New York to interview about 30 patients who were still alive. They conducted in-depth interviews about the patients' lifestyle, including homosexual behavior, drug use, and medical history.

It was quickly discovered that almost all of the patients regularly used "poppers"—amyl and butyl nitrites— as sexual stimulants. A theory was proposed that prolonged use of these nitrites might cause the new syndrome. The investigators focused on this and, within a few weeks, interviewed 416 homosexual and heterosexual men. It was quickly confirmed that use of the poppers was almost exclusively homosexual and that the heaviest users also tended to have the greatest number of sexual partners. Purchase and laboratory examination of the nitrites, however, failed to show whether the drugs could cause the new syndrome.

At this time, the fall of 1981, only 4 living heterosexual patients had been reported. Frustrated thus far, the task force designed in September a "case-control" study to seek possible causes of the syndrome in previously healthy young homosexuals. The study attempted to identify risk factors by comparing various characteristics of patients—cases—with those of healthy homosexual men—controls—with the hope of finding clues that would lead to the cause of the disease.

Using 20-page questionnaires, the investigators interviewed, in October and November of 1981, 50 homosexual men who had the syndrome and 120 healthy homosexual men, located through private physicians or venereal disease clinics in New York, San Francisco, and Los Angeles. The subjects were questioned for 60 to 90 minutes on their medical history, occupation, travel, exposure to toxic substances, use of both prescription and illegal drugs, use of inhalant sexual stimulants (poppers), sexual history, and family history. At the end of these interviews, the subjects, both cases and controls, were asked to donate biological specimens for laboratory comparisons. The task force took nearly a year to analyze the data from these sessions, using computers and sophisticated mathematical methods. They spent hundreds of hours discussing their project, from the design of the study and the questionnaire to the interpretation of results.

The most obvious difference between the cases and the controls, the study showed, was that men suffering from the new syndrome (the patients) tended to have many more sexual partners, an average of 60 per year, compared to 25 per year for the healthy homosexuals. The patients also were more likely to have frequented bathhouses, a common meeting ground for anonymous homosexual encounters. Other seemingly significant differences included a patient history of syphilis and hepatitis and more common use of drugs such as marijuana and cocaine. The use of poppers, however, appeared to be the same for both cases and controls, casting doubt on the nitrites as a cause of the new syndrome. Laboratory studies by CDC virologists, microbiologists, and immunologists of the specimens obtained from the cases and controls were pursued to determine the character and extent of the breakdown of the immune systems in patients and to search for common or variant characteristics that might yield clues to the cause of the disease.

The patients were found to have a deficiency of helper T cells, a type of white blood cell that assists the immune system in repelling invaders. Patients had elevated levels of IgG and IgA (proteins called immunoglobulins that are made in response to infection), higher concentrations of antibody to Epstein-Barr virus and cytomegalovirus, and a higher prevalence of antibody to hepatitis A. The chief conclusions of the study were that the disease could be transmitted through blood or semen, that the patients tended to have regular and anonymous sexual contacts in bathhouses, bars, and public restrooms, and that they engaged in sexual practices that produce abrasions and expose them to small amounts of blood, semen, and feces. The study also resulted in a name for the disease— acquired immune deficiency syndrome, or AIDS. Even as the task force was conducting its long investigation, AIDS was turning up in other segments of the population.

In the fall of 1981, Dr. Gerald Friedland of Montefiore Hospital in the Bronx, New York City, reported he had treated several cases of PCP and other opportunistic infections in heterosexual men and women. Their common connection was intravenous-drug abuse. Health departments in New York and New Jersey reported that a small number of inmates in state prisons had similar symptoms. Physicians began reporting a new phenomenon, a wasting disease called lymphadenopathy, which they suspected might be an early stage of AIDS. The CDC task force dispatched more epidemiologists to investigate these patients.

Meanwhile, doctors at Jackson Memorial Hospital in Miami, Florida, told the CDC that autopsy reports showed that 4 Haitian immigrants had died of opportunistic infections. A few months later, they found similar infections among several other Haitians who had recently immigrated to the United States. This added a further intriguing facet to the medical mystery. Sexually active homosexual men and intravenous-drug abusers might have habits in common that could expose them to the disease, but there was apparently little they could have in common with Haitian immigrants who, it seemed, were neither homosexual nor drug users.

The CDC sent Dr. Harry Haverkos to Miami to investigate the Haitian cases, a difficult assignment because of the cultural and linguistic barriers. Haverkos tried to concentrate on what could have exposed the Haitians to AIDS. Reports reaching the CDC from Haiti, either from local physicians or from United States doctors visiting the island nation, indicated that both PCP and KS had been found among the natives.

By July 1982, 10 months after the CDC first learned of the disease, there were 216 cases. Of those, 84 percent were homosexual men, 9 percent were intravenous-drug abusers, 2 percent were Haitians, and 5 percent were women; 88 of the patients were dead.

There had to be a common cause. Some still favored poppers, others suggested a new virus that attacked the immune system, and others favored an "immune-overload" theory. However, the Haitians remained the wild card, as they did not fit into any of the theories. Some investigators even doubted that the different groups had the same disease.

Drs. Curran, Jaffee, and others leaned toward the virus theory, and two events early in 1982 strengthened their suspicions. In January, the CDC discovered that a hemophiliac had died of PCP in Miami. However, the victim had received steroids, which weaken the immune system, had liver disease, and was dead, so the case was rejected as not fitting the CDC definition of AIDS. Then, in the spring, 2 more cases were reported, and their symptoms were similar to those of homosexual males, heterosexual intravenous-drug addicts, and recent Haitian immigrants suffering from AIDS. The most likely, and frightening, way that these hemophiliacs could have been exposed to AIDS was through the transfusion of blood-clotting factors on which their lives depend.

Hemophiliacs lack part of a blood-clotting protein called Factor VIII, which must be replaced with injections derived from donor blood. A single injection can contain Factor VIII from 2,500 donors, thus exposing a hemophiliac to the blood of as many as 75,000 people every year. It appeared that whatever causes AIDS had gotten into the Factor VIII injections.

The July 16, 1982 issue of the CDC's MMWR reported that "the occurrence among the three hemophiliac cases suggests the possible transmission of an agent through blood products." In July, the U.S. Food and Drug Administration, the National Hemophiliac Foundation, and other organizations set up studies to evaluate the risks to hemophiliacs, examine Factor VIII supplies for contamination, and try to find ways of making the injections safer. By December 1982, the 3 original hemophiliac AIDS patients were dead, and 4 more heterosexual hemophiliacs had developed opportunistic infections and symptoms of a collapsed immune system. Intensive investigations into their sexual habits, drug usage, travel, and general lifestyle failed to produce any evidence that their disease could have been acquired through contact with each other, homosexuals, drug abusers, or even Haitian immigrants. There was one common link— all had received Factor VIII concentrate.

If the hemophiliac AIDS patients made the infectious organism theory likely, the discovery of the "LA cluster" made it more so. In February 1982, Dr. Jaffee and Dr. David Auerbach, the CDC officer in Los Angeles, heard rumors that some of the gay AIDS victims in the Los Angeles area had sexual contact with each other before they fell ill. Dr. Auerbach and Dr. William Darrow, a task force sociologist, began intensive interviews of the gay population of Los Angeles and were able to establish positive links within a group of 9 of the 19 cases known in the area at the time. These homosexual men had had sexual relations with others in the group prior to their developing AIDS. Subsequent investigation enabled the task force to trace sexual connections among 40 patients in 10 cities.

A virus thus became the most likely culprit. It fit all the requirements—something transmitted sexually, especially through abrasions, carried by dirty needles, picked up in unsanitary living conditions, and able to contaminate blood. All of this was reminiscent of hepatitis B, the viral liver disease transmitted by blood, semen, and even saliva. However, there had been no proof that, like hepatitis B, AIDS could be transmitted to anyone exposed to blood and blood products, receiving blood transfusions, or treated with dialysis machines.

Then, late in the fall of 1982, the task force was tracing down reports of children who might be suffering from AIDS when they heard of a 20-month-old boy in San Francisco with symptoms of the disease. They learned that the boy had received transfusions and that one of the 19 donors was an AIDS patient they had interviewed in March. The donor had not had symptoms of the disease when he donated the blood. The CDC was later able to confirm that 2 adults had contracted AIDS after receiving blood transfusions, and 5 more hemophiliacs, including a 7-year-old and a 10-year-old, were believed to have the disease.

On January 4, 1983, representatives of every government health agency and commercial blood banks met in Atlanta to discuss ways of testing blood donors to screen AIDS carriers out of the system. Proposals included tightening federal regulations on commercial blood centers, banning donations from homosexuals and Haitians, and screening donors for a history of hepatitis B on the assumption that anyone who has had that disease might be more susceptible to AIDS. No decisions were made, and none of the proposals could be adopted because of considerable opposition.

The CDC task force opened files on two new victim groups—female sexual partners of men with AIDS, and children. By January 1983, 26 children under 5 years of age appeared to have contracted AIDS, and 10 were already dead. Although none had KS, all had PCP or similar opportunistic infections. Most were the children of Haitians, intravenous-drug abusers, or men who had homosexual contacts. There was no indication how the children might have acquired the disease. More intensive pursuit of the disease in the United States and Puerto Rico turned up 2,259 cases by late 1983, some 80 percent concentrated in the metropolitan areas of New York, San Francisco, Miami, Newark, Houston, and Los Angeles. The progression of the investigation was paralleled by the increasing rate at which cases were reported—58 before 1981, 231 in 1981, 747 in 1982, and 2,124 in 1983.

Since then the incidence of AIDS has risen to epidemic proportions. In the United States, the CDC received reports of 4,569 cases in 1984 and 8,406 in 1985. By July 1986 the cumulative total exceeded 22,000, AIDS had appeared in all 50 states, the District of Columbia, and three U.S. territories, and the rate had doubled in about 11 months.

In Europe, as of September 30, 1985, the World Health Organization (WHO) European Collaborating Centre on AIDS had received reports of 1,573 cases (half of whom have died) from 21 countries, most in England, West Germany, France, Belgium, and Italy. Czechoslovakia, Hungary, Iceland, and Poland have not reported any, and the Soviet Union recently reported cases for the first time.

About one-fourth of the earlier European cases were Africans, and all the first 40 Belgian cases had either lived in Central Africa (Zaire or Chad) or had had sexual contact with Central African residents. Of the September 1985 total, 157 (10 percent) were Africans from 22 different countries, mostly Zaire (99 cases) and Congo (16 cases). When their symptoms were first noted, 86 of them were already living in Europe, but 66 were still in Africa; the other 5 lived elsewhere. Only 11 of the Africans were homosexuals (1 of them also an IV-drug abuser), 5 had received blood transfusions, and men outnumbered women by only 2 to 1, so that homosexuality did not appear to be an important factor.

Among the European AIDS cases without African connections, about three-quarters were homosexual or bisexual men, about 7 percent were IV-drug abusers, and for about 2 percent blood transfusion was the only known risk factor. Some two-thirds were between 20 and 39 years old, and 36 were children under 15 (24 with parents who had AIDS or were members of a high-risk group, and 10 likely to have been exposed to contaminated blood or blood products).

Central African officials have been reluctant for various reasons to release information on AIDS, but U.S., European, and African investigators have reported since 1983 that the disease is widespread in 21 African countries. Studies, mainly in Zaire and Rwanda, have found that AIDS strikes men and women in approximately equal numbers and that many heterosexual men seem to have acquired the disease from intercourse with women prostitutes who had AIDS. Although the rate at which AIDS is spreading in Africa is unknown, indications are that it is common in some central but not southern African urban areas. Questions remain as to whether AIDS existed in central Africa before it appeared in the United States, and whether African and American AIDS have the same cause. Further African studies may discover clues to reasons for differences in distribution and possibly patterns of transmission.

About half the AIDS patients in the United States have already died, primarily due to opportunistic infections. PCP is the most common illness associated with AIDS (63 percent of patients have gotten it), but about 1 out of 4 get KS without PCP. AIDS respects neither racial nor ethnic boundaries (60 percent of patients are white, 25 percent black, and 14 percent Hispanic), and sex offers no sure protection (7 percent have been women). Although almost all AIDS patients are relatively young, adults who get AIDS from blood transfusions tend to be over 50.

High-risk groups in the United States have remained essentially the same since AIDS figures first began to accumulate—primarily sexually active homosexual or bisexual men (about 72 percent) and intravenous-drug abusers (about 17 percent), both also tending to be infected with hepatitis B virus—except that Haitians are no longer considered a separate group. Haitians acquire AIDS by virtue of the same risk factors as high-risk groups.

The pattern for children with AIDS in the United States resembles that for adults; differences are due to the general absence of sexual or drug-related transmission except indirectly through parents. Of 312 AIDS patients under 13 years old, 18 percent were white, 60 percent black, and 21 percent Hispanic; 55 percent were boys, 51 percent had PCP, and 3 percent had KS. One or both parents of 77 percent of the children had AIDS, 15 percent of the young patients had received blood transfusions before falling ill, and 4 percent were hemophiliacs. Almost half of the states have reported pediatric AIDS cases, but three-fourths are concentrated in New York, New Jersey, Florida, and California.

In the search for the cause of AIDS, the most important link among all patients was the peculiar breakdown of the immune system, with no indication of a genetic predisposition. By 1983 most investigators had come to the conclusion that AIDS was probably caused by a virus. Various candidates considered were hepatitis B (its spread parallels that of AIDS, but evidence of a link was not convincing), herpesviruses (they persistently infect body cells and some, like the Epstein-Barr and cytomegalovirus, are known to infect the cells of the immune system destroyed by AIDS), and others, including human T-cell lymphotropic virus (HTLV). HTLV (two forms were known) is transmitted from person to person, infects individuals in clusters (like AIDS), and is associated with the slow, long-term development of cancer. Although HTLV is not prevalent in the United States, scientists searched for some possible connection. They also speculated that the cause might be the mutation of a virus that previously affected only nonhumans, or a virus that had somehow been present in certain segments of the population without attracting medical attention.

Then in April 1984 a research team headed by Dr. Luc Montagnier at the Pasteur Institute in Paris isolated what they called the lymphadenopathy-associated virus (LAV) in six AIDS patients and five lymphadenopathy patients. In the United States, a team under Dr. Robert Gallo of the National Cancer Institute had found in AIDS patients a previously unknown form of HTLV, named it HTLV-III, and suggested that it might be the cause of AIDS. Tests proved that both belong to the same family of retroviruses (viruses that carry RNA rather than DNA genetic material), which is now called HTLV-III/LAV. Antibodies to HTLV-III/LAV were found in the blood of most AIDS patients, first in San Francisco and Paris and then elsewhere, and the virus has now been isolated from many body fluids, including blood, semen, saliva, tears, and vaginal secretions. HTLV-III/LAV is generally accepted as the cause of AIDS, but many researchers believe that the contribution of certain conditions or cofactors may be necessary.

An intense search is being carried on around the world for an AIDS cure or preventive vaccine. Meanwhile, efforts are being made to prevent spread of the disease through education in the character of AIDS and the known means of transmission. Substantial progress has been made in preventing contamination of the blood by screening blood and plasma for antibodies, treating blood products with heat to inactivate the virus, and rejecting blood and organs from donors who are infected or are members of high-risk groups.

The battle against AIDS is far from over. The Secretary of the U.S. Department of Health and Human Services prematurely predicted in April 1984 that a vaccine would be ready for testing in two years. The target date has been put off to at least the year 2000. Meanwhile, a continued commitment to research is needed, and an even greater need is cooperation between government and community organizations to disseminate information effectively to arrest the spread and to provide adequate care for AIDS patients.

3   Causes of AIDS: Etiology

EDWARD S. JOHNSON
JEFFREY VIEIRA

The understanding and conquest of recently recognized diseases such as Legionnaires' disease, toxic shock syndrome, and hepatitis B have been made possible by lessons learned in the campaigns against older infections such as cholera, smallpox, plague, and tuberculosis. Such lessons were based on the slow, painful acquisition of basic scientific and clinical knowledge.

Often, the spread of the disease was arrested long before the cause was known. A good example is cholera. After a severe outbreak of cholera in London, England, in 1832, John Snow was able to halt its advance by means of a careful epidemiologic study that demonstrated the importance of poor hygiene in spreading the disease. This was years before the germ theory of disease was proposed and before the discovery of the cholera bacillus. This pattern has been seen in the fight against AIDS. It was clear several years before the identification of the AIDS virus that certain personal and medical practices placed participants at high risk for acquiring the disease. On the basis of these observations, control measures were instituted before identification of the disease agent itself.

A decade ago Legionnaires' disease, toxic shock syndrome, and AIDS were unknown. The question that immediately comes to mind is: Are we giving old diseases new names, or are we suddenly encountering previously unknown microbes? Thanks to some far-sighted epidemiologists who had frozen serum from persons with undefined illnesses many years before, it was possible to confirm that the Legionnaires' disease bacillus had been present long before the original outbreak in Philadelphia in 1976. Likewise, the medical literature chronicles illnesses probably identical to staphylococcal toxic shock syndrome antedating the recent description of the syndrome. It is clear from worldwide epidemiologic studies that AIDS appeared abruptly in the Western Hemisphere between 1976 and 1978 and was probably present in Africa (especially central Africa) several years earlier. The discovery of the AIDS virus was made possible by worldwide concerted efforts of scientists, physicians, epidemiologists, governmental agencies, and industry.

The early 1980s saw three major hypotheses proposed to explain the new and deadly disease, first designated GRID (gay-related immune deficiency) and later AIDS (acquired immune deficiency syndrome) as it became clear that other than gay men were at risk. These hypotheses were: immune overload, multifactorial, and single agent. Other theories suggested that AIDS was an "act of God," a disease directly related to anal sex practices or bestiality, or a product of germ warfare research, among other fanciful notions.

The immune overload hypothesis was the earliest to be advanced and appeared at first glance to provide a plausible explanation for the almost unique occurrence of AIDS among gay men. Homosexual men, in particular, have a high incidence of sexually transmitted diseases (STDs). During the 1970s specialty clinics were established to treat and assess infections afflicting gays. Terms such as "gay bowel" and "gay bar syndrome" were coined to describe patterns of intestinal and anorectal disease resulting from oral-anal-genital sex, often with multiple anonymous partners. Bacteria, parasites, and viruses that were uncommon causes of disease in young, previously healthy men in developed countries were now commonly seen as sexually transmitted pathogens along with the traditional agents such as herpes simplex virus and the microorganisms of syphilis and gonorrhea. Gay men engaged in the widespread use of recreational drugs, such as amyl nitrite, butyl nitrite, amphetamines, Quaaludes, cocaine, and heroin, in conjunction with the sexual use of foreign bodies and fists for anal intercourse, and "rimming" (oral-anal sex). It was proposed that repeated infections with sexually transmitted organisms and the use of immunosuppressive drugs combined to overload and exhaust the immune system. Among infectious agents, the herpesviruses, including cytomegalovirus (CMV), herpes simplex virus (HSV), and Epstein-Barr virus (EBV), and amebas are known to cause transient immune depression.

Narcotics also suppress T lymphocytes and stimulate B lymphocytes, leading to defective cell-mediated immunity and increased production of immunoglobulins (antibodies), respectively. Amyl nitrite, or "poppers," have been used as a sexual stimulant since the 1960s. Amyl nitrite, and the related compound isobutyl nitrite, cause immunosuppression manifested by depression of helper T cells and an increase in suppressor T cells. A study reported in *Lancet* (1982) noted that homosexuals who used nitrites had more severe depletion of helper T cells than those who did not. However, conflicting reports in subsequent clinical investigations clouded the role of nitrites in the development of AIDS. Nitrite use was closely linked to other variables such as certain sexual practices, use of other drugs, and STDs suspected of being causally related to AIDS. The occurrence of AIDS among persons who did not use nitrite inhalants made untenable the theory that these agents were the cause of AIDS. However, it is still widely believed that nitrite use may act as a cofactor in the development of AIDS-related illnesses, especially Kaposi's sarcoma. Gay men are often prescribed antibiotics to treat STDs, and some of these agents, including tetracycline and metronidazole (Flagyl), are immunosuppressive in experimental and clinical settings. However, a clinically significant degree of suppression leading to disease has never been documented.

Sperm has been shown to have profound effects on the immune system. Injection of sperm into laboratory animals causes a marked depression of cell-mediated immunity. Those who practice passive (receptive) anal intercourse have significantly higher numbers of suppressor T cells and lower numbers of helper T cells than those who practice only active (insertive) anal intercourse. Microscopic tears in the tissues of the rectum during anal intercourse permit direct entry of sperm into the bloodstream. During heterosexual intercourse, in contrast, sperm is shielded from the bloodstream by the more resistant tissue barrier of the vaginal walls. Whenever sperm gains entry into the circulation it is perceived as a foreign substance (nonself), that is, an antigen, and the body produces antibody against it. Repeated exposure of the immune system to sperm is believed by some investigators to be an important risk factor in the ultimate development of AIDS in gay men. However, anal intercourse has been practiced by homosexuals and heterosexuals alike for centuries without AIDS. Thus anal intercourse *per se* is not the cause of AIDS. We now know, however, that it is an efficient way of transmitting the etiologic agent, the AIDS virus.

The multifactorial hypothesis was proposed by Dr. Joseph Sonnabend. According to this theory, an initial reversible phase of defective T-cell function is induced by exposure to infectious agents such as CMV or to immunosuppressive agents such as drugs or sperm. Reactivation of latent EBV infection in turn produces stimulation of B cells and increased antibody production. The presence of large amounts of different antibodies may then induce some of the so-called autoimmune phenomena seen in AIDS, that is, low white blood cell counts, low platelet counts, rashes, etc. Sperm antibodies may crossreact with T cells and other lymphocytes such as natural killer cells, resulting in further regulatory disturbances in the immune system. Repeated infections, recreational and prescription drug use, and environmental and genetic factors eventually lead to irreversible immune suppression, at which point the patient is defenseless against opportunistic infections and unusual tumors.

The major shortcoming of the multifactorial theory was that not all AIDS patients satisfied its requirements. Some homosexual men had developed AIDS with only limited sexual contact, and AIDS had occurred in others, such as children and heterosexual sexual partners of persons with AIDS, who lacked the multiple immunosuppressive exposures. Consequently, most investigators gravitated to the third major hypothesis, the single agent, recognizing that other factors doubtless contribute to the expression of the disease in a given patient.

Acute viral infections are known to cause transient suppression of immune function, but such defects rarely lead to the development of opportunistic infections or tumors. Therefore, the existence of previously unknown viruses or mutant forms of known animal or human viruses was entertained.

The prevalence of CMV infections among gay men was first documented in San Francisco in 1979. CMV infections were also frequent among intravenous-drug abusers and recipients of transfusions. This virus had been known to cause illnesses ranging from clinically silent infections to life-threatening disease, especially in immunocompromised persons. Patients who receive transplanted organs require immunosuppressive therapy, that is, drugs that blunt the immune system to prevent rejection of the organ. Because of their immunosuppression, such patients tend to develop CMV infections. These infections may be newly acquired or may represent reactivation of a latent infection. In such a setting of chronic drug-induced immune suppression and reactivated viral infection, opportunistic infections and tumors may occasionally follow. This was the proposed sequence in AIDS, according to some scientists. CMV would act as the primary cause of AIDS and immune suppression, with subsequent development of unusual infections and malignancies. Alternatively, another agent might cause the suppression, and then CMV would itself be an opportunistic disease-causing agent.

Like CMV, EBV produces illness that ranges from subclinical to severe and life threatening. EBV has been implicated in malignancies such as Burkitt's lymphoma and nasopharyngeal carcinoma (cancer in nose and throat). The prodromal (early, and possibly anticipatory) symptoms of AIDS are similar to those of infectious mononucleosis (caused by EBV), with malaise, fever, sweats, swollen glands, enlarged spleen and liver, and some changes in the immune system that may superficially mimic those seen in AIDS. EBV is common in all the risk groups for AIDS—in gay men in particular some studies have found that nearly 100 percent had past EBV infections. As with CMV, however, there was no evidence of a mutant form of the virus or other cogent explanation for a change in the virus's disease-producing potential. As an opportunist itself, however, EBV has been associated with lymphoma, interstitial lymphocytic pneumonia, and lesions in the mouth (hairy leukoplakia) characteristically seen in persons with AIDS.

The high rate of hepatitis-B infections in gay males and intravenous-drug abusers raised the possibility of a causative role. The discovery of the so-called delta particle or agent, a defective virus requiring a simultaneous hepatitis-B infection for its own growth, further intrigued some investigators. Epidemiologic and virologic studies have since excluded the possibility that either agent causes AIDS. Nonetheless, the hepatitis-B model of transmission by blood and contact with the body fluids of an infectious individual provided a useful guide for designing transmission control measures.

Much excitement was generated by the discovery of retroviruses in AIDS patients. Some of these viruses had been associated with tumors in animals (feline leukemia) and man (T-cell leukemia/lymphoma). Central to the eventual identification of the AIDS virus was the pioneering work of Dr. Robert Gallo of the National Cancer Institute in the United States and Dr. Luc Montagnier of the Pasteur Institute in France.

Retroviruses are tiny, RNA-containing viruses first discovered in 1909 and shown by 1911 to have tumor-causing potential. In 1976, Dr. Gallo discovered a T-cell growth factor (TCGF), now called interleukin-2 (IL-2). IL-2 is necessary for growing T cells in the laboratory and thus for isolating the retroviruses that may infect those cells. On the basis of the breakthrough with IL-2, Dr. Gallo was able to isolate the first human T-cell leukemia virus (HTLV-I) in 1982. HTLV-II was later isolated from a patient with a rare blood disease (hairy-cell leukemia). The occasional isolation of these HTLVs from patients with AIDS was of interest but, since they were not present as often as CMV, EBV, and hepatitis B, they were not likely to be the cause of AIDS. The observed selective T-cell destruction leading to severe immune depression was characteristic of retroviral infections and led researchers to seek an as yet unidentified retrovirus. Using recently developed cell culture techniques, Dr. Gallo and Dr. Montagnier simultaneously isolated viruses from patients with AIDS. Dr. Gallo, using the then existing nomenclature for retroviruses called his discovery HTLV-III (human T-cell lymphotropic virus type III). Dr. Montagnier named his isolate LAV (lymphadenopathy-associated virus) because it was isolated from an enlarged lymph node of an AIDS patient. Another group from Los Angeles, California, soon thereafter isolated another strain of the virus and called it ARV (AIDS-related virus). Evidence shows conclusively that HTLV-III, LAV, and ARV are the same virus although there are minor differences noted in some of the surface antigens. In order to standardize terminology and yet not display favoritism toward one group of researchers, an international committee has recommended calling the virus HIV (human immunodeficiency virus).

The origins of the AIDS virus are unknown, but recent studies in Africa suggest a possible ancestral tie between HTLV III/LAV and monkey retroviruses, so-called simian T-lymphotropic viruses

(STLV). STLV-I infections have been known to exist in African monkeys for many years and have been associated with the development of tumors in these animals. Like HTLV viruses, STLV preferentially infects T lymphocytes, and STLV-III, like HTLV-III infects and destroys T cells. In some strains of monkey, STLV-III produces a disease that mimics AIDS in humans, while in others the virus remains dormant, producing no recognized disease. Recently, investigators from France, the United States, and Africa working independently were able to isolate a new strain of HTLV, called HTLV-IV by Dr. Max Essex from the Harvard School of Public Health, from asymptomatic prostitutes in Senegal in west Africa. HTLV-IV is similar in structure to both the human disease-causing AIDS virus and the simian AIDS virus. Among the interpretations of these data is the suggestion that the human and simian AIDS viruses are mutants of the same nonpathogenic virus, possibly HTLV-IV. Alternatively, HTLV-III and HTLV-IV may be mutant strains of simian viruses, in one case becoming a deadly pathogen, and in the other a harmless parasite. Clarification of the relationship between various simian and human retroviruses may help improve our understanding of the way both cause disease. In addition, nonpathogenic viral strains may be useful in the preparation of an AIDS vaccine.

Overwhelming serologic, virologic, and epidemiologic evidence confirms that the AIDS retrovirus, HTLV-III/LAV, causes AIDS. Cofactors undoubtedly play a part in determining the manifestations of disease in a particular patient. As the epidemic goes on, and more and more patients develop AIDS, so too the clinical picture changes. Since the discovery of HTLV-III/LAV and the production of a sensitive and specific blood test for antibody to the virus, a classification system has been devised to reflect the full spectrum of infections, from acute, mononucleosis-like illness, through an asymptomatic period during which the victim is infectious to others, to a period of generalized enlargement of lymph nodes and a syndrome of fever, weight loss, intermittent diarrhea, and other systemic symptoms (pre-AIDS/ARC), and finally full-blown disease with severe opportunistic infections or malignancies. HTLV-III/LAV has been directly implicated in the development of certain complications of AIDS, most notably neurological signs such as dementia and peripheral nerve damage, where the virus directly infects and damages nerve tissue. The role of cofactors in determining who will develop full-blown disease, what signs and symptoms will appear and the pace of immune function deterioration remains an important area for future investigation.

The epidemiology of AIDS in the developed world (United States and Europe) is well delineated. In the underdeveloped world, however, particularly Haiti and central Africa where AIDS is widespread, our knowledge of the risk groups and modes of transmission remains fragmentary.

In the areas of immunology and virology, progress has been rapid and gratifying over the past three to four years. In that short time scientists have identified the virus that causes AIDS, probed and mapped its gene, traced the path it takes from first entrance into the bloodstream to infection of T lymphocytes and ultimate destruction of T cells and depression of T-cell immunity. Work on antiviral drugs, immune stimulatory agents, and a preventive vaccine lags behind progress in basic science but is nonetheless being actively pursued in many countries. Although the pace may appear slow to the unfortunates who suffer from this rapidly progressive, fatal disease, given the complexities of the task the progress to date has been unprecedented.

SUMMARY

The story of the discovery of the AIDS virus, through careful description of a clinical syndrome manifested by immune depression and resulting infections and malignancies, testing of theories of causation, and ultimate isolation of a virus that satisfactorily meets criteria for the etiologic agent, is an example of international scientific cooperation at its best. In the same spirit, efforts are going forward to develop effective viral inhibitors, immune system modulators, and therapies for the specific infections and malignancies complicating AIDS. Prospects for the early development of a vaccine appear remote due to the ability of the virus to mutate, thereby changing its identifying surface coat and eluding destruction by vaccine-induced antibody. The relationship of cofactors to the acquisition, maintenance, and progression of AIDS-virus infection remains to be elucidated. Until such time as effective prevention or treatment is available, disease transmission can be reduced by avoidance of certain risk-taking behaviors, notably intravenous-drug abuse and promiscuous sexual activity, both heterosexual and homosexual, which promote the sharing of potentially infectious secretions among individuals. The screening of blood and blood products, organs for transplant, and other biologic materials for HTLV-III/LAV infection has gone a long way to prevent their spread of the disease, although the technology is not yet foolproof.

As we often see in the aftermath of disasters, the lessons learned in dealing with the crisis, gaining an understanding of its origins, and rectifying its causes provide benefits to both sufferers and society in general. So too with AIDS. Ultimately, research will provide an answer to the questions of AIDS prevention and treatment. In addition, knowledge gained in immunology, virology, and other branches of science will assist research on cancer and on neurologic and rheumatic diseases, thus benefiting all segments of society.

Two   The Clinical Spectrum

4   The Immunology of AIDS
HELEN L. GRIERSON

The human body is constantly bombarded by thousands of different microorganisms, such as bacteria, viruses, fungi, and protozoa, but only a few, perhaps one hundred or so, cause disease. Microorganisms that infect and cause disease in humans are called pathogens. Entry of a pathogen may produce serious illness, often death, unless the body has some means of protection.

The human body has developed two special mechanisms, innate and acquired immunities, to cope with foreign invaders. Innate immunity, which is present from birth, is nonspecific and may be effective against all invaders. Acquired immunity is very specific and depends on the proper functioning of specialized cells in the body that are part of what is called the immune system. As the name "acquired immune deficiency syndrome" indicates, people with AIDS have lost all or part of their acquired immunity and are thus extremely susceptible to diseases caused by pathogens.

To understand the malfunction of an immune system damaged by AIDS, it is necessary first to understand how the normal immune system works. This is explained in the first section below. The next section describes some of the better known disorders of immunity. The last section deals with specific changes that occur in the immune systems of AIDS patients.

THE NORMAL IMMUNE SYSTEM

Lines of Defense

Innate, nonspecific immunity includes protection provided by the skin, mucous membranes, and special chemicals within the body.

The skin presents a mechanical barrier against invasion. The respiratory system is lined with a mucus-secreting membrane whose cells carry tiny hairlike projections, called cilia, that are constantly moving. The cilia sweep foreign invaders and other substances trapped in the sticky mucus out of the respiratory system. When the action of the cilia is impaired, for example, by cigarette smoke or drugs, the susceptibility to respiratory infections is increased.

Various secretions of the body also are important defenders against infection. Chemicals in tears attack bacteria, and stomach acids may kill harmful microorganisms in swallowed food.

If microorganisms do gain entrance to the body, for example, through a break in the skin, chemicals in the blood may destroy them. If they enter in sufficiently large numbers, the second line of defense, the acquired immune system, is activated. Acquired immunity is very specific to each particular type of microorganism and develops only after exposure to that microorganism. For example, when a child is first exposed to a measles virus, the immune system becomes programmed to recognize and destroy that virus whenever it enters the body after the initial illness. Because of this specificity, immunity to the measles virus does not protect against mumps, chickenpox, or any other infectious agent. Acquired immunity is normally lifelong.

Defensive Cells and Antibodies

The immune system is complicated and far from completely understood. A basic element is the white blood cells, called lymphocytes, that circulate throughout the body in the blood stream and in another circulatory system called the lymphatic system. Collections of lymphocytes called lymph nodes (glands), connected to vessels of the lymphatic system, are located at strategic points throughout the body. Lymphocytes can leave blood vessels, travel through body tissues and between cells, enter the lymphatic system, and eventually return to the bloodstream. The lymphocytes patrol the body for foreign invaders. For example, if microorganisms enter body tissue through a cut in a finger, they are shuttled to lymph nodes in the elbow and arm pit (axilla) where they are recognized and dealt with by lymphocytes. This prevents the microorganisms from multiplying and spreading throughout the body to cause generalized disease.

The immune system is divided into two parts: the cellular and the humoral immune systems. Cells of the cellular system are called T cells, and cells of the humoral system are called B cells.

A lymphocyte becomes a T cell by passing through the thymus gland. (The "T" comes from "thymus.") The thymus gland, located in the chest just above the heart, can be thought of as a learning center. It is responsible for processing and giving functional ability to lymphocytes, which come from the bone marrow. It also secretes hormones that circulate throughout the body and help regulate T-cell function.

T cells are the controllers and regulators of the immune system. They detect structures called antigens present on microorganisms and become programmed on first encounter to respond to these antigens thereafter. Recognition of antigens is very specific; each T cell recognizes and responds to only one type of antigen. T cells are also the teachers of B cells. One group, called helper T cells, assists B cells in making chemicals called antibodies, which then attach to and kill microorganisms. Each antibody is also very specific and reacts with only the particular antigen for which it was made. Another group, called suppressor T cells, regulates the amount of antibody made by B cells. This is important to ensure that B cells do not continue to make antibody when it is not needed.

B cells also originate in the bone marrow and circulate throughout the body. Once a B cell interacts with a T cell and is instructed to make antibody, it develops into a plasma cell, the cell type that actually makes and secretes antibody, which is a B cell's main task. The antibodies are called immunoglobulins, or Igs.

Plasma cells make five different types of antibody, called IgG, IgA, IgM, IgE, and IgD. All have the same basic structure but differ in size, location, and function. IgG makes up about 80 percent of the antibodies that circulate in the bloodstream and is important because it is produced in response to most infections. (IgM is actually the antibody produced upon first exposure to an infectious agent—primary immune response—but subsequent exposure causes B cells to make IgG instead of IgM—secondary immune response.) IgG can cross the placenta and provide immunity ("passive immunity") to babies for up to five or six months after birth.

IgA is part of what is called the secretory immune system and is an important part of saliva and other secretions of the gastrointestinal tract. IgE is one of the factors involved in allergic reactions. The function of IgD is not known for certain.

Other types of cells also are associated with immune responses. Macrophages ("large eaters") are cells that circulate like scouts in search of foreign invaders. When they recognize such intruders, they communicate the information to T cells which may then either kill the invaders or direct B cells to make specific antibody. Macrophages can also themselves engulf and destroy certain types of microorganisms.

Natural killer (NK) cells, another important component of the immune system, have both specific and nonspecific functions. They can nonspecifically recognize and kill cells of the body infected with virus, thus preventing further production and release of virus. They can also recognize and kill certain types of tumor cells; for this reason they are sometimes called the first line of defense against virus and tumor attack. The origin of NK cells is not clear. Some scientists believe they may be a kind of T cell, while others think they may be another type of lymphocyte.

Other cells of the body that act nonspecifically in defending against infection include white blood cells called polymorphonuclear leukocytes. These are somewhat similar to macrophages because they also can engulf and destroy microorganisms.

WHAT CAN GO WRONG

Because the immune system is complex, many parts may malfunction. In general, there are two categories of defects: inherited or congenital (primary), and acquired. These defects may either enhance or depress immune responses. Inherited or congenital defects are present at birth, caused either by genetic errors or abnormal embryonic development. The "bubble baby" was a child born without an immune system, and thus no defenses against foreign invaders, who had to be physically isolated from sources of infection. Some children are born without a thymus gland to transform lymphocytes into T cells and are very susceptible to infection by certain types of fungi and viruses. Other children have no B cells and are especially vulnerable to certain types of bacteria normally destroyed by antibodies. The immune system can also become overactive, resulting in allergies. Loss of the ability to distinguish "self" from "not self" can cause immune reactions against the body's own tissues—called autoimmunity.

Inherited or Congenital Defects—Primary Immune Deficiencies

Instances of primary immune deficiency are rare, but serious. T cells, B cells, or a combination of both may be involved.

In primary B-cell immunodeficiency a child is unable to make antibodies and is especially susceptible to infection by bacteria. This is usually not noticed until the age of five or six months because antibodies from the mother can cross the placenta, enter the unborn baby's circulatory system, and provide protection for several months after birth.

Primary T-cell immunodeficiencies are fortunately extremely rare. They are almost always associated with a problem in making antibody, which requires both T and B cells. In congenital thymic aplasia (DiGeorge's syndrome), caused by abnormal embryonic development, the thymus gland develops only partially or not at all. Children with this disease are especially susceptible to viral and fungal infections.

Severe combined immunodeficiency (SCID) is a genetic disease that makes children especially susceptible to *Pneumocystis carinii* pneumonia and cytomegalovirus (CMV) and *Candida* (thrush) infections. These are also the three types of opportunistic infections most often seen in AIDS patients. Children with SCID are also vulnerable to many other types of bacterial and viral infections. The basic defect is thought to be a failure of stem cells from the bone marrow to develop into T and B cells. SCID infants have no immunity and usually die within the first few weeks of life.

Acquired Defects

Autoimmunity

One of the most important features of the immune system is discrimination between cells and tissues of the parent body (self) and alien microorganisms (nonself). This ability is necessary to prevent immune responses from destroying the body they are supposed to defend. Autoimmunity is a disorder in which the immune system fails to recognize parts of the body as self and treats them as alien. The severity of the consequences depends on the extent of the immune responses and the parts of the body involved. For example, autoimmune thyroiditis is a common organ-specific (only the thyroid gland is involved) autoimmune disease. Other autoimmune diseases, such as systemic lupus erythematosis (SLE), may affect many tissues throughout the body. The main problem in autoimmune diseases seems to be a defect in communication among the cells of the immune system. Either cells or antibody can cause damage, depending upon the tissue involved.

Nutrition and Immunodeficiency

Worldwide, the most common cause of acquired immune deficiency is malnutrition. It has been estimated that 500 million people, the majority of them children, suffer from malnutrition. Nutritional disorders are particularly common in underdeveloped countries but also occur in the United States, Canada, and other industrialized areas, and in all segments of the population including hospitalized patients. The prevalence, severity, and types of infections found in malnourished persons are very similar to those seen in AIDS patients, that is, opportunistic infections by agents such as *P. carinii* and other viruses, bacteria, fungi, and protozoa. Also, measles and other common childhood viral infections are more often accompanied by complications in children who are malnourished.

The most devastating effect of malnutrition, recognized for many years, is atrophy, or wasting, of the thymus gland. In fact, in 1845 a scientist wrote that "the thymus is a barometer of nutrition, and a very delicate one." The thymus not only reacts more rapidly than other organs to nutritional deficiencies but is also the slowest to recover. The number of T cells in the circulation usually decreases with the loss of weight that occurs with malnutrition. Helper cells seem to be more affected than suppressor cells, especially in children whose diet lacks sufficient protein calories. Defects in nearly all T-cell functions have been detected. It has been suggested that the diminished number and function of immune cells are due not only to the harmful effects of malnutrition on the thymus gland but to a decrease in the number of precursor cells that normally develop into T cells and to a shorter survival time of mature cells.

Overnutrition as well as undernutrition can cause immune deficiency. It has been shown that in affluent societies, obesity, a form of malnutrition, is associated with increased respiratory infections and longer hospital stays following admission for routine procedures. In animal experiments, obesity has been found to be associated with greater susceptibility to viral and bacterial infections.

Transplantation and Immunity
Candidates for an organ transplant, for example, a kidney or heart, from someone other than an identical twin, must have their immune systems suppressed to prevent rejection of the donor tissue. Deliberate suppression is a form of acquired immune deficiency, and transplant patients are known to be especially susceptible to the same kinds of infections and cancers observed in AIDS patients.

Cancer and Immune Deficiency
People who have certain types of cancers, especially of the lymphatic system, often become immunodeficient and develop serious infections. The toxic effects of drugs used to treat cancers may also contribute to the deficiency.

Other Causes of Immune Deficiency
Almost any emotional stress may lead to temporary immune suppression due, in part, to the release of increased amounts of corticosteroid hormones. Traumas, such as burns, accidents, and surgery have been known to alter immune function. Pregnancy produces a temporary immunodeficient state, particularly during the last three months. It has been suggested that this temporary immunodeficiency is necessary to prevent the mother from rejecting the fetus as foreign tissue, but it also makes the mother susceptible to various viral infections. Immunodeficiency has also been associated with viral infections, especially CMV and Epstein-Barr virus (EBV), the cause of mononucleosis. Following infection, particularly with CMV, immune responses have been shown to be moderately decreased for up to a year. Significantly, another cause of immune deficiency is the intravenous (IV) use of drugs such as heroin; IV-drug abusers are the second largest group that develops AIDS.

THE IMMUNOLOGY OF AIDS

AIDS, as the name syndrome suggests, is a complex combination of different diseases and symptoms that each contribute to the overall state of ill health. It also means that the clinical picture is not identical for all AIDS patients, and associated changes in the immune system cannot be expressed in a single, universally applicable list. However, AIDS patients do seem to fit into three general categories: some have only Kaposi's sarcoma (KS) and no other symptoms; others have only severe opportunistic infections such as *Pneumocystis carinii* pneumonia (PCP), or *Candida* (thrush); and a third group has both KS and opportunistic infections. In general, the third group suffers the most severe changes in their immune systems, and patients with KS alone, the least.

People infected with the AIDS virus may develop another immune deficiency syndrome, AIDS-related complex (ARC), rather than overt AIDS. The manifestations of ARC include enlarged lymph glands that persist for months or years and may be associated with weight loss, fever, night sweats, and general malaise. It is still controversial whether ARC is totally different from AIDS or a pre-AIDS condition. Some ARC patients (about 20 percent) later develop AIDS. The immune systems of ARC patients show detrimental changes but not nearly as severe as those of AIDS patients. Abnormalities in immune function have also been found in otherwise healthy homosexual men (a high-risk group) infected with the virus HTLV-III/LAV.

Immune Changes in Homosexuals with AIDS

AIDS is basically a disorder affecting the cellular, or T-cell, immune system and exhibits the diseases associated with defective T-cell immunity, such as viral and fungal infections and cancer. As noted before, the infections of AIDS and kidney transplant patients are very similar. Because most (70 percent) people who develop AIDS are homosexual or bisexual men, most immunological studies have been done on blood and tissues from this group.

Scientists have many different ways of testing immune function. Cells or tissues can be removed from the body and analyzed for different types of cells. For example, lymphocytes can be separated from blood samples and counted. As described earlier, there are many types of lymphocytes with different functions. Special antibodies, called monoclonal, have been developed that recognize characteristic structures on the surface of specific types of lymphocytes; when mixed with lymphocytes in a test tube, they attach only to the types of lymphocytes for which they are specific. By linking other chemicals to the antibodies, it becomes possible under a microscope to identify lymphocytes with antibodies attached so that the abundance of a particular lymphocyte type can be measured. Lymphocytes in bone marrow, lymph nodes, and other tissues of the body can similarly be typed and measured. Using this technique, it is possible to measure the percentages of helper T cells, suppressor T cells, B cells, and NK cells.

In samples from AIDS patients, it is not surprising that significant T-cell changes are seen, since AIDS is a disorder of cellular immunity. The total number of T cells may or may not be normal, but the proportion and absolute number of helper T cells are significantly reduced. This may sometimes, but not always, be accompanied by an increase in the number of suppressor T cells. The result is a decrease in what is called the T_4-to-T_8 ratio. T_4 is the name given the antigen on helper T cells recognized by its associated monoclonal antibody; for suppressor T cells, T_8 is the specific antigen recognized by its associated monoclonal antibody. This is one of the most easily performed tests for immune changes in patients with AIDS or suspected to have AIDS. However, the test cannot definitively diagnose AIDS since other diseases such as viral infections also may change the T_4-to-T_8 ratio.

Abnormal immune function in AIDS patients is not due only to fewer helper T cells. Researchers have found in tests of purified groups of helper and suppressor cells that some helper T cells show normal function while others are abnormal. This indicates that helper T cells in AIDS patients are not only fewer than normal, but some have intrinsic defects.

Other tests can analyze body fluids such as blood serum for the various chemicals and substances associated with the immune system, for example, the amounts of different antibodies (immunoglobulin levels). Normal levels vary with age. In men with AIDS and in some with ARC, immunoglobulin levels may be above normal for their ages. IgG is the most likely to be increased, although IgA and IgM may also sometimes be high. Some researchers have found that only IgA is increased in AIDS patients with KS alone. The increase in immunoglobulins raises the question as to how a deficient immune system can overreact and make larger, rather than smaller, amounts of antibody. The answer may be that the defective T-cell system fails to properly regulate the B cells, which then make antibody nonspecifically and cannot shut down antibody production as usual. This may result in a continual outpouring of antibody that does not help defend against infectious agents.

Antibodies are not always protective and, in fact, can injure body tissues. If a large amount of antigen, such as a virus, is present together with matched circulating antibodies, antigen and antibody combine to form what are called immune complexes. Immune complexes can settle out in blood vessels or joints and cause severe damage with inflammation of the vessels and arthritis-like symptoms in the joints. Homosexual men with AIDS are infected with a variety of microorganisms and many have been found to have high levels of circulating immune complexes. Since CMV is suspected to be a contributing factor in the development of KS, some scientists have suggested that CMV immune complexes may deposit in blood vessels and help to account for the high incidence of KS in AIDS patients. Other immune complexes have been found with sperm components. Antibody to sperm and to parts of sperm have been measured in homosexual men, and high levels have been found in those with ARC or AIDS. This antibody is probably formed following the introduction of sperm during anal intercourse. Breaks or lesions in the rectum can facilitate entrance of these antigens into the blood. One type of antibody, specific to a chemical called asialo GM_1 present on the surface of sperm, may be especially important. Antibody to asialo GM_1 reacts with sperm but can also crossreact with helper T cells and NK cells. Perhaps antibody to asialo GM_1 contributes to the decrease in helper T cells and the malfunction of NK cells in men with AIDS.

Other measurable substances in body fluids include lymphokines, secreted by immune system cells as one way of communicating with each other. One type of lymphokine, called interleukin-2 (IL-2), is able to cause lymphocytes to divide and proliferate, thus increasing the number of lymphocytes reactive against specific antigens and promoting a more effective immune response. In AIDS patients, IL-2 production may be defective, and IL-2 injection is a suggested treatment to enhance immune function. Another type of lymphokine, interferon, is produced during active viral infection. Interferon may increase the activity of NK cells, which can then destroy cells infected with virus. Interferon has been found circulating in the blood of some AIDS patients, indicating an ongoing viral infection.

Tests are also available to measure the functional ability, as opposed to the quantity, of immune system cells. Virtually all such tests have revealed extreme abnormalities in AIDS patients. For example, when lymphocytes from one person are placed in test tubes with chemicals called mitogens or with cells from another person, the lymphocytes normally respond by dividing. This is called a blastogenic or mitogenic response. Tests of AIDS patients imply that their lymphocytes are defective and probably unable to divide normally after stimulation by antigen. Thus, the lymphocytes are decreased not only in number but in their ability to mount an adequate immune response, leaving the way open to severe infections.

Assays for NK cell function also show abnormalities. Some patients display virtually no NK activity. Since NK cells are important in controlling viral infections, defective activity, if it exists in the body as it does in the test tube, could lead to the persistent viral infections observed in many AIDS patients.

Some evaluations of immune function, such as skin tests, can be performed on the body (*in vivo*) rather than in a test tube (*in vitro*). Nearly all AIDS patients show decreased responses to skin tests with a variety of antigens, a further indication that their immune systems are unable to respond properly to the many agents they encounter. Their immune systems are said to have become anergic.

Immune Changes in Other AIDS Groups

AIDS also strikes IV-drug users, hemophiliacs and other recipients of donated blood and blood products, female sexual partners of AIDS-infected men, and children of mothers in high-risk groups. With the exception of KS, found only in homosexual men with AIDS, the spectrum of diseases in these groups is virtually identical to that in homosexual AIDS patients. So, too, are the changes in the immune system: decreased helper T cells, a decreased T_4-to-T_8 ratio, abnormal skin test responses, increased immunoglobulins, and defective NK-cell activity. AIDS is especially virulent in children, possibly because their immune systems are immature.

SUMMARY

The immune system is a highly specialized, complex system that has developed to provide specific protection against foreign agents that enter the body. When the system malfunctions, debilitating diseases and death can result. AIDS, which occurs primarily in homosexual men, is a graphic example of what can happen when this system fails. All data indicate that the primary target of the AIDS virus is the immune system. The earliest detectable changes are in the numbers of circulating lymphocytes. The changes become worse, and eventually the immune system fails. Individuals with AIDS then become totally unable to cope with ever-present microorganisms and fall prey to serious infections and other diseases.

5

Signs and Symptoms of AIDS

VICTOR GONG

AIDS is composed of many different diseases, and its signs and symptoms vary with their type and severity. Many AIDS symptoms are common to other illnesses, such as everyday ailments like the common cold, and may be self-limiting and minor. None by itself is specific to AIDS. Any one of these symptoms should be cause for attention but not alarm. However, if symptoms persist, a physician should be consulted. Generally speaking, the following are the most common signs and symptoms of AIDS.

PERSISTENT FEVERS OR NIGHT SWEATS

Fever is frequently the first sign that something is wrong with the body, usually an infection. The body's temperature is regulated by complex brain mechanisms. Normal body temperature is considered to be 98.6°F, taken orally, but may range from 97.0°F to 99.6°F. It also varies with age, body location, and time of day. A fever is a temperature above about 100.5°F in the mouth, 101.5°F in the rectum, or 99.5°F in the armpit. Chills and sweating may accompany a fever. Drenching night sweats are characteristic of tuberculosis and frequently occur with AIDS. Many illnesses can cause fever, chills, or sweating, but persistence of these symptoms should prompt medical attention.

SEVERE FATIGUE

Everyone goes through periods of tiredness, due to a variety of stresses such as overwork, emotional problems, and dietary changes. Profound fatigue lasting longer than several weeks, not obviously attributable to such stresses or to the effects of psychiatric distress or medication, may be an early signal of a serious illness.

WEIGHT LOSS

An unexplained weight loss in less than 2 months of 10 or more pounds, or greater than 10 percent of body weight, may indicate illness. Loss of appetite often accompanies the weight loss. These symptoms may be due to many causes, such as exercise, dieting, emotional or psychological problems, endocrine (hormone) disorders, infections, and cancers, as well as AIDS, AIDS-related complex (ARC), or the lymphadenopathy syndrome (see below). If appetite does not return, and weight loss persists with no obvious cause, seek medical attention.

SWOLLEN GLANDS (LYMPHADENOPATHY)

Lymph nodes, located strategically throughout the body (for example, in the neck, groin, and armpits), are part of the body's defense against infection. They may become swollen due to infection, malignancies, or reactions to drugs, and simply indicate an active immune system at work. Glands of the groin and neck commonly become enlarged, sometimes without obvious cause. Infections, viral (for example, the flu or mononucleosis) and bacterial (for example, tuberculosis) can cause lymph node enlargement, sometimes for weeks. The condition called lymphadenopathy—enlarged, hard, sometimes painful lymph nodes in at least two parts of the body (excluding the groin) persisting for more than 3 months—may indicate AIDS or a possibly pre-AIDS condition called the lymphadenopathy syndrome.

ORAL THRUSH

Oral thrush is an infection of the tongue and mouth caused by a fungus, the yeast *Candida albicans*. *Candida* is normally present in the mouth and gastrointestinal tract but causes serious trouble only during debilitating illness, malnutrition, or the taking of antibiotics that suppress the normal balance of microorganisms and allow overgrowth of the fungus. Thrush is a persistent, creamy-white, curdlike patch that coats the tongue, surrounding throat, and esophagus (the food pipe that connects the throat to the stomach). It may be painful and cause difficulty in swallowing but rarely involves other internal organs.

Another condition similar to thrush and also seen in AIDS patients is called hairy leukoplakia. It produces lesions that are grayish white, linear, or patchy discolorations on the sides of or beneath the tongue and cannot be rubbed off.

PERSISTENT DIARRHEA

Diarrhea is frequent and loose bowel movements, usually signifying an attempt by the body to rid itself of an irritant or harmful substance. It may be due to toxins, infections, cancers, diet, emotional stress, or a host of other causes. Persistent diarrhea (longer than one week) is not normal and may lead to severe dehydration and loss of essential body salts.

COUGHING AND/OR SHORTNESS OF BREATH

An unusual pneumonia, *Pneumocystis carinii* pneumonia, often appears with AIDS. It may begin as a cough, a normal clearing action of the lung in which a reflex triggered by irritation of the airways expels debris, pus, and pathogens. The cough may produce phlegm or be dry. In AIDS, however, the cough may persist for weeks and progress to shortness of breath, indicating more severe damage to the respiratory system. A prolonged cough accompanied by fevers, chills, tightness in the chest, and increased breathing and pulse rates is an early warning of pneumonia. Shortness of breath not associated with heavy exertion, excitement, or blocked nasal passages warrants medical attention.

SKIN RASHES AND SPOTS

Lumps, bumps, and rashes on the skin always cause concern and create anxieties about possible cancer. In AIDS, the fear of Kaposi's sarcoma (KS) is especially prevalent. The lesions of KS vary. They are painless and non-itching, range in size from an insect bite to large nodules or plaques, are colored brown, blue, or purple, and may be found anywhere on the skin. Skin lesions inside the nose, mouth, or anus also may be a consequence of recurrent herpes ulcers or various malignancies other than KS.

Patients with ARC may have other subtle skin changes such as seborrheic dermatitis, more commonly known as eczema. It may appear as dandruff on the scalp or dry, itchy skin on the nose or eyebrows. Fungal infections can affect the skin in the groin or on the feet, especially in the nail beds.

BRUISING OR BLEEDING

Easy bruising and bleeding occur in some AIDS patients. Cuts may take longer to clot, mucous membranes may bleed without being injured, and even minor injuries to any part of the body may result in bruising. These may be symptoms of an uncommon blood disorder, idiopathic thrombocytopenia purpura (ITP), which has been noted in gay men at the same times and places as the AIDS epidemic, suggesting a causal relationship. In ITP, a defective immune system makes antibodies to destroy blood platelets, necessary for normal clotting. Any unusual bruising or bleeding should be reported to a physician.

NEUROLOGICAL PROBLEMS

A great variety of nervous system disorders appear in AIDS patients that may cause headaches, stiff neck, pain, numbness or weakness of the extremities, and even psychiatric symptoms such as depression, delusions, hallucinations, and paranoia. Most common in one study of AIDS patients were headache and fatigue. In one San Francisco study, half the patients with AIDS or ARC had neurological or psychiatric symptoms. The apparent benignity of some neurological complaints may lead the unsuspecting patient and physician astray. The underlying disease may be diverse, ranging from brain infections (meningitis and encephalitis) or tumors to lymphomas to brain hemorrhages.

The AIDS virus, HTLV-III/LAV, has been isolated in brain tissues in patients with AIDS and HTLV-III/LAV-related diseases and appears to reproduce readily in the brain. Some patients are infected with the AIDS virus and have subtle neurologic symptoms but no signs of immune dysfunction. The brain may therefore serve as a sanctuary for the AIDS virus, and any effective treatment for AIDS must use drugs that can penetrate to brain tissues.

Anyone with neurologic disease who also belongs to one of the risk groups for AIDS should be given an extensive neurologic evaluation, which may include CAT scans (X-ray cross sections) of the head, spinal taps, open brain biopsy, and other laboratory tests. Some of these conditions are treatable if diagnosed early enough.

6   Infections of AIDS

A.   Viral Infections
HELEN L. GRIERSON

Viral infections are probably the most common illnesses of man and other animals. Their consequences range in severity from a complete absence of symptoms to debilitation or death. Viral infections in AIDS patients and in people at risk for AIDS are especially significant for two main reasons. First, high-risk groups are known to be continually exposed to and reinfected with a variety of organisms, including viruses such as hepatitis, herpes, and cytomegalovirus (CMV). Many of these viruses can cause depressed immune function. Second, the virus associated with AIDS, HTLV-III/LAV, infects cells of the immune system and induces a vulnerability to attack by other viruses otherwise unlikely to cause disease.

Also important is the connection between viruses and cancers. Certain viruses are known to be oncogenic, that is, cancer-causing. For example, many of the viruses that plague AIDS patients have also been linked to the types of cancers AIDS patients develop. This section considers what a virus is, how the body normally defends itself against viral infections, and the viral infections most often associated with AIDS.

WHAT IS A VIRUS?

Virus is a term for a group of extremely small microorganisms that cannot grow or reproduce outside of living cells. They must enter a host cell in order to use the cell's biosynthetic machinery for their own replication. This pirating of the cell by the virus causes the initial symptoms of viral infections. Once a virus enters a cell it instructs that cell to make more virus which then leaves to infect other cells. This process continues until the infection is either recognized and halted by the host immune system or the infection becomes overwhelming and causes the death of the host.

Certain viruses, especially of the herpes family, can remain inactive, or latent, inside the host cell for long periods without causing problems. They remain integrated with the cell's genetic material (DNA) until triggered to begin replication. The previously dormant virus is then said to be reactivated. For example, the first (primary) infection with herpesvirus type I (oral herpes) is often asymptomatic. After the initial infection, the virus lives in nerve cells of the face where it may be reactivated at varying intervals and cause characteristic fever blisters (cold sores). The exact triggers of reactivation are not known, but associated factors may include exposure to ultraviolet light, fever, the presence of other infections, and immunodeficiency. The immune system of the host is normally able to subdue the reactivated virus and put it back into latency.

When a virus enters a cell and begins to reproduce, the immediate damage may vary from none to total destruction of the cell. In many viral infections, reproduction by undamaged cells quickly replaces the destroyed cells. However, destruction of the lining (epithelial surfaces) of the respiratory tract, common in some viral respiratory infections such as influenza (flu), compromises normal defense mechanisms and makes the host more susceptible to infection by invading bacteria. This is called secondary bacterial infection. Some cells, especially of nerves, are not able to reproduce and are thus not replaced after infection by a virus. The most vivid example of this is polio, where viral replication destroys the nerve cells (motor neurons) that control muscle movement and produces permanent paralysis.

HOW DOES THE BODY DEFEND AGAINST VIRAL INFECTION?

Depending upon its severity, the body's main defenses against viral infection are inflammation, antibody formation, interferon production, and cellular immunity.

Inflammation

Inflammation in blood vessels and adjacent tissues is a typical response to any type of infection. The ultimate purpose of inflammation is to remove the offending agents and to repair and heal injured tissue. Signs of inflammation include redness, heat, swelling, and pain. Redness and heat are due to locally increased fluid and leakage of cells out of the blood vessels. Pain is caused by stimulation of nerve endings due to pressure in the area.

Antibodies

Many different antibodies are formed in response to viral infections. They may be thought of as the "footprints" of a virus and tell us what type of virus we are dealing with and how long ago it was there. The antibodies include three main classes: IgM, IgA, and IgG.

As in other infections, virus-specific IgM is produced early in the disease and is a good indicator of current or very recent infection. IgA, or secretory antibodies, is an important part of the immune response to viral infections. Its presence in nasal passages, airways, and intestinal secretions defends against further infection by respiratory or intestinal viruses. IgG antibodies indicate past infection and the raising of a defense against the infecting virus.

Interferon

Interferon proteins are produced by virus-infected cells and may be partly responsible for ending an infection. They are not antibodies and are specific for the host species in which they are produced rather than for the agent that induced their formation. (Antibodies are specific for the invading agent.) Thus, human infections must be treated with interferon produced by human cells. Interferon interferes with viral synthesis and thus inhibits the spread of the infection.

Cellular Immunity

Cellular, or T-cell immunity, also helps to end viral infections. T cells destroy virus-infected cells. They also attract macrophages, which destroy and engulf infected cells and cell debris. A specific type of T cell, called a memory T cell, is produced during an immune response. Memory T cells persist in the body for a long time and "remember" a particular type of virus. Because of these cells, later exposure to the "remembered" virus evokes a speedier immune response and, if the immune system is normal, quick destruction of the invading virus. Another type of immune cell, called the natural killer (NK) cell, is the body's first line of defense against virus-infected cells and possibly certain types of tumor cells.

VIRAL INFECTIONS OF AIDS PATIENTS

Herpesviruses

AIDS induces a particular susceptibility to infection with herpesviruses. These include CMV, Epstein-Barr virus (EBV), herpes simplex types I and II, and varicella zoster (chickenpox, shingles). Herpesviruses have a unique relationship to humans in that they are able to combine with the genetic material, DNA, of certain cells of a human host and to remain latent for long periods, possibly for the life of the host. Reactivation may occur in otherwise healthy people and is common in cases of immune deficiency.

Cytomegalovirus (CMV)
CMV is a herpesvirus that infects man and other animals. It may affect only salivary glands or many organs of the body (generalized infection). CMV infection is clinically important in three main instances: in the developing fetus (congenital), as a primary infection in nonimmune persons, and reactivation of latent CMV infection in immunosuppressed patients.

Congenital CMV disease follows infection of a nonimmune mother during the early months of pregnancy. The effects on the fetus vary but may cause stillbirth or death soon after birth. Some infants who survive may exhibit no evidence of exposure; others may suffer severe damage of the central nervous system, liver, lungs, kidneys, and other tissues.

Primary infection of nonimmune persons occurs mainly in children and young adults, and produces only mild symptoms. CMV is transmitted by contaminated droplets or contact with the secretions of congenitally infected infants. Clinical symptoms are fever, fatigue, sore throat, and enlarged lymph glands, a syndrome called CMV mononucleosis. (The virus that most commonly causes infectious mononucleosis is EBV, discussed below.)

Latent CMV infections may be reactivated in immunosuppressed persons. Consequently, it is no surprise that virtually all AIDS patients have antibody to CMV, and a large percentage of homosexual men with AIDS actually excrete the virus in saliva and semen. People with normal immune systems, experiencing CMV infection for the first time, may display an immunosuppression that lasts for weeks or months. Thus, it is likely that reactivated and persistent CMV infections in AIDS risk groups aggravate the immunosuppression and increase the severity of the disease. CMV may also play a part in the development of Kaposi's sarcoma, common in AIDS patients. It has been isolated in Kaposi's lesions, and some think CMV may be oncogenic (cancer-causing). No effective methods are known for the prevention or treatment of CMV infections.

Epstein-Barr Virus (EBV)

EBV, another member of the herpesvirus family, is the most common cause of infectious mononucleosis ("mono," or "kissing disease"). It has also been associated with two types of cancer: Burkitt's lymphoma and nasopharyngeal carcinoma. EBV infects the cells of the immune system—B cells— responsible for making antibodies. B cells have specific receptors for EBV to which the virus attaches, permitting it to enter the cells and reproduce. Like CMV mononucleosis, EBV-induced mono is usually an asymptomatic or mild disease of children and young adults. Worldwide 80–90 percent of adults have antibodies specific to EBV, indicating past infection at some time.

EBV is also able to remain latent and become reactivated. Nearly 100 percent of homosexual men with AIDS have antibodies to EBV which may have been reactivated as shown by the types of antibodies found. These patients also tend to develop lymphomas (cancers) of B cells (resembling Burkitt's lymphoma) for which it has been suggested that EBV may be at least partly responsible.

Herpes Simplex Virus

The two main types of herpes simplex virus (HSV) infections are caused by HSV-I (herpes labialis—fever blisters, cold sore) and

HSV-II (genital, or venereal, herpes). As with the other types of herpesviruses, these two are notorious for their ability to remain latent and to become periodically reactivated. Cold sores are the most common HSV-I infection, and recurrences are estimated to afflict 20 to 40 percent of the population of the United States. The characteristic lesions are fluid-filled pustules at the edges of the lips, containing viral particles capable of infecting others.

HSV-II is transmitted as a venereal infection and has been associated with cervical cancer. With genital herpes, the primary infection may be asymptomatic, but characteristic lesions may later appear on the penis of males or in the cervix, vagina, and anal areas of females. However, lesions do sometimes appear soon after first infection. One of the most serious HSV-II infections is of babies during childbirth. Premature newborns and infants with debilitating diseases or immunodeficiencies are particularly vulnerable. The disease ranges from a mild illness to a fulminating systemic infection with enlarged lymph glands and necrotic lesions (areas of dead tissue) throughout the body. The fatality rate in severe cases is very high, and infants who survive often have permanent brain damage.

HSV-II infection is extremely common in AIDS patients, particularly as a recurrent ulcer around the anus in homosexual men. Because AIDS patients are immunosuppressed, they experience more episodes of viral reactivation than others with normal immune systems. Two cancers common in AIDS patients may be associated with HSV: squamous cell carcinoma of the tongue with HSV-I, and carcinoma of the rectum with HSV-II.

Varicella Zoster Virus (VZV)
Chickenpox (varicella) is a primary infection of a nonimmune host by a varicella zoster virus, contracted by direct contact with infected droplets. The virus migrates from the respiratory tract to the lymphatic system and then spreads to the lymph glands. It replicates there and enters the blood stream, to be carried to the skin and mucous membranes where it produces characteristic blisters.

In children, chickenpox is a mild illness characterized by fever, a rash, particularly on the trunk, and often blisters in the mouth. Complications are rare in children, but in adults the disease is more severe and the risk of complications such as pneumonia higher.

Shingles (herpes zoster) is caused by reactivation of VZV latent in

nerve cells from a previous attack of chickenpox. As with other
herpesviruses, reactivation is more likely in immunocompromised
individuals. Thus, shingles is common and sometimes especially
severe in AIDS patients.

Hepatitis

Hepatitis simply means inflammation of the liver. Many different
viruses can infect and damage the liver, for example, herpes virus
hominis, CMV, EBV, Coxsackie viruses, and certain insect-carried
viruses (arboviruses) found in tropical countries. However, viral
hepatitis is the term usually applied to liver disease caused by
hepatitis A or B viruses (HAV or HBV). Hepatitis caused by other
agents is called non-A non-B hepatitis.

Hepatitis-A-like illness was described by Hippocrates 2,000 years
ago. Sporadic cases and epidemics have been reported over the
centuries, and to this day hepatitis A is a common disease. HAV is
usually transmitted from person to person by the fecal-oral route
directly or through contaminated food, water, and shellfish. Infection
is most common in children, lower socioeconomic groups, and rural
rather than urban dwellers. Incubation time is 2 to 4 weeks. Since
virus is present in the blood for only a short time and in small
amounts during active infection, transmission by blood transfusion is
uncommon. Antibody is produced quickly following infection and
persists in the blood for at least 10 years, giving long-lasting
protection against the harmful effects of reinfection.

HBV differs from HAV in many ways, including virus structure,
method of transmission, length of incubation period, severity of
infection, and the existence of a chronic HBV carrier state. The
sources of HBV infection are chronic carriers of the virus and
patients with acute infection, who both carry virus particles in blood
and other body secretions. A carrier state develops in 5 to 10 percent
of infected people, resulting in an estimated 120,000,000 carriers
throughout the world. The distribution varies with geographic
location, about 0.1 percent of the population in the United States and
more than 15 percent in some tropical areas.

HBV is transmitted mainly by inoculation, for example, in
transfusions of blood and blood products from infected donors, use

of contaminated syringes and needles by drug abusers, and use of inadequately sterilized surgical equipment. A high carrier rate is found among transplant recipients, patients who have received multiple blood transfusions, and people with immunodeficiency disorders. A tiny drop of infected blood can transmit the virus, and even shared toothbrushes and razor blades are potential instruments of inoculation. In fact, since the virus has been found in urine, saliva, semen, menstrual blood, and other body fluids and secretions, oral, sexual, or intimate physical contact of any kind may transmit HBV.

The incubation period for HBV ranges from 6 to 180 days, depending upon the amount of virus transmitted. The pathological effects of HAV and HBV on the liver are virtually identical. Infection by either virus causes structural and functional damage ranging from insignificant to severe and irreversible.

Despite similarities in liver damage, the outcomes of HAV and HBV infections differ greatly. For HAV, complete recovery within a few weeks is the rule, and complications are rare. For HBV, a few patients suffer rapid and fatal liver failure; about 10 percent develop a continuing chronic infection that sometimes causes symptoms and sometimes does not. Many patients who develop chronic HBV infections do so without going through a phase of overt, acute hepatitis.

AIDS patients tend to be infected with both HAV and HBV. However, although the incidence of antibodies to HAV in such patients is similar to that seen in the general population, the carrier rate for HBV is extremely high in both AIDS patients and homosexual men with AIDS-related complex (ARC, a suspectedly pre-AIDS syndrome). Of importance to groups of patients at risk for developing AIDS is the recent development and release of an anti-HBV vaccine produced from the pooled plasma of donors who test positive for hepatitis antigen. Initial concern that the AIDS virus might be transmitted with the anti-HBV vaccine has been allayed. Several thousand volunteer health-care workers received the vaccine between 1975 and 1983, and none developed AIDS. Since the vaccine was placed on the market in July 1982, over 200,000 more have received it, and no cases of AIDS have been reported outside of high-risk groups.

Adenoviruses

Adenoviruses cause respiratory tract infections that vary in severity from the common cold to viral pneumonia. They can also cause eye infections, which frequently accompany adenoviral respiratory tract diseases. These infections are usually mild and produce few complications. However, in patients who are immunosuppressed, for example, due to AIDS or treatment for an organ transplant, the adenovirus can cause severe disturbances and spread throughout the body. There is no successful treatment for adenoviral infections.

HTLV-III/LAV

HTLV-III/LAV (human T-cell lymphotropic virus type III/ lymphadenopathy-associated virus) is a recently (1983) discovered retrovirus that is the main cause of AIDS and AIDS-related diseases. Retroviruses (containing an enzyme called reverse transcriptase) are RNA tumor viruses (other viruses have DNA genetic material) known since 1964 to cause cancers in animals after they were identified as the cause of leukemia in cats. In feline leukemia, the virus selectively infects and destroys lymphocytes, causing immunodeficiency and T-cell leukemia/lymphoma. In 1970, the first primate retrovirus was found to cause cancer in Rhesus monkeys, and in 1980, the first human retrovirus was isolated by investigators in the United States and Japan. The human retrovirus was called HTLV-I and is associated with adult T-cell leukemia. At the beginning of the AIDS epidemic, HTLV-I was suspected as a possible cause of AIDS because it was endemic in certain areas of the Caribbean, including Haiti, and many of the first cases of AIDS were reported in Haitian immigrants to the United States.

HTLV-II was isolated from a patient with hairy-cell leukemia shortly after the identification of HTLV-I, but has not been well studied. The significance of HTLV-II in causing disease is not yet known.

HTLV-III/LAV was isolated simultaneously in 1983–84 by researchers at the National Cancer Institute (they named it "HTLV-III") and the Pasteur Institute in France (they called it "LAV"). (Another group of researchers isolated the virus and named it AIDS-associated retrovirus, or ARV. To eliminate confusion, the International Committee on Nomenclature of Viruses has recommended the name human immune deficiency virus, or HIV, which better describes its clinical effects.) HTLV-III/LAV primarily infects T_4 helper lymphocytes and destroys them. HTLV-III/LAV attaches to a special structure called the T_4 receptor, which is present primarily on T_4 helper lymphocytes. After attaching to its target cell, the virus enters the cell and sheds its protein coat, exposing the viral RNA inside. The enzyme reverse transcriptase then converts viral RNA to viral DNA, which becomes part of the target cell's DNA. Viral DNA then instructs the cell to make new virus particles, which leave to infect other cells. Production of virus particles does not necessarily cause the cells to die. Recent studies have shown, however, that virus production does cause cell death in T_4 cells if they are immunologically stimulated after being infected by HTLV-III/LAV. Since any foreign agent (bacterium, fungus, virus, protozoa) immunologically stimulates cells when it infects the body, it follows that the more infections, the more T_4-cell destruction. It is the loss of these important cells that causes the profound immunodeficiency characteristic of AIDS.

It is not clear at this time if HTLV-III/LAV by itself is sufficient to deplete the body's supply of T_4 cells, or if other factors (cofactors), such as coincident viral and parasitic infection, are necessary. Also, lymphocytes may not be the only target for HTLV-III/LAV. The virus has been isolated from tissues of the nervous system and may be the cause of meningitis and other neurological disorders in AIDS and ARC patients. It is noteworthy that HTLV-III/LAV in shape, structure, and biological classification is related to the visna virus (a lentivirus, named for its lens shape) which causes a slow degenerative disease of the nervous system in sheep.

Evidence for the role of HTLV-III/LAV in AIDS was found by isolating the virus and measuring antibodies to the virus in AIDS patients and members of high-risk AIDS groups. The virus has been isolated from blood and semen and in some instances in saliva and tears. Nearly 100 percent of AIDS patients, 50–60 percent of homosexual men with ARC, and, depending upon the population studied, 17–67 percent of all homosexual men in the United States and Europe have been reported to have antibody to HTLV-III/LAV.

The virus appears to be transmitted in infected body fluids by sexual intercourse, use of contaminated needles, blood transfusion, and delivery of newborns by infected mothers. There is no evidence that it can be transmitted by casual contact. As with other viruses, primary infection with HTLV-III/LAV can cause a spectrum of symptoms whose severity depends in part on the immune status of the host. Because of the relative newness of HTLV-III/LAV, symptoms of primary infection are not well defined, but it is known that an acute mononucleosis-like illness has been described by homosexual men within days to weeks after exposure.

HTLV-III/LAV has also been isolated from asymptomatic individuals, and it is not known for certain if all who are infected will eventually develop AIDS. Of 6,875 people in San Francisco participating in a long-term study of hepatitis-B infection, 4 percent tested positive for HTLV-III/LAV antibody in 1978, which rose to 24 percent by 1980 and 68 percent by 1984; 166 of the group (2.4 percent) have been diagnosed with AIDS and another 25.8 percent with ARC. In another study, the incubation period for transfusion-associated AIDS was found to be 4.5 years, and for homosexual men with AIDS the average interval between detection of antibodies (seroconversion) and diagnosis of AIDS was greater than 3 years.

There is no known effective treatment for HTLV-III/LAV infection, and, if this virus is similar to other retroviruses, infection is often for life. Efforts to produce a vaccine are under way, but success is not expected until the mid-1990s. Until a successful treatment or vaccine is available, measures such as education of individuals in risk groups and screening of blood and blood products to prevent transmission of the virus must be taken to control the spread of HTLV-III/LAV.

SUMMARY

There is no doubt that viruses are extremely important in the etiology of AIDS. HTLV-III/LAV is the likely main cause of AIDS and AIDS-related diseases. In combination with other, opportunistic viruses, that also produce immune depression, recurrent infections, and cancers, especially in high-risk groups, it causes the irreversible immune depression characteristic of AIDS.

B.   Parasitic Infections
NIRMAL K. FERNANDO
PETER HO

PNEUMOCYSTIS CARINII

Most AIDS patients will be diagnosed as having *Pneumocystis carinii* pneumonia (PCP) when first seen by a physician; PCP is also the leading cause of AIDS deaths. PCP is an opportunistic infection whose importance has increased over the past decade, due, in part, to the advent of effective chemotherapy for cancer patients.

In the United States, PCP was not reported until 1956, when it was first noted in children with congenital immune defects. The mode of transmission and natural habitat of *Pneumocystis carinii*, the parasite microorganism that causes PCP, remain largely unknown. It has been found in the lungs of animals and of normal, healthy humans, and autopsy studies have occasionally shown the organisms in the lungs of patients who had no immune defect. However, no documented cases of PCP have been reported in adults with intact immune systems.

The severity of PCP in AIDS patients may obscure the fact that its ability to flourish is due to a weakened immune system rather than to the infectiousness of the parasite. The parasite multiplies and fills the air spaces in the lungs, provoking an intense inflammatory response and the clinical manifestation of pneumonia.

Clinical Manifestations of PCP

Most AIDS patients have already been ill for some time before they get PCP. Weight loss, low grade fever, diarrhea, and unexplained lymph node enlargement often precede pulmonary involvement, although fever and cough are the first complaints. Gradually, the cough becomes worse and shortness of breath develops, especially with physical exertion. Interestingly, a stethoscope often reveals no abnormal sounds in the lungs, even though chest X-rays may show pneumonia on both sides. A small percentage of AIDS patients with

PCP have a more rapid and severe onset with high fever, rapidly progressive shortness of breath, and profuse sweating. The pneumonia prevents the transport of oxygen from inhaled air into the blood, lowering blood oxygen to dangerous levels. The following is a typical PCP case:

A 41-year-old intravenous-drug abuser noticed weakness, easy fatigability, and a nonproductive cough in July 1983. He attributed this to a viral infection and was able to continue his activities, although he became short-winded when he jogged. His physician prescribed an antibiotic. The shortness of breath got worse and he was hospitalized in September 1983. By then he had a fever, night sweats, and a persistent cough. He was initially treated for bacterial pneumonia, and his symptoms improved slightly over the next 2 weeks. However, he then became markedly short of breath and breathed very rapidly. He deteriorated quickly and, even with aggressive therapy, died 5 days later.

Diagnosis

No characteristic symptoms are definitive for PCP. Blood gas usually shows decreased oxygen, especially after exercise. Chest X-rays are often normal at first but, as the disease advances, bilateral infiltrate (haziness on the X-ray) is the most common pattern. Interestingly, in the early stages, when the chest X-ray is normal, a simultaneous gallium scan usually shows active uptake in the lungs. (Gallium is a metallic element preferentially taken up by certain inflammatory cells in the body.) The definitive diagnosis of PCP requires the identification of the organism in samples taken from the lung.

Lung tissue is usually obtained directly by biopsy using a flexible bronchoscope. If this fails to decide the diagnosis, open-lung biopsy is the final step. In bronchoscopy, which is less invasive than open-lung biopsy, a small tube is passed down the trachea (windpipe) and into the lung. In an open-lung biopsy, a small incision is made on the chest wall, one or two small segments of ribs are cut away, and lung tissue is obtained through the incision.

Therapy

Specific antibiotics for PCP are highly effective but the underlying immunosuppression usually results in frequent relapses. Clotrimoxazole, a combination of sulfamethoxazole and trimethoprim antibiotics in a fixed ratio and commonly used to treat urinary tract infections, is also used for PCP but in much larger doses and for longer periods. The other antibiotic most frequently used for PCP is pentamidine, available only from the Centers for Disease Control, a government agency. Clotrimoxazole causes rashes more often in AIDS patients than in the general population.

In the United States, most physicians initially treat PCP with intravenous trimethoprim/sulfamethoxazole (Bactrim or Septra) since it is believed to be the less toxic of the two drugs. If the patient does not improve, pentamidine is either added to the Bactrim or substituted for it. The complete blood count and kidney and liver functions must be carefully monitored when these drugs are administered because of their known adverse effects on bone marrow (where blood cells are made) and on the kidneys and liver. Another serious, but relatively uncommon, side effect is severe hypoglycemia (low blood sugar). Also, because pentamidine given intravenously may cause an irregular heart rhythm, it is most often injected into muscle tissue. Both pentamidine and Bactrim have been reported to cause a mild and transient inflammation of the nerves (peripheral neuritis).

A major problem for AIDS patients is that both relapse and reinfection are common due to continued immunosuppression. It is unfortunate that the immunologic impairment in AIDS is not reversible, since correction of the immunosuppression would lead to spontaneous recovery from the infection. Taking medications prophylactically to prevent infections has been proposed and even practiced by some authorities, but judgment of the effectiveness of prophylaxis awaits further clinical studies.

TOXOPLASMOSIS

Toxoplasma gondii, like *Pneumocystis carinii*, is a parasite that lives in a latent, asymptomatic state in many healthy people. It is distributed worldwide and affects virtually all mammalian species. Humans may acquire the organism through contaminated food, blood transfusions, or organ transplantation, and *in utero* (transmitted to the unborn fetus via the placenta). Drinking contaminated water, or eating undercooked meat, such as pork, beef, or veal, or food contaminated by cat feces, may lead to infection. Pet cats are a well-known source of *T. gondii* infection.

Clinical Manifestations

In AIDS, this normally asymptomatic infection involves all organs of the body, with especially devastating effects on the brain (encephalitis) that have been particularly common in Haitians who have contracted AIDS. Brain symptoms include confusion, headache, weakness, dizziness, seizures, and other characteristics resembling a stroke. This type of symptom complex mimics that of a brain tumor. The patient is very sick and often deteriorates rapidly to death.

Pneumonia can also occur as the organism attacks the lungs. Thus cough, fever, shortness of breath, and an abnormal chest X-ray are helpful clues to diagnosis.

Another organ commonly affected in immunosuppressed patients is the heart muscle. Heart infection is called myocarditis (from the Latin words for muscle and heart). Changes in heart rate and rhythm, observed in an electrocardiogram, together with a general physical examination, establish this serious diagnosis. Myocarditis can result in heart failure and, if compounded with pneumonia, may be life-threatening.

Diagnosis

A definite diagnosis of *T. gondii* infection requires a biopsy of the suspected organ. The organism can then be identified by a pathologist after the tissue sample is properly processed and examined. Blood tests are usually helpful, but often show deceptively normal responses in AIDS patients. A brain scan and a CAT scan (special cross-sectional X-ray) of the head may be helpful, but are not definitive.

Therapy

Treatment consists of general supportive measures directed at the particular organ involved. For example, if the patient has a pneumonia, the antibiotic combination of sulfadiazine and pyrimethamine is given. Repetitive courses of medication are often necessary, since complete cure is never achieved. However, this antibiotic has a dangerous side effect on blood-cell production in the bone marrow so that in AIDS, when the blood count is invariably abnormal, the addition of this drug complication would be detrimental. This again indicates that the diseases to which AIDS patients are subject are very dangerous, and that some of the medications used to combat them can lead to serious complications.

AMEBIASIS AND GIARDIASIS

For over a decade before the outbreak of AIDS, physicians found in homosexuals a large number of intestinal parasites once thought to be exclusively in the domain of tropical diseases. The associated enteric infections were named the "gay bowel syndrome," and included common venereal diseases such as gonorrhea and syphilis as well as others less generally considered venereal, for example, shigellosis, amebiasis, and giardiasis. Amebiasis and giardiasis are among the most common diarrheal diseases in AIDS. They are caused by intestinal parasites that can exist in a latent, asymptomatic state or create severe disturbances. The usual mode of transmission of the organisms is through contaminated food or drink. However, in homosexuals the anal-oral route is prevalent due to the pattern of sexual practices.

Amebiasis

Amebiasis is caused by *Entameba histolytica* and is characterized by lower abdominal cramps, fever, and bloody diarrhea. Since only about 10 percent of patients become symptomatic, the infection is largely spread by healthy "carriers." In the United States in general the prevalence is 3 percent to 4 percent, but in the homosexual population of New York City the figure is closer to 40 percent. The organism is found in soil and water, but man is the principal host and source of infection.

Diagnosis is made by identifying the organism in the stool or in material scraped from the inner lining of the lower bowel. Identifying parasites in the stool requires special experience and training, since these infections are relatively uncommon in the United States.

E. histolytica may spread to the liver but rarely to other organs. In nonbowel amebiasis, blood tests are most commonly used for diagnosis although the organism can sometimes be observed in pus collected from the abscess. Diagnosis of amebiasis is not a major problem in AIDS.

A drug called metronidazole (Flagyl) has been used successfully to treat amebiasis, but, depending on the site of infections, other medications may be necessary.

Giardiasis

Giardiasis is the most common waterborne epidemic diarrheal illness in the United States. It is caused by *Giardia lamblia,* a protozoan of worldwide distribution. Campers, particularly in the Rocky Mountains, have been infected after drinking untreated water from mountain streams, but the infection has also been found all over the country. Asymptomatic carriers can transmit the nonvegetative, or cyst, form of the organism. The organism resides in the upper part of the small intestine.

Symptoms vary, but typically include an explosive, watery, foul-smelling diarrhea, abdominal distention, and flatulence. Nausea, vomiting, fever, and blood in the stools are uncommon, but belching is frequent. Some patients have chronic intermittent diarrhea and weight loss.

Treatment is with quinacrine, considered the drug of choice, or with metronidazole (Flagyl). Quinacrine may induce abdominal pains, headaches, and a yellow discoloration of the skin and urine. Drinking alcohol during medication with quinacrine produces a violent reaction characterized by nausea, vomiting, and abdominal pain.

CRYPTOSPORIDIOSIS

Cryptosporidium is a tiny protozoan parasite that causes cryptosporidiosis, a diarrhea in animals, especially calves. Mild diarrhea can afflict infected humans, but human infection usually resolves itself spontaneously. Often, the organism is not recognized as the cause of diarrhea because the illness is self-limiting and stools may not have been examined specifically for *Cryptosporidium*. In AIDS, however, cryptosporidiosis is a devastating infection characterized by unrelenting, voluminous, watery diarrhea progressing to dehydration, loss of important body salts, and malnutrition. The clinical picture is similar to that of cholera in which the patient can die from the complications of dehydration and malnutrition. With severe dehydration, the blood pressure drops, leading to a state of shock.

There is no completely effective therapy or drug at present to eradicate this parasite, although many have been tried. In limited studies, spiromycin has been shown to be effective in some AIDS patients infected with *Cryptosporidia*, but further studies are required. Spiromycin is not available in the United States, but physicians wishing to use this drug may obtain it through the Food and Drug Administration. Treatment is directed at maintaining fluid and nutritional balance by supportive measures such as intravenous infusions. Since there is no cure, diarrhea recurs intermittently.

SUMMARY

AIDS patients are susceptible to a variety of parasitic infections. Most common is PCP, which is also the primary cause of AIDS deaths. The other infections are primarily diarrheal, and many are quite common. While they may cause extreme discomfort in otherwise healthy individuals, they rarely result in serious illness. AIDS patients, however, may have infected for prolonged periods and become dangerously malnourished. Malnutrition may sometimes become severe enough to be fatal.

C.   Bacterial and Fungal Infections

JOHN W. SENSAKOVIC
EDWARD S. JOHNSON

Bacteria and fungi are among the many different microorganisms that constantly surround us. Most prominent are bacteria, single-celled organisms barely visible under the optical microscope, which inhabit the air we breathe, the food we eat (no matter how carefully prepared), and our bodies. For example, our bowels contain millions of bacteria, some beneficial (some vitamins are synthesized by bacteria), some disease-causing.

AIDS, by damaging the body's immune defenses, upsets the balance between healthy coexistence and bacterial infection. The body then becomes prey to bacteria (and other disease-causing agents) from within and without. Previously benign bacteria can turn into deadly enemies. Opportunistic infections, rare when the immune system is normal and able to fight them off, now take hold. Common illnesses that are usually mild or controllable also occur but in more severe and resistant forms.

AIDS patients and physicians sometimes find it difficult to remember that the many infections are really a complication and not the disease itself. This is because a patient may contract a life-threatening illness, for example, pneumonia, recover with treatment and apparently regain normal health and a sense of well-being, only to become sick again. Conversely, an infection in another patient may start mild but progress relentlessly until it causes death.

This deceptive variability in the response of AIDS patients to common and opportunistic infections and malignancies can divert attention away from the real culprit, underlying AIDS. Paradoxically, this diversion may sometimes help patient morale.

The following are the most common bacterial and fungal infections characteristic of AIDS, but deficient immunities make AIDS patients vulnerable to any number of different microbes.

BACTERIAL INFECTIONS

Tuberculosis

Almost forgotten in this age of antibiotics, tuberculosis has been recorded since ancient times as a feared and dangerous disease. It is caused by *Mycobacterium tuberculosis*, a bacterium that produces small masses or lumps (*tuberculum* is Latin for lump) in almost any organ of the body but usually in the lung (pulmonary tuberculosis). It is most often spread by infected sputum droplets sprayed into the air during coughing, but also appears in some unpasteurized dairy products.

Symptoms vary. Patients may have no early symptoms, but some experience fatigue, mild fever, poor appetite, and weight loss. As the disease progresses, they develop a cough, which brings up pus and sometimes blood, night sweats, chest pains, and shortness of breath. If untreated, the disease may spread to other organs, and the patient becomes emaciated and dies.

Diagnosis is by clinical examination, simple skin tests (an extract of the bacteria injected just under the skin produces a red lump if the patient has been exposed or is infected), chest X-ray, and isolation of the bacterium, usually from sputum. Many who have been exposed develop antibodies and respond to the skin test but do not develop active disease.

AIDS patients with tuberculosis give a negative response to the skin test because their impaired immunity prevents the development of antibodies. However, chest X-rays show lung scarring and other signs, and cultures of sputum grow the tuberculosis bacteria.

While tuberculosis is not considered an opportunistic infection (people with normal immune systems may acquire the disease), it often appears with AIDS and tends to be more intense and difficult to eradicate. Treatment, futile before the availability of antibiotics, consists of drugs, including isoniazid, rifampin, ethambutol, and streptomycin, given in combination because the bacteria tend to develop resistance if only a single drug is used. Treatment usually continues for at least a year.

Atypical Tuberculosis

Modern microbiological techniques have identified other forms of tuberculosis with similar symptoms but a different cause. They are called "atypical mycobacterial infections." The first cluster of atypical mycobacterial infections, caused by *Mycobacterium avium-intracellulare,* or MAI (including *M. avium* and *M. intracellulare*), was reported in New York City in October 1982 among homosexuals and intravenous (IV)-drug abusers. MAI is common in the environment, for example, in soil, water, house dust, and even in our mouths. Except in high-risk AIDS groups, it rarely causes disease in humans.

MAI infections, like typical tuberculosis, usually affect the lungs, but any organ may be involved, and patients were generally middle-aged men with illness that suppressed their immune systems. Before AIDS, the spread to other organs had been observed in fewer than twenty cases. In AIDS patients, MAI infections are more common than typical tuberculosis and are devastating, tending to spread beyond the lung to the liver, spleen, lymph nodes, bone marrow, gastrointestinal tract, skin, and brain. Symptoms may include cough, shortness of breath, general debilitation and weight loss, severe diarrhea with abdominal pains, and swollen glands (lymph nodes). Brain infection may cause headache, visual problems, weakness, and loss of balance.

MAI infections are resistant to treatment in both AIDS and non-AIDS patients. Antibiotic therapy has met with little success, only small gains being achieved with ansamycin (a derivative of the standard antituberculosis drug rifampin) and clofazimine, an anti-leprosy drug. Infections have been contained to a limited degree with combinations of four or five drugs, such as ethionamide, cycloserine, ethambutol, and streptomycin. Good results in the test tube *(in vitro)* have been reported with a "superpenicillin" called thienamycin, which is being investigated in conjunction with an already available antibiotic, amikacin, as a promising treatment. Also under investigation is transfer factor, a chemical produced by cells (lymphocytes) of the immune system that transfers specific immunological properties possessed by one cell to another, thus helping to improve a deficient immune system.

Salmonellosis

Salmonellosis, infection with *Salmonella* bacteria, is one of the most common diseases in the United States (over two million cases a year) and frequently appears in patients with AIDS or other defects in cell-mediated immunity. It may take the form of a mild inflammation of the stomach and intestines, a localized infection, a brain infection, or a severe blood infection such as typhoid fever (caused by *Salmonella typhii*). Symptoms are fever, abdominal pain, severe diarrhea, headache, and rash. The usual mild form comes from eating contaminated or improperly prepared foods, especially eggs, chicken, and duck. Homosexuals transmit it through anal-oral sex. Diagnosis depends on isolating the bacteria from blood or stools.

The intestinal infection is usually self-limiting, improving within a week with only such treatment as rest and drinking plenty of fluids. Typhoid fever is more difficult to treat because the bacteria can reside in areas of the body not easily reached by antibiotics. It requires powerful antibiotics, such as ampicillin or chloramphenicol, administered for long periods of time. Drugs such as Bactrim, Septra, and some new cephalosporins are also used.

Nocardia Infections

Nocardia are common soil bacteria that grow by branching like fungi (mold). Infections are common but usually cause severe lung disease that can spread to other body organs only in patients with defective immune systems, as in AIDS. As with other chronic lung infections, symptoms are a cough, sputum production, chest pain, fever, and weakness. If the infection travels in the blood to the brain, it may cause confusion, dizziness, headaches, seizures, and other neurologic symptoms. Because of its nonspecific nature and its rarity in severe form, the disease requires a high degree of suspicion and appropriate laboratory tests to establish a diagnosis.

Treatment of nocardial disease may be extremely difficult, often requiring prolonged administration of antibiotics, such as sulfadiazine and cycloserine. The outlook is generally poor, and is especially grim if associated with AIDS.

Listeria Infections

The bacterium *Listeria monocytogenes* infects mostly fetuses in the womb, newborns, the elderly, and patients with deficient immune systems. The very young and the very old are considered to be naturally immunologically incompetent and therefore susceptible to opportunistic infections traditionally seen in patients lacking immune defenses due to lymphoma, treatment to prevent rejection of an organ transplant, or other causes of T-cell deficiency. The very young become infected with *Listeria* during the mother's pregnancy or in passage through the birth canal. Older people become infected from inhaling contaminated dust or contact with infected animals or contaminated sewage or soil. The disease is most often a severe brain infection characterized by fever, delirium, sometimes coma, convulsions, and even shock.

Diagnosis is made by cultures of specimens such as blood and spinal fluid and microscopic examination. Treatment consists of combinations of antibiotics such as penicillin, erythromycin, ampicillin, chloramphenicol, and gentamicin. Although *Listeria* infection is rare in AIDS patients, Dr. Donald B. Louria has suggested that they are vulnerable, and the incidence of the disease may increase.

Other Bacterial Infections

Pneumonias caused by the bacteria *Hemophilus influenzae* and *Streptococcus pneumoniae* occur more often in AIDS patients than in the general population. Also, some AIDS patients with *Pneumocystis carinii* pneumonia, a type almost indicative of AIDS, have had pneumococcal or *H. influenzae* pneumonia as well. It seems possible that this conjunction of pneumonias may be due to an additional immunologic defect in AIDS patients demonstrated at the National Institutes of Health.

The T-cell defect of AIDS (see chapter 4) is accompanied by a B-cell defect that results in high levels of antibodies, but antibodies that are ineffective. Abnormal, poorly functioning antibodies may increase an AIDS patient's susceptibility to common bacteria such as *Staphylococcus epidermidis,* the most prevalent cause of hospital-acquired infection, introduced when tubes are inserted into a blood vessel or into the bladder to drain away urine. *S. epidermidis* typically causes blood infection accompanied by a high fever, sweating, fatigue, and a general decline in health.

Still other bacterial infections are likely to become associated with AIDS. Whatever the future holds, it is clear now that, since infections by bacteria such as MAI respond poorly to antibiotic treatment, successful therapy will have to reverse the immunodeficiency characteristic of AIDS as well as combat the bacteria themselves (table 1).

FUNGAL INFECTIONS

Fungi are microscopic organisms commonly found in nature in two principal forms, yeasts and molds. The simpler form is the yeasts, single-celled organisms that divide by budding small daughter cells. Yeasts are widespread in the environment and in baker's and brewer's yeasts.

TABLE 1: DRUG THERAPY OF BACTERIAL INFECTIONS

(Agents that are used alone or in combination)

Mycobacterium Avium-Intracellulare

Ansamycin/rifampin (investigational)
Clofazimine (investigational)
Ethionamide
Cycloserine
Ethambutol
Streptomycin
Amikacin
(Thienamycin—based on laboratory results only)
(Transfer factor—investigational)

Salmonella

Ampicillin
Chloramphenicol
Trimethoprim sulfamethoxazole (Bactrim, Septra)
Some new cephalosporins

Nocardia asteroides

Sulfadiazine
Cycloserine

Listeria monocytogenes

Ampicillin
Chloramphenicol
Aminoglycosides (gentamicin)

Molds are composed of branching, intertwined cells that create the characteristic furry appearance. A familiar mold is the one that grows on bread.

Most fungi, both yeasts and molds, do not cause human disease. When disease does occur, for example, fungal skin infections such as diaper rash and jock itch, it usually tends to be a nuisance rather than a threat. When fungi do cause serious infection, they do so primarily in individuals with an abnormal immune system, for example, in cancer patients or in patients receiving drugs that depress the immune system. Since AIDS patients characteristically have an impaired immune system, it is not at all surprising that they are candidates for certain fungal infections.

Candida albicans

The most common fungal infection seen in AIDS patients is due to a yeast called *Candida albicans*. Indeed, some physicians consider it a clue to the presence of AIDS if found in the proper clinical setting. Fortunately, it is not typically a serious infection. *Candida* causes a superficial infection of the mouth and throat with pain and white plaques in the affected areas. Though it may be very difficult to cure in AIDS patients and tends to recur, it rarely spreads to other parts of the body and, therefore, is not likely to be fatal. *Candida* also causes infections in patients, e.g., diabetics, who do not have AIDS, and is responsible for certain types of diaper rash, oral thrush in infants, and vaginal infections in women.

Some groups that acquire similar superficial *Candida* infections—AIDS patients and infants born with certain genetic immune deficiencies, glandular disturbances, or tumors—share in common an impaired T-cell immune system.

Cryptococcus

Another fungal infection seen in AIDS patients is due to *Cryptococcus,* another yeast common in nature, that causes disease in patients with immune defects. *Cryptococcus* produces a thick, protective capsule that enables it to resist the body's defenses. The yeast enters the body via the lungs, migrates into the blood, and spreads to other organs, especially the brain. In the brain, it causes severe meningitis, which is very resistant to therapy and often fatal.

Histoplasma

The third fungus seen in AIDS patients is called *Histoplasma*. This fungus is also very common in nature, especially in the Ohio River valley and eastern United States. People with normal immunity are commonly exposed to *Histoplasma* without developing disease. If disease does develop, it produces upper respiratory symptoms in healthy adults, but in AIDS patients it quickly involves the lung, liver, spleen, brain, and gastrointestinal tract. The increasing number of severe *Histoplasma* infections described in AIDS patients is again the consequence of their T-cell defect.

Diagnosis of *Histoplasma* infections is helped by recovery of the fungus from the blood, urine, or infected organ tissues. Amphotericin is used for treatment.

SUMMARY

AIDS is characterized by a melange of rare bacterial and fungal diseases and disorders that are consequences of the body's frail and failing immune system. Immune dysfunction does not cause the deaths, but complications of the diseases do. The clinical course in these patients is marked by recurrent, severe, multiple opportunistic infections, which present major challenges to physician and patient alike. Treatment with antibiotics may temporarily control opportunistic infections, but merely postpones, rather than prevents, the development of other AIDS-related illnesses.

7 Cancers and Blood Disorders of AIDS

MICHAEL SCOPPETUOLO

The attack of the AIDS virus, HTLV-III/LAV, on the immune system lowers the barriers not only to many opportunistic infections but also to various rare and aggressive cancers and to several blood disorders. The first malignant disease to be linked to AIDS, Kaposi's sarcoma, appeared in 1981 in young homosexual men almost simultaneously in San Francisco and New York City. The fact that a rare lung infection, *Pneumocystis carinii* pneumonia, was also being reported in men of this same group was one of the clues that brought the new disease AIDS to light.

As more cases of AIDS were diagnosed, other cancers, especially lymphomas, appeared in high numbers. Somewhat surprisingly, solid tumors, such as growths in the bowel and lung, were infrequent. AIDS also became associated with blood disorders, neither malignant nor related to the side effects of therapy, including pancytopenia, a reduction in red and white blood cells and platelets (important in coagulation), and immune thrombocytopenic purpura, a rare phenomenon in which only platelets are reduced.

CANCERS

Kaposi's Sarcoma

First described in 1872 by Moriz Kaposi, a Hungarian dermatologist, classical Kaposi's sarcoma is an infrequent skin cancer that mostly affects elderly men of Mediterranean descent (ten times as much as women), especially those of Italian or East European Jewish ancestry. The disease starts as one or more small, raised, red or purple patches, often on the foot or ankle. It progresses slowly over a course of 10–15 years, the lesions tending to grow and coalesce until they cover the surface of the lower legs.

Although the growing patches tend to remain near the early lesions, they may spread to other areas of the body such as the trunk and the hands, occasionally the eye or the lining of the mouth, but rarely a distant organ. The main problem is usually cosmetic, but the coalescing lesions may also ulcerate and become infected. Obstruction of blood vessels may prevent return of fluid to the rest of the body, leading to swelling of the legs and new infections of the lesions and surrounding tissues. If the disease lasts long enough, it eventually spreads to the lining of the gastrointestinal tract and the lymph nodes. This usually causes no symptoms and is discovered only at autopsy. About 30 percent of patients with classical Kaposi's sarcoma develop a second malignancy, most commonly a non-Hodgkin's lymphoma.

Essential treatment of infected lesions consists of antiseptic soaks and the surface application of antibiotics. Treatment of the underlying disease includes all anticancer measures, beginning with surgical removal of the lesions. As the disease spreads, this becomes impractical, and radiation is used to control the spread and ease the pain. Eventually, chemotherapy is necessary to kill the cancer cells, most often with vinblastine (Velban), but other drugs have also been used alone or in combination.

Because the patients are elderly, and the disease develops slowly, they usually die of causes unrelated to the sarcoma, such as heart disease or stroke. In contrast, AIDS patients are relatively young, and the Kaposi's sarcoma that affects them is much more severe and progresses rapidly. To distinguish the AIDS-related from the classical form, it is called epidemic Kaposi's sarcoma.

Unusually aggressive Kaposi's sarcoma has also been found in kidney transplant patients whose immune systems have been deliberately suppressed by drugs (for example, prednisone and azathioprine) to prevent rejection of the foreign tissue. The incidence in such patients is about 200 times as great as in the general population. Also, the greater the immunosuppression, the more virulent the disease. If immunosuppression is stopped, the disease diminishes. In these patients, the disease often begins as skin lesions but then spreads and eventually affects lymph nodes and distant organs. About one-third of these patients die of Kaposi's sarcoma, rather than kidney failure or infection. Depending on the severity of the disease, radiation and chemotherapy may be used to control its progress. Kaposi's sarcoma has also been reported in patients undergoing immunosuppression for disorders such as systemic lupus erythematosis and rheumatoid arthritis.

Classical Kaposi's sarcoma typically afflicts only certain elderly men. The recent epidemic type is associated with relatively young AIDS sufferers. It was also recognized in the late 1950s that the disease was widespread among Bantu tribesmen of southern Africa, and cases were reported soon after in Equatorial Africa. (Interestingly, Burkitt's lymphoma and Epstein-Barr viral infections, frequent in AIDS, are also common in this same geographical area.) The disease in Africa has three distinct forms. One resembles classical Kaposi's sarcoma in its patchy skin lesions and slow development. A second, which usually affects older people, is aggressive, grows rapidly, infiltrates deeper tissues, is usually fatal, and can kill within a year. The third form, a quick killer that affects younger people, starts in lymph glands and then invades major organs. Various types of chemotherapy have been used against these three forms with different degrees of success.

Epidemic Kaposi's Sarcoma

Epidemic Kaposi's sarcoma, more aggressive and virulent than the classical disease, affects primarily homosexual and bisexual AIDS patients, who make up about 90 percent of all AIDS patients with Kaposi's sarcoma. About half of all homosexuals with AIDS are expected to contract Kaposi's sarcoma at one time or another. Fewer than 10 percent of AIDS patients who are intravenous-drug abusers or of Haitian descent get Kaposi's sarcoma, and no case has yet been reported in hemophiliacs. However, the disease appears in about 5 percent of infants with AIDS or AIDS-like illnesses, born to parents with AIDS.

The typical AIDS patient with Kaposi's sarcoma is also susceptible to opportunistic infections. They often have histories of venereal diseases, such as syphilis, gonorrhea, venereal warts, and herpes simplex, and also frequently have rare infections such as parasitic infections of the bowel. Implicated in the greater incidence of Kaposi's sarcoma are the use of certain recreational drugs (especially amyl nitrite), anal intercourse, and fecal contamination. (Tearing of the rectal lining is a suspected factor in causing Kaposi's sarcoma, and the use of condoms is a recommended protective.)

Almost all patients with epidemic Kaposi's sarcoma have antibodies (detected in blood tests) to the AIDS virus, HTLV-III/LAV. Some also have a particular immunologic abnormality that may make them more susceptible to the sarcoma, and many have been previously infected by certain viruses: Epstein-Barr, hepatitis A and B, and cytomegalovirus. These may contribute to the development of Kaposi's sarcoma, but no specific agent has yet been shown to cause the disease directly.

Unlike the classical form, which is usually confined to the lower extremities, epidemic Kaposi's sarcoma can produce its purplish raised lesions over many areas of the body simultaneously, including the trunk, the mucous lining of the mouth, the lymph nodes, and various internal organs. Eventually, usually in the terminal phase of the disease, it affects the lung and its lining membrane.

In the beginning, the epidemic Kaposi's sarcoma patient usually shows no signs of AIDS, but then tends to contract various opportunistic infections, oral thrush (a fungal infection), or shingles, and eventually full-blown AIDS. Only about 10 percent die of Kaposi's sarcoma alone, most succumbing to an opportunistic infection or another malignancy. A patient with only Kaposi's sarcoma has an 80 percent chance of surviving for two years, but an accompanying opportunistic infection reduces the chance to 20 percent.

Epidemic Kaposi's sarcoma spreads so rapidly and involves so many areas of the body that surgery is not a practical treatment. Nuclear radiation or X-rays may be used for local problems. Low-dose radiation can often relieve the pain of bone and skin lesions, control bleeding from fast-growing or ulcerated skin lesions, reduce swelling caused by obstruction of fluid flow, and sometimes help affected mouth tissues. However, chemotherapy is the mainstay of treatment.

Drugs used in chemotherapy to kill rapidly growing cancer cells also affect rapidly growing normal cells such as those in hair follicles, the blood, and the gastrointestinal tract. This causes major side effects such as hair loss, lowering of the blood cell counts, nausea, and vomiting. The most common drugs used against epidemic Kaposi's sarcoma are vinblastine (Velban) and etoposide, or VP-16 (Vesped). About 90 percent of patients with classical Kaposi's sarcoma improve with vinblastine, in contrast to only a 30 percent response among those with the epidemic form. V-16, which acts very much like vinblastine, is more effective. About 75 percent of patients with epidemic Kaposi's sarcoma benefit from V-16, and in 25 percent all disease disappears. However, the response lasts only about nine months. Other drugs have been used, such as bleomycin, actinomycin-D, and adriamycin, with varying degrees of success.

Because the response to single drugs varies and is short-lived, combinations have been used. A combination of adriamycin, bleomycin, and vinblastine approximately equaled the single drug V-16 in effect, achieving improvement in 80 percent of treated patients and total disappearance of the disease in 25 percent. However, again the improvement lasted only nine months.

No drugs, alone or in combination, have been shown to give a survival advantage. They can relieve symptoms and improve cosmetic appearance by reducing disfiguring lesions, but patients do not live longer. New drugs and combinations are being tested at most major cancer research centers.

Since AIDS is a disease of altered immunity, drugs that affect the immune system have been tried to control epidemic Kaposi's sarcoma. The first was interferon, which seemed a promising possibility because it has been shown to inhibit viral growth and reproduction, and both AIDS and Kaposi's sarcoma may have a viral cause. In extensive tests, about 40 percent of all patients improved, without the major side effects of chemotherapy. Side effects were present—low-grade fever, weakness, and muscle ache—similar to the flu. Although interferon had a beneficial effect on Kaposi's sarcoma lesions, it had no major effect upon the underlying immune defects found in AIDS. Opportunistic infections were still frequent and the primary cause of death. Interleukin-II was also tested (AIDS patients are deficient in natural interleukin-II production), but results were disappointing. For example, ten patients with epidemic Kaposi's sarcoma in one study showed no response at all.

It is apparent that the various forms of Kaposi's sarcoma are similar but differ in many respects. Men are more susceptible than women to all forms. The fact that men of Mediterranean ancestry seem to be especially prone to both classical and epidemic forms suggests a common genetic origin. The fact that certain viruses (Epstein-Barr and cytomegalovirus) seem to be associated with both the epidemic form and the forms found in Africa and in kidney-transplant patients suggests a causal agent. Yet, no single cause has been identified to date.

It seems likely that a genetic predisposition allows some agent (a virus or a combination of environmental substances) to start the disease. In the classical form, which strikes otherwise healthy people, an intact immune system may control the severity of the disease. In the epidemic form, or in immunosuppressed kidney-transplant patients, the weakened immune system cannot prevent the tumor from growing without inhibition. Unfortunately, this likelihood is scientifically unproven. In fact, interleukin-II, which is supposed to correct the immune defect of AIDS, produced no benefits for epidemic Kaposi's sarcoma, and drugs that produce such benefits failed to correct the immune defect. So the puzzle of what causes Kaposi's sarcoma continues, but once deciphered it might unlock the key to the causes of other forms of cancer.

The various forms of Kaposi's sarcoma most likely represent different parts of the spectrum of the same disease whose severity depends on the degree of immunosuppression. Since the disease seems so closely linked to the status of the immune system, there is reason to hope that correction of the basic immune defect of AIDS will also control Kaposi's sarcoma.

Lymphomas

The most common of the other malignancies associated with AIDS is the group called lymphomas. Lymphomas are cancers of lymphocytes, white blood cells active in the body's immune defenses, and are of two types, Hodgkin's and non-Hodgkin's, distinguished by their appearance under the microscope. Hodgkin's disease is characterized by a distinctive cell (called Sternberg-Reed), and all others are collectively called non-Hodgkin's. Non-Hodgkin's lymphomas are more prevalent in AIDS patients, but Hodgkin's disease has also been reported. Since the immune system is supposed to exercise protective surveillance against cancers, it is possible that the AIDS virus in destroying immunity is also responsible for various lymphomas. Other cancers do appear with AIDS, but whether this is due to a cause-and-effect relationship is uncertain.

In keeping with the idea that the immune system not only protects against infection but also suppresses cancer growth, and that cancers flourish when the immune system becomes overtaxed or blocked, the incidence of cancers is higher in the presence of diseases that cause immune defects. For example, both congenital and acquired immunodeficiency are associated with a large number of tumors, mostly non-Hodgkin's lymphomas. Chemotherapy drugs that suppress the immune system are associated with a relatively high incidence of lymphomas and leukemias. Steroids and other drugs that do not specifically harm body cells but do suppress the immune system are also associated with a relatively high incidence of cancers, especially cancers of the skin and lip, lymphomas, and Kaposi's sarcoma.

AIDS patients suffer from probably the most severe immunodeficiency known today, and homosexuals and hemophiliacs seem to be especially susceptible to non-Hodgkin's lymphomas. While lymphomas usually begin in the lymph glands (or nodes), about 90 percent of the lymphomas in AIDS patients begin outside the lymph nodes, about half in the brain, a third in the bone marrow, and a quarter in the bowel. AIDS-related lymphomas also tend to be more aggressive and less responsive to treatment, only about half the patients showing any benefits at all from therapy, and half of these rapidly relapsing after initial improvement. In contrast, 75 percent of non-AIDS lymphomas respond to treatment, and remission lasts much longer.

The most common non-Hodgkin's type, normally a relatively rare disease, is Burkitt's lymphoma. First observed in Africa and associated with the Epstein-Barr virus, it usually affects the lymph nodes in adolescents and is readily cured with chemotherapy. An American form is known that also affects the young, but is usually not so responsive to chemotherapy and is not associated with the Epstein-Barr virus. Burkitt's lymphoma in AIDS patients is extremely virulent and usually widespread, affecting many lymph nodes, the bone marrow, and brain membranes. Malignant cells contain the Epstein-Barr virus and exhibit genetic changes. It is possible that the disease starts with infection by the virus, and then the genetically altered cells reproduce, win out over normal cells, and aggressively advance the disease. Treatment usually involves chemotherapy but with mixed results. Patients respond but relapse quickly, and the disease resists further treatment and is usually fatal.

Other lymphomas also occur with AIDS. Lymphoblastic lymphoma (lymphoblasts are the immature precursors of mature lymphocytes), an aggressive disease even in non-AIDS patients, resembles acute leukemia (cancer of blood-forming tissues) and is treated the same way. Lymphomas that start in the brain are rare but do appear in AIDS patients. The finding of Epstein-Barr virus in malignant cells suggests a causal agent. As mentioned before, Hodgkin's disease has appeared in AIDS patients. It is believed to be an overreaction of the T cells of the immune system to a malignant process. However, the AIDS virus destroys T cells, so the relationship between Hodgkin's disease and AIDS is unknown.

A nonmalignant involvement of the lymph nodes is also associated with AIDS and the AIDS-related complex (a group of AIDS-like illnesses in patients who may have antibodies to the AIDS virus and the reversal of the ratio of helper-to-suppressor T cells in the immune system, characteristic of AIDS, but not AIDS itself). This is called the lymphadenopathy syndrome, an enlargement of lymph nodes all over the body accompanied by flu-like symptoms, such as fatigue, fever, sweating, and weight loss, and often minor bacterial infections, fungal skin infections, and oral thrush. Fewer than 10 percent of the patients have developed full-blown AIDS, and about 25 percent developed Kaposi's sarcoma. No special therapy is recommended as yet, and patients are usually treated as required to relieve symptoms.

Solid Tumors

Solid tumors (growths in major organs such as the bowel, lung, and breast) rarely occur with AIDS, except for a two-to-threefold increase in tongue and anal cancer since 1981. More solid tumors would not have been surprising, since the AIDS-damaged immune system cannot provide its postulated protection against cancers. However, studies have revealed an increase in tongue and anal malignancies in homosexuals as far back as 1970. Also, some evidence suggests a virus as the cause. It is possible that local abrasion due to oral and anal sex may make as important a contribution as a depressed immune system.

BLOOD DISORDERS

Pancytopenia

Pancytopenia (below normal levels of red and white blood cells and platelets) in AIDS patients seems to be related to the basic immune defect rather than to cancer in the blood-producing bone marrow, side effects of chemotherapy, or other infections. Examination of bone marrow specimens shows apparently normal numbers of precursors to the three types of blood cells, so it is possible that the AIDS virus may play a role in suppressing the body's ability to upgrade the precursors into mature blood cells.

Pancytopenia appears in varying severity. The white blood cell count may be only slightly diminished or so low that the patient is deprived of the normal white-cell protection against disease and is left vulnerable to various bacterial and fungal infections. The red blood cells, which carry oxygen from the lungs to the rest of the body, may be so depleted as to require replenishment by transfusion. Since the mechanism underlying the pancytopenia is unknown, no specific treatment can be prescribed. The usual treatment is supportive care to correct any of the consequences of reduced blood cell counts.

Immune Thrombocytopenic Purpura

In immune thrombocytopenic purpura, only the blood platelets are destroyed, reducing the blood's ability to coagulate normally. Patients are susceptible to bleeding, and may develop small, discolored, hemorrhaging patches all over the body, and possibly tiny spots of bleeding. The disorder is sometimes related to an underlying Kaposi's sarcoma but other times is directly related to AIDS, with no evidence of cancer or bone-marrow suppression due to chemotherapy. No specific cause is known, but a virus or a hidden lymphoma is suspected. Treatment is with drugs, most commonly prednisone and vincristine (Oncovin). Vincristine is preferred because prednisone is a steroid that can aggravate the immune depression already present in AIDS.

SUMMARY

AIDS not only incurs a great risk of opportunistic infections but also cancers and blood disorders that may often otherwise be rare. Kaposi's sarcoma, normally a relatively mild skin disease of elderly men, is an aggressive cancer of AIDS patients that can spread rapidly to other organs of the body. Even so, most patients die of opportunistic infections or other malignancies rather than Kaposi's sarcoma. Lymphomas, particularly Burkitt's lymphoma, also become more virulent in AIDS patients and can kill in a short time. Solid tumors are not as frequent with AIDS as might be expected in view of the loss of capacity of the immune system. Although cancer treatments by radiation and chemotherapy are used, they are generally either minimally effective or provide only temporary benefits. Blood disorders involving diminishing numbers of red and white blood cells and platelets (pancytopenia), or platelets alone (immune thrombocytopenic purpura), are also associated with AIDS. They may or may not be related to simultaneous cancers, such as Kaposi's sarcoma or lymphoma, and are treated with transfusions to replenish lost blood cells, other supportive care, or drugs.

It is hoped that in the future the basic immune defects in AIDS patients can be corrected and an effective cure found for their cancers.

Three   Groups at Risk

8 Children with AIDS and the Public Risk
ARYE RUBINSTEIN

A RATIONAL PERSPECTIVE

The main question that still torments the scientific community, the mass media, and the public is the possible spread of the AIDS virus to the general population. The Centers for Disease Control (CDC) recently predicted that the cumulative number of AIDS patients may exceed 250,000 by 1991. What are the chances that this tenfold increase will also entail a spread beyond the known major risk groups?

AIDS is undoubtedly an increasingly alarming public health issue. However, the nationwide rise in numbers of AIDS cases has been accompanied by a greater understanding of routes of transmission, so that a fairly reliable epidemiologic picture of this dreadful disease can be described.

Who are the major risk groups for AIDS? The largest and best studied includes homosexual and bisexual males. Over the years their national share of the total AIDS population has remained fairly constant at about 70 percent. The disease is increasing in intravenous-drug abusers, and a further increase is projected. The risk factors for these two major AIDS groups are well recognized and indicate possible means of control. For example, by not sharing needles, refraining from homosexual contacts with infected males, and limiting the number of homosexual partners, these two groups can theoretically decrease the spread of the disease among themselves.

In the United States, women were, and still are, much less frequently affected by AIDS than are men. They now comprise around 7 percent of the total number of AIDS patients. The emergence of AIDS among women was not a surprise to AIDS experts. Women acquire the disease as frequently as men from the use of intravenous drugs and from sexual contact with high-risk males. The fear of a major AIDS epidemic, which abated somewhat when the disease seemed confined to relatively few groups, was revived when it became clear that the risk to female sexual contacts was higher than predicted and when the disease also appeared in other patient populations, such as recipients of blood and blood products, recent Haitian immigrants, heterosexual male partners of infected women, children of high-risk parents, and individuals outside of any recognized risk group. A close look at all available evidence does not now justify this fear. The following consideration of relevant aspects of disease transmission and lessons learned from the study of children with AIDS, their siblings, and their families provides a model for predictions of future spread and prospects for containment of the disease.

EPIDEMIOLOGY

The number of AIDS patients who do not belong to the two major groups at risk make up no more than 6 percent of the total. This percentage has so far remained fairly constant, which suggests that new surprises are unlikely. If the AIDS virus had extensively contaminated blood supplies in the United States, or if the disease was highly contagious, many more AIDS patients outside the risk groups would have been expected.

In 1985, on the basis of known cases, the risk of acquiring AIDS in the United States through transfusions of blood or blood products was 1 or 2 per million transfusions. The experience abroad has been similar. This risk is extremely low compared to risks of other transfusion reactions. Theoretically, the most vulnerable patients are recipients of multiple transfusions and those whose immunity is suppressed, for example, cancer patients and recipients of kidney transplants. (Transplant patients are given potent drugs that destroy their immunity to prevent rejection of the alien tissues. Cancer chemotherapy also causes immunodeficiency.) These patients frequently receive multiple transfusions, and yet only a few have contracted AIDS. Among hemophiliacs, who necessarily receive blood products from a large donor pool, infection is much more frequent (over 80 percent in some areas). However, only a relatively small percentage of infected hemophiliacs have come down with the disease. Infection by blood and blood products is now significantly curtailed by the advent of new serological tests (available in all U.S. blood banks), which can detect the presence of antibodies to the AIDS virus in potential donors and in donated blood. Although these tests do not capture all donors at risk of having the AIDS virus and thus do not completely eliminate the risk of transmission by blood, newer, more sensitive tests that detect the AIDS virus itself will soon be commercially available. Blood and blood products will then no longer be a possible means of inciting an epidemic.

It has been postulated that the epidemiology of AIDS mimics that of hepatitis B. Both diseases are transmitted by needle sticks, blood transfusions, and sexual contact. Since hepatitis B is quite ubiquitous, widespread infection of the population by the AIDS virus might have been expected, and the number of AIDS patients would be 10 or 100 times greater than it is now. The fact that such a widespread infection did not occur suggests that the AIDS virus has extremely low infectivity. This is confirmed by the very few infections reported in health-care workers who are frequently exposed to and infected by hepatitis B.

Several medical centers have been studying health-care personnel who have had close contact with AIDS patients, particularly those inadvertently stuck with a needle used for an AIDS patient or otherwise exposed to AIDS blood, for example, through a skin abrasion. It has to be remembered that the exposure of health-care personnel to AIDS patients was not controlled by significant precautionary measures until late 1982. Blood was often drawn without gloves, secretions were not specially handled, and blood-count samples were spread thinly on glass slides without protection. Moreover, many patients underwent surgery or were examined with bronchoscopes before it was known that they had AIDS. During bronchoscopy, a tube is passed down the airways to the lungs, and the examiner is exposed to secretions and blood coughed up by the patient. If AIDS were highly infectious, these health-care workers would have been likely victims. However, only four who were not apparent members of recognized high-risk groups have so far contracted the disease. These four aroused a near panic among health-care workers, which subsided when the cases were statistically compared with an estimate of how many cases might have been expected merely on the basis of chance.

In mid-July 1983, the total number of AIDS cases reported to the CDC was 1,902, of whom 110 could not be assigned to any designated high-risk groups, including four health workers. In 1986, with the total having risen to over 25,000 AIDS patients, the percentage of unexplained transmission has remained the same, and no new infection among health-care workers has occurred. According to the 1980 census, the U.S. population of ages 18–64 totaled 137.2 million. This age span encompasses almost all employed persons and virtually all AIDS cases. The National Center for Health Statistics reports that in 1980 approximately 7.23 million persons were employed in the health industry. If this figure bears no relationship to the risk of AIDS, that is, AIDS infections are assumed to happen merely by chance, then the number of health workers expected among the 120 "unexplained" AIDS cases would be $110 \times 7.23/137.2 = 5.8$, which exceeds the 4 cases observed. In effect, this means no increased risk for health-care workers. Encouragingly, continuing nationwide studies have confirmed this finding of little risk to health-care workers at least up to 1984.

These findings do not justify a cavalier disregard for prudent precautions. Two instances of transmission of the virus from a patient to a person administering intensive care illustrate the point. The first occurred in England, where a woman provided home care to a Ghanaian man who was found after he died to have had AIDS. The woman recalled having chronic eczema (a skin inflammation) and small skin cuts while caring for the patient. She was found to have developed antibodies to the AIDS virus. The second case was a mother caring for her child who had contracted AIDS from a transfusion. The child had had several surgical operations, and his mother had provided nursing care that involved extensive unprotected exposure to body secretions and blood. The mother drew blood, removed intravenous lines, emptied colostomy bags, inserted rectal tubes, and changed nasogastric (nose-to-stomach) feeding tubes. She remembered no needle stick injuries and had no other risk factors for AIDS. During her care of her child, blood tests revealed that she had developed antibodies to the AIDS virus and was thus probably infected although she is still healthy.

Such examples are extremely rare, and both involved unprotected contact with blood and body secretions of an AIDS patient. They therefore do not at all indicate the possibility of widespread infection to the general population, but they do stress the necessity for precautionary measures recommended by the CDC for health-care workers.

AIDS IN CHILDREN

Perhaps most perplexing was the spread of the disease to children. In 1979, we encountered a child with recurrent infections that suggested immunodeficiency. A series of immunologic tests revealed abnormalities different from any known congenital (inborn) immunodeficiency. The infections were also accompanied by unusual markedly enlarged lymph nodes and swelling of the salivary glands. The most puzzling finding was that the mother had the same symptoms and the same immunodeficiency. In 1981, when AIDS was reported in adults, we realized that the child and his mother had AIDS.

Since 1981, the number of infants with AIDS has increased sharply. By June 1982, we had treated 7 such infants, by January 1983 the number was 13, and at present over 150 children infected by the AIDS virus are being treated in our clinic. Nationwide, the CDC has received reports of over 300 children with AIDS.

As with all other newly discovered patient populations at risk for AIDS, the disease in children soon reached news headlines, and the alarm sounded again. When we and others found families with more than one affected child, the alarm grew to panic. "Here is the proof for the spread of AIDS to the general population" and "AIDS may spread from child to child by casual contact" were some of many fearful statements publicized.

It took months to resolve the mystery of AIDS in children. Our medical center is located in a geographic area where AIDS is widespread among intravenous-drug abusers. The mothers of most infants with AIDS admitted to intravenous-drug abuse. Others had had sexual contact with infected men. When these women were examined, many were found to have an immunodeficiency identical to that of their infants. Moreover, several eventually developed the clinical symptoms characteristic of AIDS and died. These findings clearly linked the disease in children to that in their mothers.

When did the children acquire AIDS from their mothers? Retrospective analysis suggested that it was at an average age of six months. In adults, the incubation period for AIDS is estimated to be between six months and several years. The general rule is that incubation periods of infections are shorter in immunodeficient patients, who cannot prevent invasions by microorganisms, such as viruses and bacteria, and often are unable to inhibit their reproduction or to destroy them. As a result, the organisms have free access to the body and multiply much faster.

Newborns are physiologically immunodeficient and more prone to infection. Thus, a shorter incubation period for the AIDS virus, probably a few months, might be expected. Since the disease in infants starts in the first months of life, we suspected that AIDS could have been acquired in the womb or during or shortly after birth. During birth, the newborn has ample contact with maternal blood and can acquire AIDS from infected blood as do hemophiliacs and intravenous-drug abusers. If, however, the disease is acquired in the womb, the AIDS virus must be able to penetrate protective barriers into the placenta. For a long time we were unable to determine definitively whether children acquire the disease before, during, or after birth. As time passed, new facts shed light on this enigma.

Some infants with AIDS never left the nursery or were placed in foster care shortly after birth. Contact with their mothers was limited to the first days of life. We studied the foster parents and found them to be immunologically competent and healthy. However, the natural mothers had symptoms suggestive of AIDS and/or were immunodeficient. This convinced us that AIDS was transmitted from an infected mother to her baby during or before birth.

Observation of a family of intravenous-drug abusers strengthened this conviction. Early in 1984, we diagnosed AIDS in a 22-month old child whose mother was an intravenous-drug-using prostitute who was pregnant again when we first studied her. When her baby was born, we watched carefully for symptoms of AIDS. The baby's psychomotor development appeared abnormal from birth. Within two weeks, the first bacterial infections were noted, followed by fungal blood infection and meningitis at four months. Although its immune system appeared to be normal when tested soon after birth, the fact that the older brother had AIDS made us suspect that the disease in the newborn was also AIDS and that an immunodeficiency might develop at any time.

A fungus infection in the blood at four months was a bad omen. Soon after, laboratory tests showed a progressive deterioration of the immune system and a disease pattern developed similar to that of the mother and older brother. It was clear that the baby could not have acquired the disease from his older brother since there had been no contact between them. Did the baby acquire the disease at birth or in the womb? If he acquired it at birth, the incubation period could have been only a few days or at most two to three weeks. This is unreasonably short and inconsistent with previous data on adults with AIDS.

Since 1984 we have studied many more babies born to AIDS-infected mothers and identified the AIDS virus in the babies' blood at birth. Moreover, many of the babies had a distinctive facial appearance, which indicated that AIDS infection early in pregnancy had damaged developing organs. Also, birth weights and body lengths were often far less than normal for the babies' gestational ages. Many AIDS babies also did not exhibit normal psychomotor development from birth, indicating damage to the brain in the womb.

This information slightly allayed anxiety concerning the risk of AIDS to the general public. However, as often before, disturbing new questions soon arose. Scientists claimed that a mother who acquires an infectious disease during one pregnancy seldom transmits it to children of subsequent pregnancies. For example, if a woman has one baby with congenital cytomegalovirus infection or congenital toxoplasmosis (a parasitic disease), she is highly unlikely to have another baby with the same infection in her next pregnancy. This also applies to congenital rubella (German measles) syndrome. The reason is that once a woman has had the disease, she develops immunity, and the mother's immunity thereafter prevents infection of the fetus. If this is true of AIDS, then of two infected siblings the older may have acquired it in the womb while the younger may have acquired it by contact with the older sibling. Since the AIDS virus has been isolated from body secretions other than blood, including tears, urine, and saliva, of adult AIDS patients and healthy homosexual men, the question is: Can secretions from one child infect a sibling? If so, the possibility must again be considered that the general population may acquire AIDS by intimate, but nonsexual, contact with AIDS patients.

Several studies of household contacts of AIDS patients have been completed in the last few years. One, covering 101 household contacts, found little or no risk of transmitting the AIDS virus to close nonsexual household contacts. Moreover, we have been unable to document disease transmission between children with AIDS and more than 100 other, healthy children in the same households. When our social workers and nurses visited the homes of children with AIDS, they were impressed by the unusually close contact between family members. In many instances, children with AIDS were born to families of low socioeconomic background who lived under poor hygienic conditions. A mother and several children often lived in one room. The child with AIDS was sometimes not toilet trained and regularly shared utensils or a bed with siblings. This was not casual contact, but an extremely intimate physical closeness that might be expected to facilitate transmission of disease. In spite of this, no disease was transmitted.

Over a five-year period, we examined all members of families in which more than one child had AIDS. When a second or third child developed AIDS in a family with a previous AIDS child, it was always a younger, never an older, sibling, suggesting transmission of AIDS in the womb. Moreover, we studied over 100 household contacts of AIDS patients for clinical or immunologic signs of AIDS. No foster parents, no older children in the family, and no unrelated playmates of children with AIDS developed AIDS. Also, none had antibodies to the AIDS virus in their blood.

This information indicated it was extremely unlikely that one child with AIDS could infect a brother or sister by casual contact. So how can we explain the fact that several children of the same family had

AIDS? Can an infected woman after all transmit the virus in consecutive pregnancies without ever developing immunity to protect her fetus? Several studies have confirmed this supposition. Not only can an infected woman transmit the AIDS virus repeatedly in a series of pregnancies, but she may not even exhibit any disease symptoms. That is, a woman can harbor the AIDS virus, look healthy, and yet infect her baby in the womb.

Can such a woman also transmit the virus to her husband who is not infected? Recent studies indicate that she can, through sexual contact. In fact, in Africa men and women are infected in almost equal numbers. Moreover, two investigators have reported isolating the AIDS virus in vaginal and cervical secretions. Nevertheless, and fortunately, female-to-male sexual transmission in the United States seems, for unknown reasons, so far to be infrequent, and the presence of the virus in female genital secretions is not sufficient evidence of its transmissibility through these secretions. More importantly, the fact that infected healthy women transmit the disease to the fetus in the womb is solid evidence for the infectiousness of healthy disease carriers. In fact, the future distribution of AIDS in the U.S. population may depend on this pool of infectious healthy carriers.

PROSPECTS FOR THE FUTURE

Is there any reason to fear that the demographic picture of AIDS may change in the future? Although at present it appears that surprising changes are not likely, some observations may point to a grimmer outlook than indicated by past epidemiological studies.

First, the number of people with AIDS continues to increase among intravenous-drug abusers. Extensive efforts to reach this risk group with cautionary information have not been significantly successful. While homosexuals have been receptive to a variety of precautionary measures and changes in lifestyle, intravenous-drug abusers have not. As a consequence, they may constitute an increasing reservoir of AIDS-infected men and women in the United States.

Second, studies in Africa, the United States, and Europe have shown that all AIDS viruses are not exactly the same. One variant in Africa seems to have been relatively benign. It infected a large segment of the population but caused little disease. On the other hand, the virus isolated in the United States and France tends to cause disease often, after long incubation periods. Which virus appeared first, the African or the European-American? If the African virus was first, it may be that it changed with time (mutated) from benign to virulent. If so, can the present U.S. virus mutate further to become more easily transmitted and suddenly spread to the general population?

There is as yet no conclusive answer to these questions. On the one hand, the AIDS virus has been shown to mutate rapidly. The virus in one infected individual may differ somewhat from the virus in another in the same environment. On the other hand, no new, more virulent AIDS viruses have been detected. Therefore, it is fair to say that the general public is not now at risk. AIDS today is associated with the high-risk sexual and drug-taking practices of particular groups and, to a much smaller extent, with special circumstances such as blood transfusions (now safer than ever) and births to infected mothers. Nevertheless, AIDS tomorrow may behave differently than AIDS today. Therefore, it is essential to keep a close vigil on this devastating disease.

SUMMARY

AIDS has become the major health concern of this decade. In the United States, homosexual and bisexual males make up the largest population to develop AIDS. The incidence of AIDS in both male and female intravenous-drug abusers is, however, still increasing, while new AIDS cases among hemophiliacs, transfusion recipients, and homosexual males have decreased. The decrease among hemophiliacs and transfusion recipients is due primarily to testing of donated blood for antibody to the AIDS virus. The decrease among homosexual males is due to successful education about unsafe sexual practices. The increase among male and female intravenous-drug abusers and their sex partners has also led to a growing number of children with AIDS. The most common way for a child to contract AIDS, now that the blood supply is not an important source of the AIDS virus, is from an infected mother during pregnancy. Much evidence indicates the transmission of the AIDS virus from an infected woman to her developing fetus early in pregnancy. Since newborn infants do not have a fully developed immune system, they develop AIDS much sooner than an adult would. All studies of household contacts of both pediatric and adult AIDS patients, and of health-care workers, support the CDC's finding that AIDS is not contracted by casual contact, but is acquired only through sexual contact with an infected person, use of intravenous drugs, or intimate contact with blood, blood products, or body secretions from an infected individual. AIDS continues to increase, with intravenous drug-abusers forming the fastest growing reservoir of infected men and women in this country. Although the general public is not now at risk for AIDS unless they engage in high-risk sexual practices or intravenous-drug abuse, the AIDS virus is known to mutate rapidly. It is therefore essential to watch changing disease patterns very carefully, since the AIDS virus, which is weakly infective today, may become more highly infective tomorrow.

9

AIDS and the Blood Supply

ROBERT L. HIRSCH

FEARS ABOUT BLOOD

Early evidence suggested that blood might play a role in transmitting AIDS. Because AIDS was deadly, and little was known about its cause, diagnosis, treatment, and prevention, a fear of any and all contact with blood gripped both the general public and health-care workers. Some patients were reluctant to accept needed blood transfusions; others requested blood only from family or friends; hospital and laboratory workers were afraid to give appropriate and much needed personal care to AIDS patients or to perform tests on their blood samples; and even loyal donors stopped giving blood.

Identification of HTLV-III/LAV (human T-cell lymphotrophic virus type III/lymphadenopathy-associated virus) as the primary causative agent of AIDS, and the development of a test that detects antibodies to the virus, led to studies that confirmed the role of transfusions in transmitting the disease but found no evidence of transmission by casual contact with AIDS patients. This provided the basis for rational procedures to minimize the risk of getting AIDS from exposure to blood or blood products. An understanding of the cautions taken in collecting, handling, and administering blood for therapy should allay exaggerated public fears and prevent inappropriate responses from causing blood shortages, resistance to needed blood transfusions, and inadequate care of AIDS patients.

SHARED NEEDLES—INTRAVENOUS-DRUG ABUSE

AIDS transmission by blood was first suggested by the fact that about 17 percent of all AIDS patients are intravenous (IV)-drug abusers. Injectors of illicit, habit-forming drugs often share needles and syringes without cleaning or sterilization between uses, which allows blood containing a disease-causing agent to pass from person to person. The spread of hepatitis B, malaria, and other blood-borne infectious diseases by this route has been well documented. It is now clear that IV-drug abusers also transmit AIDS by this route rather than through any other shared group characteristic.

BLOOD AND BLOOD PRODUCTS—TEN MILLION PINTS A YEAR

More than ten million pints of blood are collected each year in the United States. Each pint is referred to as a unit. Most units are subdivided by mechanical means (for example, centrifuging) into two or more components such as red cells, white cells, platelets (involved in coagulation), and plasma (the liquid part). Each component is considered a blood product, and the amount of each product derived from a given unit of whole blood is called a unit of that component. Every unit of blood or blood product is completely identified and can be traced back to the donor, the donor's medical history, the time, place, and circumstances of the donation (equipment, personnel), and all other significant details.

Components are transfused as single units or, in the case of platelets or white blood cells requiring larger doses, as pools of six to twenty units (representing as many donors). A few patients may receive as many as several hundred blood products a year (units of various components), but the average is about three. Although blood-borne diseases can be transmitted by blood transfusion, the risk is very much smaller than in indiscriminate drug abuse, thanks to the care exercised in selecting healthy donors.

However, before 1983 not enough was known about the natural history of AIDS to select donors appropriately, and no reliable tests were available to screen blood for possible AIDS contamination. From mid-1981 to mid-1984, during which time about 45 million units of blood components were transfused, 52 cases of AIDS were verified in patients who had received transfusions but belonged to none of the recognized high-risk AIDS groups (such as homosexuals, bisexuals, and IV-drug abusers). It was assumed that the transfusions were the source. Thus, the risk of contracting AIDS by this route was about one in a million component units, or blood products. Since an average patient received three, this amounted to about one of every 333,000 patients transfused.

This ratio is very small compared to other transfusion risks. For example, it is estimated that one in ten transfused patients is exposed to hepatitis, of whom about 500 each year develop jaundice, but many more become hepatitis carriers or develop a chronic illness that may take months or years to be recognized. Since most transfusions are given when urgently needed to counteract rapid blood loss, make operations safe, or keep people with chronic anemia alive, the risk of disease must be weighed against expected benefits.

Even at the beginning of the medical experience with AIDS, it was clear that the benefits of transfusions outweighed the risks. Fortunately, donor screening and blood treatment have now made transfusions even safer, further reducing the risk-to-benefit ratio.

Coagulation Products for Treating Hemophilia

Plasma contains a number of proteins—blood products extracted by more complex means than those used to separate primary components—that are useful for treating patients. To prepare these products in therapeutically significant quantities, many units of plasma are pooled from which the various products are segregated and concentrated into small volumes. As a result, a patient treated with one of these products (called blood derivatives as distinguished from components) may receive material contributed by many donors. For example, hemophiliacs may receive a blood product, cryoprecipitate, derived from the contributions of 6–12 donors, or another, Factor VIII, from the plasma of 2,500–10,000 donors. Moreover, both treatments are given many times a year to stop or prevent the recurrence of bleeding, exposing hemophiliacs to blood derivatives from many thousands of donors, as compared with three donors for the average transfused patient.

Consequently, it is not surprising that hemophiliacs show proportionately more evidence of exposure to hepatitis B, and that most hemophiliacs in the United States have developed antibodies against AIDS. But, for both hepatitis B and AIDS, only a few of those exposed develop the disease. The 75 cases in hemophiliacs reported to date represent only 1 percent of the total number of U.S. AIDS cases. The factor, or factors, that protect some exposed individuals from manifesting the disease is not known.

The rate at which new cases of AIDS among hemophiliacs have appeared has begun to decrease. While general steps taken to make all blood products safer have helped, much of the decrease is due to special treatment of Factor VIII concentrate. Since 1985, this blood product has been subjected to a controlled cycle of temperature and time designed to destroy the AIDS virus without reducing the effectiveness of heat-sensitive Factor VIII. It is not yet clear that viral inactivation is total, but a substantial reduction in the number of live virus particles has been demonstrated. A promising method of inactivation is about to be introduced, using solvents and detergents rather than heat, that does not compromise the effectiveness of Factor VIII.

Serum Albumin—The Lesson of Pasteurization

Two other blood products are prepared from large pools of plasma: serum albumin and gamma globulin. Serum albumin is not sensitive to moderate heat and is routinely pasteurized at 60°C for 10 hours. (Pasteurization is named for Louis Pasteur, the famous French scientist who discovered this method of sterilization for material that should not be boiled.) This treatment kills most known species of viruses. No case of any infectious disease, viral or otherwise, has been reported in patients receiving albumin exclusively. Nor has any case of AIDS occurred among albumin recipients who were not at increased risk of developing AIDS for other reasons.

Gamma Globulin—A Safe Product

Gamma globulin contains many antibodies that the donor's body developed to guard against infections. The antibodies develop either in response to a disease, such as measles or hepatitis, or the administration of an immunizing vaccine. No one has been reported to have contracted any disease, including AIDS, from gamma globulin, even though it cannot be pasteurized. Just why this is true is not known. It is thought that, because it is made from a pool of plasma from so many different donors, it probably contains anti-bodies to all known viruses. These antibodies combine with and inactivate the viruses, including the AIDS virus, rendering them noninfectious. Also, the chemical treatment used to separate the gamma globulin from the rest of the plasma may either inactivate the virus directly or eliminate it with the other unwanted parts of the plasma.

Hepatitis Immune Globulin and Hepatitis B Vaccine—Risks vs. Benefits

The fear of getting AIDS from blood products created a problem with two other blood products, hepatitis B immune globulin (HBIG) and hepatitis B vaccine (HBV), recently developed to combat hepatitis B infections.

HBIG is gamma globulin made from pools of plasma obtained solely from donors who have had hepatitis B and developed a high concentration of antibodies against the hepatitis B virus. It is given primarily to health-care workers accidentally exposed to the virus while handling infected blood, for example, through needle sticks or cuts from broken glass. It confers temporary protection and prevents the infection from developing. HBV is prepared from plasma obtained from hepatitis B carriers and contains the virus itself. It is treated to kill the virus, which prevents it from causing the disease, but still induces those injected to produce their own anti-bodies. Vaccination with HBV provides lifelong protection against hepatitis B.

Since the major source of plasma containing hepatitis B antibodies or live hepatitis B virus has been male homosexual donors, some people who should receive protective injections have been reluctant to accept them for fear of contracting AIDS. The truth is that no gamma globulin, including HBIG, has been associated with AIDS, so the risk is small or nonexistent. The benefits of preventing hepatitis B, which may result in chronic illness or death, far outweigh the risk. In the case of HBV, treatment to kill the hepatitis B virus was shown to be effective enough to kill all known viruses. Again, protection of health-care workers, who are constantly ex-posed to hepatitis B, is a benefit that exceeds any possible risk.

MAKING BLOOD SAFE

Exclusion of High-Risk Donors

Potential blood donors are carefully screened to exclude anyone who is not in excellent health. All are informed of the general criteria before they come to donate and are questioned in detail by a health professional at the blood collection site about past diseases and symptoms of current ailments. Blood pressure, pulse, temperature, and blood hemoglobin level are measured. This system has been working well for many years. Volunteer donors can be relied on to answer health questions truthfully, and the blood supply has been remarkably safe.

With AIDS it became apparent that additional screening was needed. The first step was to stop collecting blood from members of known high-risk groups as well as potential donors with AIDS symptoms, on the assumption that their blood might transmit the disease. In 1983 the Food and Drug Administration, the agency that regulates blood transfusion practices on a national scale, defined those at increased risk as "persons with symptoms and signs suggestive of AIDS, sexually active homosexual or bisexual males with multiple partners, Haitian entrants into the United States, present or past abusers of intravenous drugs, and sexual partners of individuals with AIDS or at increased risk of AIDS." "Males with multiple partners" was revised in September 1985 to read "individuals who have had only a *single* homosexual experience since 1979," because of a report that some bisexual or homosexual men whose blood contained AIDS antibodies thought they were acceptable donors because they were no longer sexually active. Educational programs and materials were prepared to inform such people that "until the AIDS problem is solved or definitive tests become available" they should refrain from donating. The second step was to add to the donor health history examination specific questions about the symptoms of AIDS, such as night sweats, unexplained fevers, unexpected weight loss, swollen glands, and Kaposi's sarcoma (a skin tumor frequently associated with AIDS). Persistent cough and diarrhea were later added to the list. None of these symptoms is exclusive to AIDS since one or another may be a consequence of other ailments and disappear upon recovery, but it seemed wise to postpone donations until the donors were free of symptoms.

Screening donors for AIDS raises a special problem. For personal reasons, many may be extremely reluctant to acknowledge belonging to a high-risk group, such as homosexuals, so that it is very important to do the health screening in private. However, even private screening may not give sufficient assurance of confidentiality to convince hesitant donors not to give false information. As an additional safeguard, the donor may, in private, check a form that identifies the donation by number but not name to indicate whether the blood should be used for transfusions or only for research purposes. The donor then gives blood and departs, and the blood, if not destined for transfusions, is removed from inventory at a remote station where the donor cannot be identified. An alternative method gives the donor the option of making an anonymous telephone call several hours later to specify how the blood is to be used, giving only the number identification. Studies at a large regional blood center have indicated that the combination of informational brochure, additional health questions, and confidential exclusion of donated blood is working effectively to reduce the risk of transmitting AIDS by blood transfusions.

Blood Test for AIDS Antibody

The first breakthrough in the search for a test to identify possibly infectious blood came when an association was noted between AIDS and the family of human T-cell lymphotropic viruses (HTLV). The first virus in this family, called HTLV-I, was discovered in patients with human T-cell leukemia. The second, HTLV-II, appears to be associated with a variant of this leukemia. Subsequently, two research groups independently isolated a third (called HTLV-III by one group and lymphadenopathy-associated virus, or LAV, by the other) from the T cells of patients with AIDS, patients with diffuse persistent lymph node enlargement (thought by some to be a pre-AIDS condition), and a few patients without symptoms in high-risk AIDS groups. In one donor-recipient pair, HTLV-III/LAV was isolated both from the high-risk donor, who developed AIDS long after donating the blood, and from the recipient who developed AIDS seven months after the transfusion. The recipient was not a member of any high-risk group.

A rapid, reliable, practical blood test for the AIDS virus would be ideal for screening potential blood donors; such a test is routinely used to screen for the hepatitis B virus, with excellent results. However, present tests for HTLV-III/LAV are neither rapid nor practical. They are impractical principally because the virus is present in the blood only from time to time. The hepatitis B virus is always there. However, antibodies developed against the AIDS virus after exposure are continually present, and rapid, reliable, and practical tests for AIDS antibodies have been performed on all donated blood since mid-1985.

It is very important to understand the significance of antibody test results. First and foremost, positive results do *not* necessarily indicate a current AIDS infection. Presence of the antibody indicates *only* exposure to the virus at some time in the past. Many who test positive appear to have fought off the virus without manifestations of illness, but the antibody may persist for years, even a lifetime, as in the case of measles or mumps. However, it is not known whether the virus has been completely eliminated from the body or remains, making the person a carrier. Nor is it known whether the person will ever develop the disease, signs and symptoms appearing weeks, months, or years later. The test merely identifies blood that contains antibodies and may or may not contain the virus. Nevertheless, since blood that tests positive is a *potential* transmitter of AIDS, prudence insists that no such donations be used for transfusion, however few are actually dangerous.

Second, the limited reliability of the test must be considered. There is no single test, but a hierarchy of several tests, for the antibody. Blood is first assessed by a test that is extremely sensitive but not very specific; that is, it responds not only to the HTLV-III/LAV antibody but to other substances in the blood. The latter response is known as a false positive. Also, for as yet unknown reasons, the test fails to catch a very few samples that do contain antibodies, resulting in rare false negatives. Correction of false negatives must await further research. Blood that tests positive is discarded to be on the safe side, but positive results can be, and all are, confirmed by different kinds of test. Confirmation tests are too slow to be practical for screening but are useful to check screening results because they are very specific. This means that they rarely give false positives because they react only with HTLV-III/LAV antibodies. The confirmation test most commonly used today is called the Western blot, but others are under study. Confirmation tests help to determine what is told to the donor.

An important issue in blood testing for AIDS antibodies concerns the rights of the donor: should the donor be told explicitly that the test will be performed? Should any result other than a clear-cut negative be revealed? Exactly what should the donor be told and what advice given? Equally important is the donor's right of privacy and strict confidentiality in the recording, storage, and communication of all test data.

Virtually everyone agrees that the donor must be informed beforehand of the mandatory test so that donating is also the giving of consent. However, notification of a positive test result is sometimes questioned because there is no known cure for AIDS and little that the donor can do once informed. On the other hand, public health officials rightfully point out that the antibody-positive donor must be advised not to donate again and to take other steps to prevent possible spread of the disease. Such steps include modifying or stopping sexual contact between males, refraining from the use of intravenous drugs and shared needles, using condoms, and notifying health-care professionals of positive blood test results prior to any needed medical treatment.

Donors who test positive initially but negative on a confirming test are not now being informed, because of doubts about the significance of the test results. For confidentiality, all test records are stored separate from the general records of blood collection organizations, in locked or encoded computer files. Some questions arise about the possible need of local, state, or federal public health authorities for test information and their legal right of access, but as yet there are no requirements to reveal these results to anyone except the donors. Lastly, blood collection agencies have established special procedures for notifying donors. These procedures respect privacy, are sensitive to the potentially traumatic nature of the news, and try to deal with the uncertainty about what the donor should do next.

Test Results
The test for AIDS antibodies provided a tool for comparing the number exposed to the HTLV-III/LAV virus with the number of

reported cases of AIDS. Some 2.5 million blood donors throughout the United States were screened in mid-1985, shortly after test kits became available. Three samples in a thousand (0.3 percent) gave positive results when tested twice with the same screening test. Results of follow-up confirmation have not yet been published, but several blood centers report approximately 7 confirmations per 10,000 tests. This suggests that about 7,000 of the approximately 10 million healthy adults who volunteer to donate blood each year may have been exposed to AIDS. Because of the long incubation period of the disease, several years of experience are needed to learn how many will develop AIDS and how many will prove to be immune.

Autologous Blood Transfusions—Donating for One's Own Use

Fear of contracting AIDS has renewed interest in providing blood for oneself (*autologous*—derived from the same person). People in otherwise good health who are scheduled for elective surgery donate blood in advance, to be placed on reserve for use during the operation. It is even possible to collect up to three or four pints of blood this way through a complex procedure of collecting a unit volume, then later returning it to the donor and drawing off more than was returned. While this technique reduces the risk of exposure to most hazards associated with blood transfusion, it is applicable only when the individual is healthy, not anemic, and there is time to make the arrangements. Most people who need blood transfusions are not in this category. A further disadvantage is the complicated clerical procedures required, which significantly increase the risk of errors. In blood transfusion therapy there is no room for errors.

Because red blood cells can be stored frozen for several years, it is theoretically possible to donate blood while healthy and have it stored until needed. Although possible, it is completely impractical; it would require vast storehouses of frozen blood, some of which would never be used.

Fallacy of the Dedicated Donor

Another attempt to protect against AIDS from blood transfusions is the "dedicated donor" recruited from among relatives and friends of the patient in the belief that blood from such a donor is necessarily safer than blood from strangers. The three major U.S. blood banking organizations—the Council of Community Blood Banks, the American National Red Cross, and the American Association of Blood Banks—have issued a joint statement pointing out the fallacy of such reasoning and agreeing to oppose the practice.

The main fault of dedicated donors is that they often are too dedicated. Friends or relatives may be as likely as others to be in poor health, to be secret members of a high-risk group, to have been exposed to communicable diseases, or to have a disease or condition that they do not want to reveal. Yet they may be so concerned about the welfare of their relative or friend who requires a blood transfusion and so eager to help that, consciously or unconsciously, they do not answer the health history questions truthfully. In an effort to do good, they may actually do harm. The safest donor is the true volunteer who gains no advantage from donating—neither money, special privileges, days off, nor the chance to do a friend a favor. Another important reason for not earmarking specific donations for specific patients is the extra steps and bookkeeping required in collecting, testing, storing, and distributing the blood. Each additional step carries an inherent risk of error. It bears repeating that there is no margin for error in blood banking.

THE SAFETY OF DONATING BLOOD

A Roper public opinion poll reported that 91 percent of all Americans know about AIDS, about 50 percent think they can get AIDS from receiving a blood transfusion, and 26 percent believe they can get AIDS from donating blood! The fact is that one simply cannot get AIDS from donating blood. No AIDS patients are present at the donation site. Workers and donors who are there are in the best of health. The staff who collect the blood have been specially trained in techniques to prevent the spread of any disease. The equipment used to draw blood is disposable, delivered in sealed, sterile containers, used only once, and discarded under special sanitary conditions. Needles inserted into the donor's vein receive particular attention; after use they are cut off the tubing and placed in strong, covered containers to prevent handlers from being stuck with a used needle. On the rare occasion that blood spills or contacts a reusable instrument, it is immediately removed with solutions that thoroughly disinfect the area. The best evidence of safety is the record of the nursing staff. Collectively, they have been exposed to tens of millions of blood donors and blood donations, and not one case of AIDS has been reported among them.

These strict hygienic measures have been in force for years at blood collection facilities and have protected both donors and staff. Giving blood is safe.

SAFETY OF HEALTH-CARE WORKERS
ATTENDING AIDS PATIENTS

Another concern is the safety of personnel caring for AIDS patients. To date, no case of AIDS has been reported among health-care workers—doctors, nurses, orderlies, laboratory workers, or other hospital employees—who were not members of a high-risk group and therefore exposed to infection elsewhere. This strongly indicates that AIDS is not being spread through the air when patients cough or sneeze, by touching patients, or by eating food they have handled. On the basis of these findings, hospitals have issued clear guidelines that AIDS patients need not be placed in strict isolation. Special precautions are necessary only when drawing or handling blood samples, to avoid being stuck by a needle or cut by broken glass contaminated by blood from an AIDS patient. Transmission of hepatitis B by a needle stick is quite common; such transmission of AIDS is very rare. Only two cases have been reported in the United States and one in England, but these few are enough to warrant caution.

SUMMARY

Identification of the virus HTLV-III/LAV and development of a test for the antibody to that virus confirmed early speculation that AIDS can be transmitted by blood transfusion. The risk appears to be less than one in a million transfusions. The risk for hemophiliacs is higher, probably due to repeated injections of Factor VIII (for blood coagulation), which is prepared from pools of plasma obtained from 2,500 to 10,000 donors. Even so, only a very few hemophiliacs have developed AIDS, and treatment of Factor VIII now further reduces now further reduces the risk. No AIDS has been associated with serum albumin or gamma globulin, two other plasma proteins prepared from large pools. This is probably due to pasteurization of the former and the abundance of antibodies in the latter.

Careful screening of donors eliminates blood donations from members of high-risk groups. Strict confidentiality protects donor privacy. Autologous blood transfusion to avoid receiving infected blood is possible but seldom practical. Blood from dedicated donors, chosen by recipients for their exclusive use, is not considered as safe as blood from anonymous, volunteer donors, who are more likely to answer health screening questions freely and honestly.

A blood test for AIDS antibodies has been used to screen donated blood since March 1985. This is *not* a test for AIDS; rather it detects evidence of exposure to AIDS at some time in the past. It is not known whether someone, apparently healthy, whose blood tests positive has successfully fought off the virus and no longer harbors it in blood or other body tissues, is a carrier without symptoms but capable of transmitting the virus, or will develop AIDS in the future. All blood that tests positive is destroyed, and, if the results are confirmed by a second test, donors are notified and advised not to donate again. Some 7 out of 10,000 healthy adult volunteer blood donors test positive.

There is no way to contract AIDS by donating blood. All equipment, including needles, is new, used once, and safely disposed of. The effectiveness of strict hygienic measures used by all blood collection agencies is demonstrated by the freedom of agency staff from infection after participating in many millions of blood donations.

Also, AIDS is not spread by ordinary contact between health-care workers and patients. However, as mentioned above, care must be exercised to prevent being stuck by a needle or cut by broken glass contaminated by blood from an AIDS patient. Although transmission of the virus in this way is very rare, it has been reported.

10   The Haitian Link

JEFFREY VIEIRA

During the summer of 1982, physicians in Brooklyn, New York, and Miami, Florida, reported observations on 40 Haitian immigrants with unusual or opportunistic infections and/or Kaposi's sarcoma (KS). The patterns were strikingly similar to those found earlier in homosexuals and intravenous-narcotics abusers with acquired immune deficiency syndrome (AIDS). Meanwhile, reviews of hospital records and autopsy materials in Haiti indicated that the first cases of AIDS encountered there coincided with the first cases seen in homosexuals in New York and Los Angeles. Since Haitians lacked any of the then recognized risk factors for AIDS (for example, homosexual promiscuity and intravenous-drug abuse), they were classified by the Centers for Disease Control (CDC) as a separate high-risk group.

Since 1982, studies of Haitians with AIDS in the United States and in Haiti have identified some of the risk behaviors in this group and have provided some of the first convincing evidence for heterosexual transmission of the disease. In response to these findings and political pressure by the Haitian community, Haitians are no longer classified as a discrete risk group by the CDC.

CLINICAL PICTURE OF AIDS IN HAITIANS

Clinically, AIDS in Haitians is similar to AIDS in others at risk for acquiring the disease. Enlarged lymph nodes (lymphadenopathy), fever, weight loss, and chronic diarrhea, which have become known as the AIDS prodrome, or AIDS-related complex (ARC), are almost universal precursors of the disease. These signs and symptoms may persist for weeks to months before development of an opportunistic infection or malignancy.

Parasitic infections of the lung due to the protozoan *Pneumocystis carinii* and infection of the mouth and esophagus (oroesophagitis) due to the fungus *Candida albicans* are the most common opportunistic infections encountered in Haitians with AIDS, whether in the United States or Haiti. Certain infections appear to be particularly common in Haitian patients, reflecting their prevalence in the Haitian environment. Widespread *Mycobacterium tuberculosis* (TB) occurs in about 50 percent of Haitians with AIDS (unpublished figures, New York City Department of Health). Because TB also occurs in persons with normal immunity, it is not considered an opportunistic infection by the CDC definition. However, AIDS patients with TB can be differentiated from otherwise healthy TB patients by significant depression of the cell-mediated immune system. This defect is demonstrated by a reversal of the ratio of helper T to suppressor T cells and by the absence of local swelling in skin tests when antigens (PPD, Tine, mumps, *Candida,* and Trichophyton) are injected under the outer layers of the skin. Homosexuals and drug addicts with AIDS also develop mycobacterial infections, but these are usually caused by one of the so-called atypical mycobacteria, particularly *Mycobacterium avium-intracellulare.* As many as 20 percent of Haitians with AIDS develop lesions in the brain due to the parasite *Toxoplasma gondii* (unpublished figures, New York City Department of Health), which may take the form of meningitis, confusion and behavioral changes, or signs of stroke. The infection usually represents reactivation of latent (dormant) toxoplasmosis, rather than a new infection, due to the loss of effective cellular immune surveillance. In contrast to their incidence in Haitians with AIDS, *T. gondii* infections have been reported somewhat less frequently in non-Haitian AIDS patients.

Intestinal infections with parasites, such as amebiasis, giardiasis, and cryptosporidiosis, may cause significant sickness as a result of dehydrating diarrhea and malabsorption of nutrients. Virtually all AIDS patients in Haiti develop chronic diarrhea, often due to one or more of these parasites.

The laboratory blood test results characteristic of AIDS—anemia, decreased numbers of white blood cells (especially lymphocytes), decreased numbers of functional helper T cells, and reversal of the helper/suppressor T-cells ratio—are found in all Haitians with AIDS. As with homosexuals and many narcotics addicts, blood tests for syphilis and viral infections (Epstein-Barr, cytomegalovirus, herpes simplex, hepatitis A, hepatitis B) are often positive. About 40–45 percent of all AIDS patients die within the first year, but the one-year mortality for Haitian-Americans with AIDS approaches 60 percent and is over 70 percent in Haiti. This unfavorable prognosis is attributable to several factors. Malnutrition in rural Haiti is common. Recurrent or chronic parasitic infections combined with protein-calorie malnutrition cause debilitation and impair immune defenses against serious infection. A minority of Haitian-Americans were malnourished prior to the onset of AIDS, but undernourishment and consequent exhaustion become the rule as the disease progresses. Also, although basic medical care is free in Haiti, the cost of medications is usually borne by the patient or the family. Because most patients with AIDS require prolonged therapy with antibiotics, which are frequently expensive, some can afford only short-term medication while others receive none at all. The high incidence of toxoplasmosis affecting the central nervous system, with a mortality rate over 75 percent, also increases the overall death rate.

HAITIAN BACKGROUND

AIDS is caused by infection with human T-cell lymphotrophic retrovirus (also called lymphadenopathy-associated virus) HTLV IIII/LAV (possibly with other contributing conditions). The virus has been isolated from blood, semen, breast milk, tears, saliva, and vaginal secretions, among other body fluids. It is known to be transmitted by sexual contact, by exposure to infected blood (intravenous-drug users and transfusion recipients), and to children in the womb of an infected mother. To explore various theories of transmission among Haitians in particular, it is useful to consider the social, economic, and cultural climate of Haiti.

Haiti occupies the western half of the island of Hispaniola in the Caribbean. It is the most densely populated and poorest nation of the Western Hemisphere, with a population of about 6 million. The

natives are descended from central and western African blacks of
various tribal origins brought to Haiti (then Saint Domingue) as
slaves in the sixteenth and seventeenth centuries. French is the
official language, but Creole, a dialect unique to Haiti, is spoken by
all natives.

Haiti is predominantly agrarian. Apart from a small middle and
upper class of professionals and skilled technicians, the majority of
the population achieves only a meager existence as common laborers
or farmers. The mean annual income is less than $350. Since the
mid-1960s thousands of Haitians have emigrated to the United States
and Canada to escape political repression (the Duvalier dictatorship
has been ousted, but conditions are not yet stable). More recent
emigrants have been motivated by unfavorable economic conditions.
Most Haitians settled in Miami, New York, and Newark, with
smaller enclaves in Boston, Los Angeles, and Montreal. Haitians in
the United States are estimated to number between 0.5 and 1 million,
about 100,000 having arrived since 1978, but this figure is imprecise
because many are unregistered. Roman Catholicism is the Haitian
state religion, but a sizable Protestant following exists. Voodoo, a
synthesis of Catholicism and African tribal rituals, flourishes in rural
Haiti and is practiced by many Haitian-Americans. A small number
practice magic or spiritual rituals, whose details are not openly
discussed by Haitians, especially to white foreigners.

At first, AIDS among Haitians was puzzling because the Haitian
lifestyle seemed to lack the characteristics associated with vulnerability. Yet, the prevalence of antibodies to HTLV-III/LAV among
Haitians in the United States is about five times that in the general
American population. Studies in the United States and Haiti have
now demonstrated that Haitians probably acquire AIDS in the same
ways others do—homosexual/bisexual activity, transfusions, children born to infected mothers, and promiscuous heterosexual
contacts.

For economic reasons, some Haitian men resort to prostitution,
pandering to vacationing homosexuals, many from the United
States. Carrefour, a suburb of Port-au-Prince, the Haitian capital, is
the center of prostitution, both male and female. It is probably no
coincidence that Carrefour is also the center of the AIDS epidemic in
Haiti. Although 98 percent of the population lives in rural areas, they
account for fewer than 5 percent of the AIDS cases.

In a society so staunchly Catholic, and in which the macho image is avidly cultivated, the stigma of homosexuality is a formidable disincentive to candor in the discussion of sexual habits. Thus, it is likely that the prevalence of homosexuality in Haiti is underestimated. (Heterosexual promiscuity by bisexual males may also explain the relatively high incidence of AIDS among Haitian women.) In the United States, despite concerted efforts to elicit histories of homosexuality, fewer than 5 percent of Haitians will admit to such relationships at any time during their lives. Having distanced themselves from the poverty that promoted homosexual prostitution, and having assumed a more conventional lifestyle in the United States, most are understandably reluctant to make such admissions. There is no evidence to implicate intravenous-narcotics abuse as an important means of AIDS transmission among Haitians, probably due to both cultural taboos and the prohibitive cost of drugs and paraphernalia.

Sexual transmission of AIDS between men and women seems to be more common among Haitians in Haiti and in the United States than among non-Haitian AIDS patients. (Interestingly, in the central African countries of Ruanda, Zaire, and Zambia the vast majority of cases appear to be related to promiscuous heterosexual activity rather than homosexuality, blood transfusions, or drug abuse. In some areas of central Africa, 10–20 percent of the general population are infected with AIDS, and up to 80 percent of prostitutes.) Which particular heterosexual practices transmit the virus is not established, but anal intercourse used as a means of contraception is suspected to put women at risk. Also, because of the expense and scarcity of medical supplies, some physicians in Haiti may reuse needles and syringes without adequate sterilization, raising the specter of iatrogenic (physician-induced) transmission of disease. However, no such cases have been proved.

Many Haitians use potions and concoctions from herbs and roots whose chemical composition and potential for suppressing the body's immune system are unknown. Antibiotics available over the counter are also sometimes used indiscriminately to treat recurrent infections. Such antibiotics may be immunosuppressive but, like the potions used for many years without apparent ill effects, are unlikely to be the primary cause of severe immune depression in AIDS patients. Magic rituals sometimes transfer blood and secretions from person to person. Women have been known to add menstrual blood to the food and drink of their partners to prevent them from "straying." Worshippers of Erzulie, a benign deity, engage in rituals during which the hougan, or priest, may engage in intercourse with other male worshippers. Although such practices may be suspect, present ignorance about the prevalence and forms of Haitian rituals requires that suggestions of disease transmission by this route be considered purely speculative.

Transfusion-related AIDS among Haitians has not been documented. In Haiti, 20 percent of patients questioned had had blood transfusions from 1.5 to 6 years prior to the onset of the disease, but no reliable transfusion history is available for the majority of Haitian-Americans.

The antigenic-overload hypothesis suggests that a combination of factors (multiple viral, parasitic, bacterial, and fungal infections, and exposure to recreational and prescription drugs) may contribute to immune depression and eventual predisposition to opportunistic infections and malignancy. Since venereal diseases and intestinal parasitic infections are common in Haiti, they may be a cofactor with the virus HTLV-III/LAV in the onset of AIDS. Poor sanitation and overcrowding in the cities of Haiti also favor the spread of infections from person to person or by insect carriers such as flies and mosquitos. However, these theoretical modes of transmission would not be expected to play an important role in the temperate climate of the United States, nor is there evidence of their spreading AIDS in the tropics.

SOCIAL AND ECONOMIC IMPACT

The original reports of AIDS among Haitian immigrants were sensationalized and misrepresented in the popular press. Some news broadcasts pictured scantily clad black natives dancing frenetically about ritual fires, while others caricatured Haitians with AIDS as illegal aliens interned in detention camps. The majority of Haitian AIDS patients fit neither of these stereotypes, but the impression often left with the public was that AIDS was pervasive throughout the Haitian community. Unlike the homosexual or drug addict, the Haitian was highly visible and could be singled out by ethnic and cultural features.

Unfounded anxiety over the risks of acquiring AIDS by casual contact resulted in widespread discrimination against Haitians in housing and employment. Many were dismissed from their jobs, while others were not given fair consideration for positions for which they were qualified. Parents expressed fears that their children might contract AIDS from Haitian domestics or from Haitian classmates in school. The Haitian community responded with appropriate concern for the health of its members and with understandable anger at what they considered unfair and racist treatment. In Haiti, aside from its local public health consequences, AIDS has had an adverse impact on one of the major sources of Haiti's foreign exchange, tourism. In the aftermath of the reports of AIDS in Haitian-Americans, the tourist trade to Haiti declined by 20 percent. Although the picture has improved somewhat, AIDS anxiety is still expressed by some travelers to Haiti. Dialogues between Haitian and American physicians have helped to cool tempers and to educate both the Haitian and non-Haitian communities about AIDS in general and about the scope of the problem among Haitian-Americans in particular.

SUMMARY

AIDS is a new, lethal viral disease characterized by severe defects in the immune system with a resulting variety of unusual infections and malignancies. Originally, Haitians were labeled as a discrete group susceptible to AIDS due to unrecognized risk factors. It is now conceded that they acquire AIDS by the same behaviors as others in known risk groups. There is no evidence to implicate a racial or ethnic predisposition, and suggestions of contributing factors in Haitian culture are merely speculative.

11

AIDS in Prisons

ISABEL C. GUERRERO
ALAN C. KOENIGSFEST

AIDS among prison inmates presents special problems arising from the conditions of controlled confinement and the character of the prison population. The number of inmates with AIDS also reflects the way AIDS is distributed in the population at large.

Since its recognition in 1981, AIDS in the general population has appeared almost entirely in well-defined risk groups: homosexual or bisexual men, abusers (largely heterosexual) of intravenous (IV) drugs, and recipients of blood or blood products, especially hemophiliacs. (Others, in smaller numbers, include prostitutes, wives or lovers of high-risk men, and children born to infected mothers.) The disease is also geographically concentrated in a few large cities on the East Coast, where it primarily affects IV-drug abusers, and the West Coast, where homosexual AIDS cases predominate. As pointed out in a Centers for Disease Control (CDC) publication, the relatively high incidence of AIDS in prisons is not surprising since many inmates had been convicted of criminal offenses related to IV-drug abuse, and IV-drug abuse is a predisposing factor for AIDS. Nor is it surprising that the incidence is particularly high in New Jersey and New York prisons since these two states have reported 62 percent of all AIDS cases related to IV-drug abuse in the United States.

Data on the incidence of AIDS in U.S. correctional institutions have not previously been accurately determined. For example, a questionnaire survey by the National Institute of Justice (U.S.

Department of Justice) and the American Correctional Association reported a cumulative total of 766 AIDS cases in prison (over 70 percent of them in New York, New Jersey, and Pennsylvania) but did not have the data on changes in prison population with time, necessary to calculate annual incidence rates.

Information solicited from health administrators in New York (state and city), Florida, and California, and compared with available data from New Jersey, all areas of high AIDS incidence, provides a more useful indication.

	No. of Inmates (Approx.)	No. of Cases (1984–1985)	Rate per 100,000	(Total Cases 1981–1985)
New York City	11,000	50	454	(150)
New Jersey	12,500	33	264	(76)
New York State	36,000	50	138	(266)
Florida	28,000	14	50	(37)
California	50,557	25	49	(25)

The figure for New York City prisons is misleading because it was based on a very transient population, including individuals jailed for only one or two days. State figures were based on relatively stable prison populations. When only stable populations are considered, New Jersey prisons rank first, with an annual prison incidence of AIDS 66 times as great as in the general community. (These are AIDS cases diagnosed, not contracted, in prisons.)

Correctional facilities all over the country share similar security, medical, ethical, and legal problems in dealing with AIDS, combined with the concerns of prison staffs and inmates about the deadly disease. Consideration of New Jersey's experience as the site of highest prison incidence of AIDS will illustrate the circumstances and difficulties and may be helpful to others.

AIDS IN NEW JERSEY PRISONS

The N.J. Department of Corrections started watching for possible AIDS in inmates in 1981 and by 1985 had hospitalized 98 patients with conditions suggesting immune deficiency. AIDS was confirmed in 76, AIDS-related complex (ARC) in the other 22.

Almost all the confirmed AIDS cases (95 percent) had *Pneumocystis carinii* pneumonia (PCP), and a few (5 percent) had other severe opportunistic infections, but none had Kaposi's sarcoma. Ninety-three percent were men and 7 percent were women, somewhat like the proportions in the general population. Ninety-four percent were heterosexual IV-drug abusers; 5 percent were homosexual or bisexual (much less than in the outside community); 76 percent were black, 24 percent white (9 percent Hispanic); and half were between 30 and 39 years old. The large number of IV-drug abusers indicates the effects of both geographical concentration and the tendency for drug abusers to be arrested for crimes punishable by imprisonment. Most of the inmates had lived in areas, such as northern New Jersey counties, which reported a relatively high incidence of AIDS to the state health department.

The number of inmates with AIDS reported each year is increasing. Also, of the 76 known by the end of 1985, 62 (82 percent) have died, including all those diagnosed before 1984.

Although almost all these inmate patients (95 percent) were diagnosed while in prison, between 1 month and 5½ years after entering (an average of 18.9 months), no case of an inmate being infected in prison has been documented. No cluster of cases traceable to a common source, such as a needle or a tattoo machine, has appeared in any prison. During 1981–1985 no inmate was diagnosed with AIDS who had served more than 10 years and had no known risk factors. Nevertheless, as the years pass and AIDS continues to spread, new infections are likely to occur in prison.

Hospital Care

When inmates are diagnosed as having AIDS, they are hospitalized. Before April 1986 no AIDS cases in remission were returned to prison. In April a 14-bed infirmary unit was opened at a major New Jersey state prison to provide medical care and secured housing for such inmates within the prison but not as part of the general prison population.

The length of time spent in the hospital before death or parole has ranged from 1 to 601 days (average 85 days). One inmate had a sudden fever, cough, and shortness of breath, diagnosed as pneumonia, and died of respiratory failure within a day of admission. The longest hospitalization also involved pneumonia, PCP, which went into remission several times with treatment until the inmate succumbed to a fatal resistant infection. Only 2 of the 76 confirmed AIDS patients were paroled, and were in remission when discharged.

These hospitalization times do not include recurring illnesses, such as bronchitis, bacterial pneumonias, and pulmonary tuberculosis, for which most of the inmates were in and out of the hospital before the onset of serious opportunistic infections, such as PCP, atypical mycobacterial, or severe fungal infections, indicated full-blown AIDS. If these times are taken into account, the hospital stays are even longer.

Long stays in the prison hospital can be oppressive. Inmate patients, apparently lucky to have their infections go into remission, may actually suffer more from an intensification of the depression and isolation already associated with AIDS. They may now be housed in a prison infirmary unit but are still not mixed with the general prison population because correctional authorities fear they would be exposed to assault by other inmates who dread the disease. In the hospital prison unit they are confined to private rooms with secured windows and doors. They are allowed only books, typewriters, and games, and are provided with television to give some relief from perpetual boredom. Usually, each is alone in one room because non-AIDS patients refuse to share quarters with AIDS patients, which accentuates feelings of ostracism and solitude. Attempts are made to alleviate the depressing atmosphere, including frequent visiting privileges for relatives, hospice programs, and counseling for families. Unfortunately, most inmate patients do not have relatives who visit or write, and children in the family are sometimes not permitted to visit inmates with AIDS.

Very ill AIDS patients are retained even after they are due for parole unless the family is willing to assume further hospital expenses and is ready to provide a home environment. This has not happened very often. No inmate has been granted medical clemency because of a diagnosis of AIDS. If an AIDS patient is well enough to be paroled, arrangements are made for future follow-ups in a clinic or hospital in the home community, and the wife or other relatives is advised of the health risks and appropriate hygienic measures.

As a ward of the state, an inmate who dies of AIDS is subjected by law to an autopsy. Since one Medical Examiner's Office, whose jurisdiction included a hospital prison unit, has been reluctant to perform autopsies on AIDS patients, some bodies have had to be autopsied by the county medical examiner where the prison that first received the inmate is located. Families notified of an inmate's death have shown responses varying from grief to indifference to anger, anger at the Department of Corrections for allegedly allowing the inmate to acquire AIDS or anger at the inmate for having exposed relatives to a fatal illness.

Medical Costs

Inmates, relatives, and sometimes the community have a misconception that an inmate's health care is neglected. The public does not realize that an inmate receives more adequate medical, dental, and nursing care than is available to many economically deprived members of the community who have no medical insurance. Also, the care of inmates who have, or are suspected to have, AIDS or ARC is expensive.

On the basis of available information for 36 inmate AIDS patients, hospitalization costs ranged from $310.50 for a one-day stay to $104,295 (averaging $31,426), varying with the severity and length of illness. The expense mounts if intensive care, surgery, or special treatment such as hemodialysis is required. Physicians' fees ranged from $170 to $7,940 (averaging $2,714) per patient.

Custodial expenses ranged from $184 to $67,904 (averaging $25,993), including salaries and overtime pay for correction officers who guard the inmates. Each inmate patient who leaves the hospital prison unit, for example, to enter the intensive care unit, requires two correction officers per eight-hour shift.

Since AIDS was first recognized in prison inmates, the N.J. Department of Corrections has spent $4 million on care for inmate patients diagnosed to have AIDS. Expenses for inmates hospitalized but not confirmed to have AIDS have not been accurately calculated but are projected to be enormous and may double the total cost.

PRISON PROBLEMS

AIDS Risks

The prison population in all states consists of a concentration of groups at high risk of AIDS, particularly IV-drug abusers. In New Jersey, about 70 percent of the inmates were involved in criminal drug use. They have usually been detoxified in county jails so they are no longer suffering from drug withdrawal when they enter state prison. However, despite strict and punitive state prison policy, inmates manage to abuse drugs, although to a lesser degree than in the free community. Illicit drugs and paraphernalia are smuggled in by couriers during personal visits. Since the practice continues, the risk of transmitting AIDS through shared needles and syringes is present.

Inmates may also increase their risk by the use of illegal tattoo machines. To date, however, there is no evidence of the disease having been transmitted in prison through the sharing of tattoo machines with inmates who have AIDS.

Some risk is associated with homosexual practices, but this may be small since only 4 percent of inmates with AIDS admitted to being homosexual or bisexual. Gay inmates are usually well known to prison staff and other inmates and generally become attached to a lover or friend who offers protection. Also, forcible sodomy and other sexual attacks are not as frequent as outsiders may believe, at least in New Jersey prisons.

AIDS Diagnosis

AIDS in prison may be more difficult to diagnose than in the outside community. In the early days of experience with AIDS, prison physicians unfamiliar with the new disease sometimes made misdiagnoses. The difficulties were increased by the nature of the inmates, who are mostly young, malnourished, and chronically ill with seizure or psychiatric disorders. Their unkempt appearance, uncooperativeness, and characteristically hostile and manipulative attitudes interfered with physical examinations, the obtaining of reliable medical histories, and the assessment of medical problems.

Fear and Administrative Problems

An inmate who merely develops suspect symptoms and receives a medical checkup is automatically labeled an AIDS carrier by other inmates and nonmedical staff. Even if discharged from the hospital as AIDS-free, the inmate becomes an administrative problem because other inmates refuse to room with someone they fear is tainted.

Other problems arise if an inmate is chronically ill with ARC infections and is in and out of the hospital, but is always returned to the general prison population. If the inmate then develops an opportunistic infection that results in a diagnosis of AIDS, both inmates and staff accuse the medical department of lying, neglect, and indifference for apparently exposing them to a fatal disease.

Such fear and suspicion in the nonmedical correctional staff contribute to the difficulties of dealing with AIDS in prison. Correction officers belong to one of the strongest labor unions in the state. Union concerns about the occupational risk their members may face in contacts with inmates having ARC or AIDS have become contract issues regarding salary adjustments, changes in work conditions, and employment guarantees for members who contract AIDS. Fortunately, very few officers have refused to perform their duties related to inmates suspected of having or diagnosed to have AIDS, but episodic disruptions of prison operations have occurred, sometimes almost to the point of a staff walkout.

A correctional employee diagnosed to have AIDS encounters special difficulties. Like an inmate, such an employee who is well enough to go back to work will be subjected to harassment and ostracism by fellow employees and inmates. However, unlike an inmate, the employee must undergo investigation to determine the source of the infection. An employee with AIDS, whether or not a member of a known risk group, is entitled to disability compensation and coverage by medical insurance. Compassion for the employee must be the paramount consideration, and employment status and medical benefits must be appropriately protected.

AIDS Prevention

The confined, secured environment of prisons, where law enforcement is the rule, raises unique difficulties. Risk reduction measures applicable in the outside community are not feasible in prisons. For example, the use of condoms is strongly advised for high-risk homosexual and bisexual groups, but the provision of condoms is contrary to prison policy, which prohibits and punishes homosexual practices. Similarly, IV-drug abusers in the community are advised to sterilize needles and to avoid sharing them with others. This cannot be tolerated in prison where the use of unprescribed drugs is forbidden.

Such discrepancies between recommended public health measures and prison practice have evoked the legal issue of inmates not being informed about condom and needle recommendations that might help them avoid the consequences of their risky habits. The N.J. Department of Corrections now faces a suit by inmates who claim that their risk of developing a fatal illness has been increased by prison restraints. Nevertheless, departmental policy is strict and clear: Any inmate caught engaging in homosexual acts or using illicit drugs will be punished.

HTLV-III/LAV Blood Tests: Dilemma and Controversy

The availability of blood tests for HTLV-III/LAV antibodies (a sign of exposure to the virus associated with AIDS, not proof of active disease) has caused confusion and controversy in correctional facilities. The issues are the desirability of mass screening, the applicability of the test, and the medical and legal implications.

Some usefulness is generally accepted with little dispute:

To help the medical evaluation of unexplained illness among inmates in high-risk groups.

To prevent transmission of AIDS to newborns during birth. The test would be given to pregnant female inmates who show any symptoms of AIDS infection, have a history of IV-drug abuse, have been prostitutes, or were sex partners of men in high-risk groups or showing evidence of infection.

To test prison staff or inmates accidentally exposed to blood, blood products, or other body secretions of inmates in high-risk groups, for example, in cases of needle sticks or cuts with sharp instruments by medical, nursing, or dental personnel, or in instances of violence, human bites, or personal assaults.

To find the common source of clusters of AIDS cases or to investigate continuing transmission of infection. Such investigations must be done by experienced personnel under the guidance of an epidemiologist. Otherwise, antibody testing would be haphazard and unscientific. Done properly, such testing can accumulate information on the prevalence of exposure to guide the formation of public health policy.

Mass screening is controversial and poses a dilemma for corrections departments. Proponents argue that identifying and segregating inmates who test positive will prevent disease transmission in prison and also forestall negligence lawsuits. However, correctional systems generally lack sufficient medical facilities and separate accommodations to make this feasible, and none has had the opportunity to budget for the necessary additional construction. This is certainly the case in New Jersey, where a large number of inmates are expected to test positive. Even if segregated housing were available, a major obstacle would be the recruitment of staff willing to work in such a volatile environment, highly susceptible to the outbreak of violence.

Some community groups have suggested house arrest as a possible alternative. A criminal who tests positive would be confined to home, rather than prison, and wear a radio collar to enable the police to monitor any movement outside the house. This seems less a solution than an indicator of the magnitude of the problem.

Mass screening may also provoke hysteria among the prison staff and inmates. Confidentiality of test results is difficult to achieve in prison. Inmates who test positive cannot be relied on to keep it to themselves, but are likely to use the information for self-serving purposes such as acquiring medical clemency, special diet, various privileges, and more favorable housing. On the other hand, non-medical prison officials may use such knowledge to intimidate inmates for the maintenance of peace and security.

The absence of protective segregated housing would subject inmates known to test positive to ostracism, harassment, and even violence from other inmates. Staff would be reluctant to be near them. Affected inmates might press legal suits on the basis of alleged discrimination that violates their constitutional rights by forcing them to live under conditions worse than administrative disciplinary detention. An inmate in disciplinary detention is isolated in a cell and denied the privilege of participating in prison activities like sports, movies, school, and eating with others. If segregated because of AIDS, the inmate would not only be isolated but treated differently by correction officers wearing masks, gowns, and gloves that promote additional anxiety.

RECOMMENDED ACTIONS

AIDS-related problems in both the closed prison environment and the open community stem from the lack of a clear understanding of the disease. Experience and scientific studies indicate that the virus is transmitted by sexual contact and in blood and blood products, not by casual contact. It is ignorance of this that causes irrational reactions. To dispel ignorance, prison facilities must undertake an intensive educational program to enlighten both staff and inmates. If a facility cannot assemble a training team from its own physician and an employee who is a skilled educator, it can tap resources provided by the local or state health department. Instruction must be repeated often, in words simple enough to be understood even by the poorly educated, and updated continually to keep pace with the latest discoveries.

New Jersey has successfully established such an educational program on AIDS, consisting of lectures, videotapes shown regularly to staff and inmates, and leaflets. Leaflets are given promptly to all new inmates. Before the program was initiated, inmates were threatening disorder, and staff were on the verge of staging walkouts, even asking to wear space suits when transporting an inmate suspected of having AIDS. After the program was under way, and after conferences with labor union and inmate representatives, attitudes changed markedly for the better toward both the disease and inmates who had AIDS.

Another essential is a central hospital facility and a central clinic. The hospital's purpose is definitive diagnosis and treatment of inmates requiring hospitalization and the gathering of useful epidemiologic information (data related to the cause, incidence, and distribution of AIDS in the population). The clinic, with an epidemiologist or internist on staff, will provide a well-planned, uniform medical evaluation of inmates referred by prison physicians. Such evaluation would make it unnecessary for prison physicians to order excessive and expensive tests and also determine appropriate hospitalization for all sick inmates, most of whom will not have the signs and symptoms of AIDS. This coordinated system can considerably reduce the financial burden of prison hospital care.

Since AIDS weakens or destroys the body's immune defenses, it leads to the development of various communicable diseases, a serious problem in the closed, densely populated prison environment. To combat the possible spread of such diseases, corrections departments must institute effective infection control. The infection control program instituted by the N.J. Department of Corrections involves isolation and other precautionary measures as needed, but also has other important features. Inmate care is managed according to symptoms, not disease, so the stigma of labeling is avoided. For example, an inmate being moved to the hospital is not designated as having or not having AIDS but is accompanied by appropriate instructions, such as the wearing of masks if the inmate has a cough. Since correction officers are told the symptoms and necessary precautions but not the diagnosis, they do not have the opportunity to breach confidentiality. In particular, establishment of an infection control program has been necessary to contain the epidemic of contagious diseases like tuberculosis, which is becoming more associated with AIDS. Infection control guidelines were established for an accurate epidemiologic investigation, contact follow-up, and specific preventive therapy for tuberculosis.

The rising number of AIDS cases (new cases each year are double those of the year before) demands expansion of hospital bed capacity. Also, since patients in remission are not returned to the prison population, a unit outside the hospital is needed to house them for protective custody.

Until a cure or preventive vaccine is discovered, the number of AIDS patients in prisons will continue to rise. An imperative action against spread of the disease is education to modify behavior that contributes to the risk, specifically to stop drug abuse and to counsel other high-risk groups against destructive habits.

Taking these recommended actions can help not only to control AIDS but to prevent prison disorder, even riots, and threatened employee walkouts. It may not forestall all malpractice suits, but will diminish the culpability of prison physicians and correction authorities. The enormous amount of money already spent on the care of prison inmates with AIDS testifies to the fact that they are not being neglected. The more dedicated and comprehensive the AIDS program implemented by correctional agencies, the fewer the taxpayer dollars required to treat inmates and to repair the damage caused by ignorance, misinformation, distrust, and violence.

Four Society's Response to AIDS

12 Ethical Issues in AIDS

THOMAS H. MURRAY
GRETCHEN M. AUMANN

To understand the ethical issues posed by AIDS, we must see it as contrary to the general trend in modern medicine, a menacing anachronism. To a society and its health-care professions grown accustomed to the idea that the fight against disease is being progressively won, the appearance of a virulent and as yet intractable new disease is an astonishing rebuke.

In this century, health care has advanced from providing largely care and comfort to administering cures, beginning with the availability in the 1940s of penicillin and other antibiotics and the development of remarkable medical devices. Until then, bacterial pneumonia and other infections were often lethal, and the weapons of medicine were meager. Suddenly, physicians acquired the means to treat those infections and often to defeat death itself, and refinements in the skills of curing mingled with the start of a new technical era— the era of control. We can, and at times literally do, control the functioning of body organs. The ventilator, which does the breathing when the lungs and muscles cannot, and the artificial kidney and heart are some of the best known examples of our increasing ability to at least postpone death. It is now possible even to keep vital functions operating in the body of what was once a living person, and physicians have been known to refer to mechanical life support when the patient's brain has ceased to function as "ventilating a corpse."

These dramatic and newly acquired abilities to cure and control bring in their wake many ethical dilemmas. The moral problems created by AIDS for the most part escape familiar categories, compel us to remember the earlier days of medical care, and require us to face old problems with new understanding. The root of most contemporary dilemmas in medical ethics is our power to cure and control; in the case of AIDS almost the opposite is true—here it is our powerlessness and ignorance. Indeed, as we endeavor to learn more about this disease, both the information gained and the process by which we gain it raise new and complex ethical issues.

The ethical problems raised by AIDS fall into four categories:

Moral responsibilities of health professionals
Moral responsibilities of researchers
Moral responsibilities of people with AIDS or infected by the AIDS virus
Moral responsibilities of society

MORAL RESPONSIBILITIES OF HEALTH PROFESSIONALS

Few physicians and nurses today remember that in the era of care and compassion, before the discovery of antibiotics, medicine and nursing were often dangerous professions. When disease and contagion were poorly understood, and no effective treatments were available for infection, those who cared for the sick risked illness and death themselves.

Though the time of greatest danger is past, hospitals are still among the most dangerous work environments, principally due to the hazards of anesthetic and sterilizing gases and the chance of infection. These risks are usually regarded as routine and barely noticed. The fear inspired in some physicians and nurses by the advent of AIDS is therefore all the more troubling.

It must be said that there is no reliable information on the number of doctors and nurses who have refused to care for AIDS patients. In all likelihood, the vast majority of health professionals have behaved appropriately and accepted their responsibility to care for these patients. Still, the publicized cases of refusal, and the experiences and impressions of AIDS patients and of professional colleagues, indicate that some doctors and nurses have failed to show the courage and dedication we have come to expect of them. Dr. Joseph Sonnabend, a physician and researcher treating AIDS patients in

New York City, bemoaned this: "All down the line there are frightened people. There are doctors and nurses refusing to treat sick people. I don't know why they went into the field in the first place."

Documented examples are less common. One is the sad case of Morgan McDonald. McDonald was an AIDS patient in a hospital in Gainesville, Florida. The hospital discharged him and arranged for him to be flown by chartered jet to San Francisco, where he was quickly admitted to San Francisco General Hospital. Mervyn Silverman, Director of Public Health for San Francisco, has quoted parts of a letter written by an attorney for the Gainesville Hospital, which said, among other things: "The attending physician has determined you're no longer in need of acute hospital care; that you're utilizing hospital space and resources that should otherwise be available to acutely ill patients." The hospital's letter advised McDonald that he should be examined every two weeks and offered to transfer him anywhere in the continental United States. The letter also said, "Basically, regardless of your decision as to where you would like to go, you will be discharged on October 8, 1983." McDonald died 16 days after being flown to San Francisco. Silverman called the entire incident "a little bit baffling and a little bit tragic."

The response of nurses to AIDS has varied from refusal to care for patients, to guarded concern, to freely volunteering to work exclusively with AIDS patients in some of the AIDS centers around the country.

Having to care for an AIDS patient can be a frightening prospect, but reluctance to treat AIDS may sometimes have reflected prejudice rather than justifiable fear. Dr. James W. Curran of the U.S. Public Health Service's Centers for Disease Control (CDC) wrote, "The past year has also been characterized by unwarranted hysteria over AIDS. Particularly disturbing are stories, although they are infrequent, about inadequate care given to patients with AIDS and the use of the syndrome as an excuse to justify discrimination." Some people may tend to focus their fear of AIDS on the issues of homosexuality and illegal drug use. Since the great majority of people with AIDS are already regarded with some suspicion, health professionals must make a special effort to disentangle feelings of personal discomfort or disapproval from the reasonable precautions they should follow to avoid contracting AIDS themselves.

For all the fear and worry, very few cases have been confirmed of health workers contracting AIDS from treating AIDS patients. In five separate studies, 1,498 health workers were tested for antibody to the AIDS virus, HTLV-III/LAV (a sign of infection, but not necessarily of disease); of these, 674 (45 percent) had been exposed by needle sticks, cuts, or mucous membrane contact. Twenty-six tested positive on first blood tests, but all but 3 of them were members of known high-risk groups who may have been infected elsewhere. The danger appears to be real, but minimal. Health professionals have a duty to exercise great care in handling blood and sputum samples from AIDS patients and, in general, to follow appropriate guidelines for infection control, such as those published by the CDC.

The final judgment on doctors and nurses must be that their avowed obligation to care for the sick extends to AIDS patients, regardless of personal fears or prejudices. The moral force of a professional commitment means nothing if it applies only when safe and convenient. People with AIDS often need intensive medical and nursing attention and deserve the same quality of care given any other patient. Exaggerated fears of a minimal danger of contracting AIDS are no excuse for failing to live up to professional vows.

Professional responsibility not only forbids the denial of treatment to AIDS patients, but includes the duty to respect the confidentiality of information patients may disclose. It is implicitly understood that physicians and nurses may and should share such information for the purpose of aiding medical treatment. Ruled out, though, are gossip, careless chatter in elevators and hallways, and other violations of patient privacy that do not contribute to patient care.

One important exception to the usual practice of respecting confidentiality is a state requirement that the disease or condition be reported. In virtually all states, gunshot wounds, suspected child abuse, and some sexually transmitted diseases must be reported. AIDS is now a reportable disease in over thirty states.

Caring for patients with AIDS also raises ethical dilemmas about when, and when not, to provide life-sustaining treatment such as mechanical ventilation and cardiopulmonary resuscitation. As the number of AIDS patients increases, more health professionals are being faced with these questions. The issue of withholding, withdrawing, or providing life-sustaining treatment is familiar to a great many health professionals but more frequently becomes a problem only for very old or very young patients. For the most part, AIDS patients are of a young age when we do not "expect" people to die and frequently are the same age as their health-care providers. This makes it more difficult to fulfill the health professionals' duty to discuss their patients' diagnoses and prognoses with them. Some AIDS patients become mentally incapacitated and unable to participate in treatment decisions. In many states, a court appointed guardian, usually a parent or spouse, can make these decisions. However, homosexual men, who constitute a significant proportion of all AIDS patients, may not have a legal spouse and may not want a parent to determine their care; they may prefer a lover or a friend to do so. Unless legally empowered, for example, by a durable power of attorney for health-care decisions, the patient's lover or friend may not be able to make these decisions. As difficult as these issues are to address, health professionals must discuss them with their patients to reach a shared decision on desired care.

Caring for AIDS patients represents an "extraordinary paradigm of a problem that is very much traditional in medicine." The reaction of health professionals to this problem will greatly inform the public's understanding of how deep a moral commitment contemporary physicians and nurses actually make.

MORAL RESPONSIBILITIES OF RESEARCHERS

There is a pressing need for continued research on AIDS to develop effective treatment and prevention. Money has been allocated, and scientists are naturally attracted to attack a new puzzle like AIDS, but an important impediment to AIDS research has surfaced. Scientists sometimes need to gather very sensitive information from the subjects of research, but potential subjects are reluctant to reveal intimate details for fear they might be used against them, their friends, and their social contacts. Doubts about the protection of the confidentiality of research records have seriously inhibited cooperation by subjects most necessary to, and most likely to benefit from, AIDS research. Particularly affected is research on the epidemiology of AIDS. Epidemiologists must often ask very personal questions, for example, about sexual practices and drug use.

All research on human subjects poses dangers. The three greatest concerns are respect for the rights of individuals, protection against unjustifiable harm, and the honoring of privacy. Subjects' rights are respected by requiring their informed consent in advance of conducting research and prohibiting research on unknowing, incompetent, or coerced individuals. Unjustifiable harm is avoided by having a group of disinterested persons—the local Institutional Review Board—judge whether the risks of research are excessive. Privacy is honored by ensuring that personal information learned is kept in confidence. The special problem in AIDS research is a heightened need for confidentiality because some of the most needed information is precisely the most sensitive and potentially damaging that people can reveal about themselves.

The primary risk factors for HTLV-III/LAV infection are sexual contact with infected persons, especially male homosexual contact, intravenous-drug use, and having received blood or blood products (before widespread antibody screening of the blood supply and special treatment of blood products). Thirty states in the United States have antisodomy laws (some recently enacted), and illicit drug use is illegal, by definition, in all states. Thus, the people in the two highest-risk groups have reason to fear they are jeopardizing themselves by cooperating with researchers and revealing their names, residences, and other information.

Still, the need for research is apparent, and many researchers and government officials recognize the problems. Dr. Edward N. Brandt, Jr., Assistant Secretary of Health and Human Services, has said, "In investigating this disease, we've needed to examine and understand gay lifestyles. We've had to probe. Every disease raises the problem of confidentiality. But this disease raises it much more."

Representatives of the gay community, especially, have raised questions about the confidentiality of research data. In "Who Knows What About Us?" six men (C. Collins, T. Sweeny, J. Boring, and others), identifying themselves with the gay community, pointed to demands such as that by the conservative columnist—now Presidential advisor—Patrick Buchanan that homosexuals be banned from jobs involving food, health care, and contact with children. They described scenarios in which federal or state agencies, such as the FBI and Drug Enforcement Administration, might try to obtain information about persons with AIDS, and concluded that "we as a community can no longer trust that the good intentions of others will adequately safeguard the confidentiality of information volunteered in good faith for research."

Despite grave reservations about giving sensitive information to researchers, some representatives of the gay community acknowledge the importance of research. Jeffrey Levi (see chapter 15) of the National Gay Task Force summed it up well: "We could not be more interested in the gathering of information about AIDS. But we also firmly believe that reporting mechanisms must guarantee confidentiality."

The conflict could not be clearer or more tragic. The groups most at risk for contracting AIDS, with the most to gain from research, are at the same time hesitant to cooperate. Their hesitation is understandable in light of the casual attitude researchers have too often taken toward confidentiality of data. Also, except in a very few special categories related to drug addiction and crime, most research data are not well protected by either state or federal law. For the most part, the confidentiality of research records in the United States relies on the integrity of researchers, including their courage in facing possible imprisonment should a court rule that records must be disclosed.

One possible path out of this ethical morass is technical. There are many ways to disguise the identities of individuals in research. Names can be coded, parts of names deleted, and elaborate schemes erected to make it virtually or completely impossible to identify the subjects of research. However, no technical solution will work in all cases, and, even under the best of circumstances, coding subjects' names would add to the expense and effort of research.

The problem must be solved in a way that wins the trust and promotes the candor of subjects suspicious of researchers and research agencies. A solution of sorts was proposed by a group organized by The Hastings Center. The group, which included AIDS patients, representatives from the gay and Haitian communities, researchers, public health officials, and experts in law and ethics, published guidelines for protecting confidentiality in AIDS research that are acceptable to all of the involved communities. One feature of the guidelines is a review board to address unresolved and newly emerging issues. This board would include representatives from all constituencies participating in the project.

MORAL RESPONSIBILITIES OF PEOPLE WITH AIDS

AIDS poses a particularly severe moral challenge to the group most at risk—homosexuals. Among at least some homosexuals, promiscuity is a prominent feature of their lifestyle. It is likely that the very promiscuity that bolsters their sense of identity and raison d'être is also probably their greatest threat. The issues confront both those who are not infected with the AIDS virus and those who are. Prudence alone requires that the uninfected reconsider whether the pleasures of promiscuity are worth the risk. But is there a moral issue beyond this commonsensical advice? An increasingly popular theme is that people are responsible for maintaining their own health.

Rene Dubos argued that the great advances in health in the past century have been due more to public health improvements, such as sanitation and safe water, than to technological medicine. Certainly, medicine must be given its due, but it is a delusion to think we can keep doing things that make us ill and rely on medicine to restore us to health. The analogy in the contemporary United States to the improvement of sanitation and water cited by Dubos is probably the preservation and improvement of health by means of sensible diet, regular exercise, avoiding stress, stopping smoking, and getting enough rest, which together may be more beneficial than the most sophisticated medical remedies. Likewise, the most effective way to prevent the spread of AIDS is to avoid risky activities.

Does this imply a *moral* obligation to conduct our lives so as to avoid risks to health? The question of personal responsibility for individual health is far from settled. At one extreme, surely we are not required to avoid everything that poses the slightest risk. If there is any moral issue here, it must take into account the extent of the risk and the severity of the possible impact on health. At the other extreme, blatant carelessness that is almost certain to severely damage health may amount to immoral irresponsibility.

Where AIDS and sexual promiscuity are concerned, the health risk, while undoubtedly present and dire in consequence, is not yet known with enough certainty to permit the judgment that promiscuous people are taking *immoral* risks with their health. Nor is it clear what would follow from such a judgment. Denial of medical care? We do not deny medical care to people who overeat, smoke, or drive without fastening their seat belts. Happily, at least for homosexual men, who are at risk for AIDS, studies have shown beneficial changes in sexual behavior, such as fewer partners and use of condoms, which have resulted in declining gonorrhea rates.

For those with HTLV-III/LAV antibodies in their blood, who might transmit the virus to others, the moral questions are more compelling. Most important is the question of their responsibility to protect others. Some in the gay community regard calls for more "responsible" sexual behavior as a threat to the community's existence and values, while others argue that it is both prudent and ethical to show restraint in a time of crisis. Since members of the gay community are at great risk, the debate has a special poignancy.

Actually, the issue of responsibility to refrain from spreading a sexually transmitted disease (STD) is an old question. Persons with a nonlethal STD such as syphilis are already legally (and morally) required to have their contacts notified for treatment if necessary. However, the relative lethality of AIDS casts this issue in a new light. As there is no known cure for AIDS as yet, can we say that there is a moral responsibility to notify contacts of infected people? One potential benefit of notifying contacts is that, should a cure become available later, they will be alerted to seek help if needed. Another benefit would flow from notification of new potential contacts who could be protected by appropriate caution.

Also to be considered, however, is the shock and subsequent psychological stress of learning that one has been exposed and may be at risk for AIDS. Since a positive HTLV-III/LAV antibody test indicates only exposure to the AIDS virus, not necessarily disease, and is not absolutely reliable, should all contacts be tested, risk being distressed by a possibly false positive (or reassured by a false negative), and suffer the attendant social and psychological difficulties? The tension between personal freedom and public good makes for difficult choices.

Concerns about "irresponsible" behavior by AIDS-diagnosed persons have led to actions and policy that put personal freedom in great jeopardy, actions that have included police surveillance of individuals such as Fabian Bridges. Bridges, a male prostitute, traveled from Cleveland, Ohio, to Houston, Texas, where the city health director placed him under twenty-four-hour police surveillance, supposedly because Bridges planned to continue plying his trade. When Bridges did not do so, police convinced him to seek psychiatric or physical treatment at a hospital. Because he was not acutely ill, either mentally or with AIDS, Bridges was released and again placed under police surveillance. More than a week after his arrival in Houston, the conflict between Bridges' personal liberty and the public's health was finally settled, with a little effort and creativity, by a representative of the Gay Rights Coalition who provided room and board for Bridges until his death two months later. Further investigation revealed that Bridges had had a subnormal IQ (in the 70s) and apparently no idea of the implications of his disease. With a fearful public and perplexed officials, balancing the interests of infected individuals with the interests of public health is likely to remain difficult for some time.

MORAL RESPONSIBILITIES OF SOCIETY

Among the many debates inspired by AIDS, one of the most problematic is between those who believe that society is not doing nearly enough to study and control AIDS and those who believe that society is doing too much.

The question has no simple answer because there is no simple way to judge the ethics of resource-allocation decisions, especially when health is at stake. One commentator has suggested that we could save more lives for the same money by giving air conditioners to the elderly poor than by doing research on AIDS. Whatever the truth of that suggestion, the fact is that allocation decisions often defy moral logic. We spend nearly 200 million dollars to build an artificial heart, but cut preventive medicine programs, which cost a tiny fraction of that per person, even though those programs largely benefit the neediest.

If nothing else, the controversy over public money and AIDS may alert us to the moral confusion surrounding how we spend health dollars. Lacking a simple guide to how much money should be spent on AIDS, we can venture a complex principle—all members of the human community deserve efforts to spare them from disease and avoidable death. If that requires an intensive effort against AIDS, so be it. But we cannot stop there. The same logic applies to other health needs and other underserved people. People with AIDS are not the only relatively powerless group; the effort made for them should also be made for the poor, the elderly, and children.

A profound moral problem is raised by HTLV-III/LAV antibody testing. Identification in 1983 of the HTLV-III/LAV virus and its relation to AIDS was followed rapidly by the development and licensing of a blood test, ELISA (enzyme-linked immunosorbent assay), which specifically detects antibodies produced by the immune system in response to infection by the AIDS virus. Since AIDS transmission by blood transfusions had been confirmed (recipients, especially hemophiliacs, contracted the disease although they had no other known risk factors), ELISA was first used to screen donated blood and plasma to insure an uninfected supply.

ELISA indicates only previous infection by the virus. The clinical relevance of test results is uncertain. For example, a positive result (the presence of antibody) does not guarantee the eventual development of AIDS or other disorders of the immune system. Conversely, a negative result is not definitive. If confirmed, it most likely means no previous exposure to the virus, but might mean exposure too recent for antibodies to be produced in detectable quantities.

Actually, seronegativity (negative test result) and seropositivity (positive test result) represent a continuous range of test values, from low to high reactivity. Calling a result "positive" signifies a social as well as a scientific judgment. Since AIDS is lethal, a conservatively low threshold is chosen to indicate "positive." This risks classifying as seropositive people who may not actually have AIDS antibodies or be infectious, to prevent missing people who are infectious. Moreover, the tests are not absolutely specific and may be affected by substances in the blood other than antibodies to the AIDS virus, which contribute to "false" positives. False positives can be further confirmed or refuted by repeating ELISA, by using the more complicated Western blot test, or by other new tests now being developed that will detect actual viral proteins rather than antibodies to the virus. False negatives, say in blood for transfusions, risk contaminating the blood supply.

Mandatory HTLV-III/LAV antibody screening of all blood and plasma donations was instituted in July 1985 to protect people from contracting AIDS via transfusions. (See chapter 9.) At that time the American Red Cross introduced a policy of notifying donors with positive test results confirmed by retesting with ELISA and Western blot and advising them to seek medical attention. Names are kept on the Red Cross's national deferral registry. Those who test positive only once are not notified, but their names are placed on a local deferral registry, and any blood they subsequently donate is disposed of.

The widespread availability of an inexpensive test for HTLV-III/LAV infection has spawned a remarkable variety of schemes for testing various groups. The United States military now tests all new recruits and proposes to test all current employees. Proposals have been floated to test food handlers, prostitutes, hemodialysis patients, prisoners, health or life insurance applicants, teachers, and employees of particular firms, among others. These screening proposals are often accompanied by plans to "solve" problems by, for example, firing or not hiring people, issuing cards "certifying" people as HTLV-III/LAV-free, setting up separate facilities (dialysis machines, prisons), or denying access to services or benefits.

For the most part, these screening proposals are ill-conceived and raise serious moral problems. Could they be described as having "evolved in a rapid, haphazard, often poorly planned fashion, generated in large measure by public clamor and political pressure"? This judgment was part of an assessment made a decade ago by a National Academy of Sciences panel, not about HTLV-III/LAV screening, of course, but about screening black populations for the genetic anomaly known as sickle-cell trait. It points up difficulties common to all mass-screening programs. We can summarize the moral issues by saying that responsible screening programs must ask and satisfactorily answer five questions:

1. For whom is the testing being done—the person tested (first-person benefit) or others (third-person)?

   Other than informing those who wish to know, HTLV-III/LAV testing today confers few benefits on the person tested. Justifications are usually made in terms of benefit to third parties.

2. Is testing voluntary or mandatory?

   Voluntary testing raises few moral problems. Most of the difficult questions come with mandatory testing.
3. What will be done with the information?

   What acceptable social goals can be achieved through screening? At what ethical and economic costs? The history of genetic screening is rife with cases where no thought was given to this question.
4. Will this screening program permit us to reach the desired goal?

   What are the acceptable realistic goals? Will this program achieve them?
5. Is this the least intrusive and restrictive means to the goal?

   It is not enough to reach the goal if we could have done so with less harm.

There is nothing magical about these particular questions, but they bring to light key ethical issues. Consider two of the proposals: using the ELISA test to screen the blood supply, and screening food handlers.

1. In both proposals, testing is not intended to protect the person tested. Since no effective treatment exists for HTLV-III/LAV infection, the primary beneficiaries will be third parties. This is in contrast to most genetic screening programs, which were and are intended to benefit the person tested.
2. Both programs involve mandatory testing, thereby raising the specter of coercion. Since blood donation is mostly voluntary (although people may feel some pressure to donate as part of some work or other group), people may avoid the test simply by not donating blood. Particularly among unskilled workers and in times of high unemployment, the choice of work may be much less voluntary, making the use of the test more coercive.
3. Screening blood aims to minimize the danger of transmitting infection, an acceptable, realistic goal. Considerable thought was given to minimizing possible harm to donors. Screening food handlers is intended presumably to protect those who

consume the food. The harm done to those tested, in an affront to privacy and the possible loss of job and livelihood, seems large in proportion to the uncertain and improbable benefit sought.

4. Screening blood donors greatly reduces the chance of transmitting the AIDS virus via the blood supply and restores confidence in the safety of donated blood. Since there is substantial evidence that transmission of the virus through food is highly improbable, perhaps even impossible if a few commonsense precautions are observed, a program of mass testing and worker certification serves no reasonable goal.

5. Testing already-donated blood is not particularly intrusive, and donors are not restricted more than necessary to achieve the desired goal. Requiring blood tests of food service workers, forcing them to carry cards certifying they are uninfected, and firing those found to be infected are highly intrusive and terribly restrictive. Even if there *were* evidence that the virus could be transmitted through food, less intrusive and restrictive means to protect consumers are available (for example, the Centers for Disease Control guidelines). Without such evidence, screening food handlers may assuage irrational fears, or satisfy punitive feelings toward homosexuals, drug users, or the ill, but it does not serve any morally defensible public policy goal in a morally acceptable manner.

Even acceptable screening programs involve legitimate concerns over the proliferation of lists of people with HTLV-III/LAV infection or risk factors for infection, particularly when individuals do not know they are listed. In the wrong hands, such lists may lead to job and social discrimination, loss of insurance eligibility, and other hidden injuries.

All members of the human community deserve efforts to spare them from disease and premature death as a fundamental human right. Their humanity likewise entitles them to equal consideration and respect. What awful lessons are we teaching our children and others when we give in to mass hysteria based on rumor? When we keep children from schools attended by a child suffering from AIDS, when we talk of quarantine and health cards for people in high-risk groups, or when we claim that AIDS is a judgment from God, we reveal uncomplimentary aspects of our reasonableness, compassion, and courage. Fortunately, once people have understood the scientific facts about AIDS, they have responded well, even nobly at times.

SUMMARY

At least four groups have special moral responsibilities with respect to AIDS. First, health professionals, particularly physicians and nurses, have the same duty to treat AIDS patients and respect their right to confidentiality as they have toward all other patients. The risk of contracting AIDS in the line of duty appears to be highly exaggerated, but, even if not, the obligation would still exist. Second, scientists doing research on AIDS have an especially strong obligation to respect personal confidentiality. Failure to fulfill this obligation may both invalidate present research and make it more difficult to gain the confidence of subjects for future research. Third, people infected by the AIDS virus have a moral responsibility to take reasonable precautions to protect their own health and the health of others, which may mean modifying sexual behavior and refraining from donating blood. Fourth, society has the same obligation to people with AIDS as it has to others who need assistance in the maintenance of health and treatment of illness. Society must take great care in fashioning public policies towards AIDS to assure that those policies are scientifically well informed and ethically acceptable.

13   The Public Health Response
MERVYN F. SILVERMAN

Other epidemics in recorded history may have attacked faster and taken many more lives, but AIDS presents a unique challenge to the public health and medical community, political leaders, and the general public. Its devastating impact on the physical and mental health of the stricken is described elsewhere in this book. This chapter concerns the response of public health authorities and citizen groups, using the city of San Francisco as an example.

The public health response has varied across the United States, depending on the number of AIDS cases, the size and resources of the city or town, the quality of public health departments, the abilities and predispositions of political authorities, the nature of press coverage, and the habits and prejudices of the community. San Francisco may not be representative, because it is exceptional in many ways, but its experience sharply illuminates various aspects of the problem, forceful actions that can be taken, and sometimes unforeseen dilemmas.

THE SAN FRANCISCO EXPERIENCE

Although San Francisco's relatively large homosexual population contributed to the city's relatively high incidence of AIDS, it was also the reason that the Department of Public Health had an effective Gay-Lesbian Coordinating Committee before the AIDS outbreak, which gave it an advantage over health departments elsewhere in dealing with the epidemic. In 1981, when cases were first being recognized and their number was clearly growing, the Committee was already at work on a document to describe the mysterious new disease and to assess the resources available to meet the needs of AIDS patients, the worried well, and the medical community.

As the problem worsened, it became obvious that the city government alone could not do all that was needed, and also that people in the community by themselves could not be expected to initiate, plan, and implement the response to AIDS. The idea of a cooperative, collaborative arrangement was proposed, that is, a partnership. The Department also realized that this was a new kind of health crisis, needing a new approach, and that different inpatient and outpatient services would have to be created.

By July of 1981, a reporting system and a registry of AIDS cases were established, each case being investigated and each person with AIDS symptoms being interviewed whenever possible. Liaisons were formed between the Department of Public Health, local hospitals, private physicians, and the Centers for Disease Control (CDC) to share information and coordinate the response to the disease as much as possible. As cases multiplied, the mystery persisted about the origin, causative agent, and means of spread of AIDS. In October 1982, a multidisciplinary outpatient clinic was created at San Francisco General Hospital (Ward 86), where screening, diagnosis, follow-up, education, and counseling could be provided. This was the first time various medical specialties were made available at an outpatient clinic instead of patient referrals to individual specialized clinics. As the number of cases and the pressure on Ward 86 increased, a screening clinic was organized at a city public health center from which only those who appeared to have AIDS were sent on to Ward 86.

It was clear very early that the only defense against the new disease was education, the dissemination of information about possible routes of transmission and ways to protect against infection. In cooperation with gay organizations, especially the AIDS Foundation, and businesses in the community, over a half million pieces of literature were distributed to both the gay and general populations within the first year. During 1982 to 1984, over 500 training sessions, educational programs, and forums were provided. A telephone hotline was installed, which has received tens of thousands of calls, and signs were posted in buses and bars and on billboards.

Public service announcements to both the gay and straight communities were aired on radio and television.

In the summer of 1983, an AIDS activity office was established to
coordinate the range of services being provided, to identify service
gaps and make plans to fill them, to oversee, monitor, and support
AIDS-related contract services, to anticipate funding requirements,
and to maintain and expand the Department's contacts. In July of that
year, the first dedicated inpatient AIDS ward in the country was
established at San Francisco General Hospital (Ward 5B). It started
with only 12 beds, and not without some trepidation. The Director of
Health, author of this chapter, and others feared that a dedicated ward
might lead to further isolation of already ostracized patients and
create a leper-colony atmosphere. Fortunately, the doubters were
convinced otherwise. Even before the ward opened, more staff
offered to serve than there were vacancies to be filled. Like the
outpatient clinic, Ward 5B, too, was designed to be multidisciplinary. The Shanti Foundation assigned a volunteer to each entering
patient, and the volunteer served as a patient advocate with the social
service agency and also provided important emotional support. This
ward exemplified the close cooperation between the community and
the hospital.

The Department funded counseling services by both professional
and lay practitioners, on both an inpatient and outpatient basis, for
people with AIDS, the worried well, loved ones, and others.

It should be understood that most of these service activities were
performed by agencies within the community. The Department has
functioned primarily as a source of funds and an overseer.

Prior to the summer of 1983, the first AIDS-prevention poster was
created with such basic statements as "Limit Your Number of
Partners, Don't Share Body Fluids, Use a Condom, and Reduce
Drug Use." What in retrospect seem like benign bits of information
drew critical reaction from both the right and the left of the political
and social spectrum. Many in the gay community, local and national,
felt the statements were too blatant and might cause an antihomosex-
ual backlash just when gay groups were making great strides in
fighting discrimination. They felt that a public focus on gay sexual
practices might appear as blame and thus increase homophobia.
Others felt the advice did not go far enough, that sexual partners

should be strictly limited to one or none and drug users told to stop immediately and totally.

By late summer of 1983, despite the campaign of education and distribution of information, anxiety in both the gay and straight communities remained extremely high, intensifying almost daily. No matter how much the Department of Public Health tried to calm fears, public anxiety mounted. This fact clearly demonstrated that:

Government, whether local, state or federal, is all the same, and suspect, in the public view.

Government, which previously minimized the risks of Three Mile Island, Love Canal, and other potential health hazards, was now trying to allay public fears about a disease for which there was no cure or preventive vaccine, whose incubation period could be years, whose cause was then unknown, and, furthermore, which seemed universally fatal.

Little wonder that the public was on the verge of hysteria. To cope with the public reaction and to make sure that the best services were being provided, it was necessary to establish an AIDS medical advisory committee. Certainly, with so many other factors creating anxiety, what was not needed was conflicting opinions by uninformed physicians to feed the fire. The committee included physicians from San Francisco General Hospital, the University of California (San Francisco) Moffitt Hospital, the Veterans Administration hospital, the Blood Bank, the local medical society, and practicing physicians both gay and straight. It reviewed and digested the latest information and reached a consensus on an enlightened response to the community concerns and questions.

Also established was an advisory committee representing the providers and recipients of services within the community. Effective education programs soon diminished public anxiety, and the attitude of San Francisco citizens to AIDS and to those who have the disease has since been remarkably rational and compassionate.

By the beginning of 1986, almost 1,700 cases of AIDS had been diagnosed in San Francisco, and over 900 had died. Ninety-eight percent of all cases were gay or bisexual, 90 percent were 20 to 49 years old, and 88 percent were white males. Only about 5 percent were black or Hispanic. Survival time after diagnosis was 0 to 60 months, half living less than 13 months. For half the survival time, on average, patients were in fairly good health, but 40 percent of the time they were chronically ill or debilitated, and the last 10 percent were in their terminal stages. To meet the varied needs associated with different stages of the disease, existing services were expanded or enhanced, and others were added. Obviously, these services were made possible only by the concerted efforts of responsive legislative and executive branches of government and a supportive community.

AIDS screening was performed at one public health center and the Haight Ashbury Free Clinic; 480 patients made 940 visits each year. The Ward 86 outpatient clinic was expanded and reached over 1,500 registrations per month by early 1986. Shanti continued to provide emotional support, education, and advocacy. Under contract, the University of California, San Francisco, Department of Psychiatry, provided mental health services, including crisis intervention, psychological assessments, short-term therapy for those on waiting lists for psychotherapy, and educational support groups to promote healthy lifestyles for people with AIDS. In over 2,600 hours of services, 228 clients were accommodated.

To prevent San Francisco General Hospital from becoming dedicated solely to AIDS patients, it was felt that other hospitals should assume their fair share of the burden. Accordingly, a registry was compiled of physicians willing to serve patients referred by the Ward 86 outpatient clinic. It then became possible for AIDS patients to be treated with various experimental drugs, and, when hospitalization became necessary, be admitted by their private physicians to private hospitals, thus achieving broader distribution. By mid-1986 San Francisco General was receiving only 35 percent of all AIDS inpatients.

Early in the course of the disease, the Ward 5B 12-bed dedicated inpatient unit became inadequate, so additional steps were taken to meet patient needs. In the spring of 1986 an expanded inpatient unit was created to serve 20 patients. A contract was made with a local hospital to provide skilled nursing services with a guarantee of 4 beds for AIDS referrals. To make outpatient care more available to patients who could benefit from such care, public health nurses began making health assessments and referrals of people with AIDS and AIDS-related illnesses (ARC) in their homes and were seeing 150 clients with over 3 visits per client. The Department also contracted with Hospice of San Francisco for registered nurses (RNs), licensed vocational nurses (LVNs), medical and social workers, home health aides, and attendants; patients not needing inpatient care were given supportive services in their own homes.

Emergency housing, which had been provided for several years, was expanded with the leasing of residences, each sheltering four to six persons for two weeks, although some have stayed as long as two months. This program has served about 84 individuals per year. Because many needed more than mere shelter, the long-term housing program was also expanded to give displaced people with AIDS a home environment rather than just a roof over their heads. Shanti has enlarged its program of general emotional support for AIDS patients, families, and loved ones and includes hospice counseling on death and dying. Some 220 Shanti volunteers have given more than 70,000 hours of counseling and personal conference each year, which has had an enormous beneficial impact on the mental health of all affected by AIDS. Shanti has also provided 30,000 hours per year assisting people with AIDS in the tasks of daily living, such as transportation, shopping, cleaning, cooking, and laundry.

San Francisco, unfortunately, serves as a magnet for teenagers who have left home and are often found in the streets hustling as male prostitutes. A youth outreach service has been funded to provide individual counseling and health education, and special training is offered to those who will work with these youngsters. Although the vast majority of older gay and bisexual men were aware of the threat of AIDS and were taking major steps toward reducing their risk, many were not aware of the availability of peer support for them. The Stop AIDS Project, initiated in January 1983, offers small-group discussions for these men that reinforce the idea of safe sex and assures them that this is the prevailing practice in their community. The staff of Substance Abuse Services also has been helped with their assessment and referral of people with AIDS who are also intravenous (IV)-drug abusers.

Finally, the AIDS Health Project makes psychological and general health assessments, emphasizing the modification of habits that tend to reduce the body's immune defenses. This had led to the forming of support groups that focus on the prevention of depression, the management of stress, and the promotion of safe sexual practices.

Obviously, other communities, with and without the financial and technical support of government, have tried to meet the needs of people with AIDS and those at risk. Fortunately, many communities not yet hard hit are preparing in advance to adequately meet the challenge so they can respond in a proactive rather than reactive manner.

With the background of San Francisco's experience, some of the important issues that have made AIDS so complex and problematic can be reviewed.

SPECIFIC ISSUES

The Media

The news media have often responded well and served as an important means of informing the public. One TV station in San Francisco, KPIX Channel 5, went so far as to establish an AIDS Team, which not only followed the epidemic but reported it in a balanced and responsible manner. Unfortunately, some attempts by the media generated more confusion than clarity. The action of one San Francisco newspaper had particularly regrettable consequences.

During the early period of the epidemic, it became necessary to house AIDS patients on an emergency basis in a motel. The proprietor was kind enough to provide individual rooms with private baths and separate entrances at a very reasonable rate. The media in general were aware of the motel's location but did not consider it appropriate or newsworthy to reveal it. The newspaper in question disagreed, contending that the public had a right to know that the motel was being used for this purpose. Appeals from the Director of Health and the Mayor could not dissuade the newspaper from publishing the story. The information could serve no useful purpose, either for San Franciscans, who did not normally frequent the motel, or for out-of-town visitors, who would be unlikely to have read the article in what was a local San Francisco paper. The city's concern was that those with AIDS, displaced from their previous residences and relocated, would be thrown out of yet another home. The story was printed, the occupants were again displaced—this time by the motel owner—new locations had to be found, the motel owner suffered a loss of business, and the public's "right to know" was upheld. Sadly, this did nothing to further the public's health but served only to further stigmatize those with AIDS and create more public anxiety.

The announcement by Rock Hudson that he was suffering from AIDS stimulated a veritable media explosion of AIDS information, as well as sensationalistic exploitation, throughout the nation. Magazine and newspaper editors who had not previously considered AIDS newsworthy now featured it on front pages and in cover stories on an almost regular basis. Someone else's disease had become everyone's fear.

IV-Drug Abuse

AIDS in IV-drug abusers, though not a major problem on the West Coast, has plagued New York and New Jersey. The incidence of new cases of AIDS among IV-drug abusers now equals and may even surpass that among homosexual and bisexual men. The reason is simple: sharing of unsterilized needles and syringes. Present law ensures that the problem will get worse. Since drug abuse is illegal by definition, reaching and gaining the cooperation of individuals about a problem created by their illegal acts is at best very difficult. The ban on the purchase of needles and syringes in many states, which induces the reuse and sharing of possibly contaminated drug equipment, guarantees more AIDS and more AIDS deaths. It is tragic that addiction, really a medical condition, is still seen as a criminal problem. By such a view, society is sentencing many drug abusers to an early death.

Prostitution

Society has also failed to respond properly to the issue of prostitution, a transmission route for AIDS. This too is illegal, and prostitutes, like drug abusers (many prostitutes also have drug habits), are also outcasts. Very few programs offer alternatives to women who depend on prostitution for their income. Social attitudes can be callous, as well as shortsighted. For example, a prostitute who was ill was brought to the clinic at San Francisco General Hospital on a Friday for testing. She may have had AIDS. Because it was late in the day, testing was postponed until the following week. The woman left the clinic, stating clearly that, with or without diagnosis, she had to work the streets over the weekend and into the future to support her child and herself.

Some cities have tried to place prostitutes under house arrest if they were thought to have AIDS. This is not only a poor solution, since society must then support these women as long as they live (perhaps several years), but also an ineffective public health measure. Since many prostitutes carrying the virus have not been identified, isolating one with AIDS does not protect the unwary clients of the others.

Isolation

Politicians and some members of the public have demanded draconian actions such as legislation to quarantine everybody with AIDS. This would not only be ineffective for protecting the public health, it would be hopelessly impractical, since thousands would have to be isolated and cared for at public expense. Ironically, most individuals with overt AIDS become less able to infect others because their destroyed immune systems no longer offer a fertile breeding ground for the virus. On the other hand, others (over a million) have already been infected but not identified and pose an even greater risk to sexual partners who do not protect themselves or associates who share their needles for injecting drugs. Since there is no practical way to test them all and reliably detect all infections, the spread of the disease cannot be stopped by any conceivable isolation plan. Such a plan would be physically and economically impossible.

AIDS is a disease of "consenting adults." As such, it would be far better to emphasize public education, specifically to change the two highest risk behaviors—the intimate sharing of body fluids during sexual relations and the sharing of IV needles and syringes.

Schools

An important problem that surfaced in the summer of 1985 was that of schoolchildren with AIDS. Unfortunately, some communities did not make the necessary effort to educate parents, teachers, children, and the public at large about AIDS and how it is spread. Thus, when it was announced that children with AIDS might be allowed to attend school, the public outcry might have been expected from those who were misguidedly concerned about the health of other children in the same classroom. In spite of the overwhelming evidence that AIDS was not being transmitted casually, or even by intimate but nonsexual contact, many still saw an unnecessary risk to their children. At the same time, many of these same individuals also did not wish to have AIDS or explicit details about its spread discussed in the classroom. What was often lost in the debate were the needs of the child with AIDS. If teachers, parents, and other students are not well informed about AIDS, the child will be further traumatized by insensitive teachers and taunting classmates.

Civil Rights

Many people seem convinced that there is an inherent conflict between the actions of public health officials and the preservation of civil rights and liberties. However, the evidence is abundant that public health officials have generally acted in the public interest by giving public health the highest priority while ensuring that civil rights and liberties are not unnecessarily compromised. Actually, the conflict was largely between public health officials and some political figures who responded to public demands that "something" be done about AIDS by adopting conspicuous and strong, if unwise, positions to show that they were, indeed, doing "something." Homophobic politicians also grasped the opportunity to exploit prejudices against homosexuals. Unfortunately, these positions often called for quarantine, the inappropriate use of blood tests, and other actions whose ramifications will be felt long after AIDS has become medical history.

One particularly troublesome area of conflict was gay bathhouses. This issue drew the attention of politicians, the news media, and the medical and legal professions. Bathhouses and other similar facilities promoted and profited from multiple, anonymous, and unsafe sexual encounters that fostered the spread of AIDS. Because a change in behavior by high-risk groups was of paramount importance, the San Francisco Department of Public Health judged that initial requirements were a strong and effective educational program and a working partnership between the Department and the gay community. It rejected hasty action to regulate sex-related facilities like bathhouses as reducing the chance of success because it was anticipated that it would not be recognized as necessary and would alienate those whose cooperation was most needed. Furthermore, it was feared that such premature action would be an empty gesture likely to be overturned by the courts at that time. By the spring of 1984, however, widespread changes in sexual behavior were taking place, the level of public knowledge about AIDS was high, and new scientific information suggested a definite association between attendance at these facilities and the spread of AIDS.

The Director of Health could no longer allow the operation of facilities that advanced the spread of AIDS. After an attempt at licensing regulation failed, the only course left open was to inspect such facilities and close those that still encouraged unsafe practices.

The courts ultimately allowed the facilities to reopen but put into effect previously proposed regulations: turn up lights, open up closed-off areas and make other changes in the physical structure, and forbid sex between individuals. Other communities have simply closed such places. Regretfully, these actions by local governments stemmed from the failure of high-risk groups to take the necessary actions to prevent establishments supported solely by them from continuing to facilitate the spread of AIDS. Strong action by the affected groups would have had a substantial educational impact on those most at risk.

Antibody Blood Test

An issue that may not be resolved for years to come concerns the proper use of the blood test for antibodies to the AIDS virus, HTLV-III/LAV. The Secretary of Health and Human Services announced in April of 1984 that a blood test would be available that indicates the presence of infection with the virus HTLV-III/LAV (which had just been identified). As the time for licensing the test approached, it became evident to many in the public health community that use of the test only to screen blood donors might not reduce contamination of blood bank supplies, the expected benefit, but might actually increase contamination. Early reports had indicated as many as 4 percent or more false negatives (failures to detect existing infection), and studies had suggested that members of high-risk groups who had not been donating blood might do so to find out if they had been exposed to AIDS. If high-risk individuals in San Francisco had received the test as prospective blood donors, and 4 percent were erroneously found acceptable, they potentially would have added 1,000 contaminated units to the blood supply.

As President of the U.S. Conference of Local Health Officers and a representative of the American Public Health Association, the author met with U.S. government officials to urge a delay in the licensing of the test until alternative testing sites were established and funded where high-risk individuals could be tested without having to offer to give blood, thus reducing the risk of contaminating the blood supply. Although the request was initially rejected, the government eventually did provide funds, and alternative testing sites were created, but unfortunately not until some time after the test was licensed and in use at blood collection centers. California therefore found it necessary to pass a law forbidding the disclosure of test results obtained through blood banks until alternative sites had been established and operating for three months, thus discouraging blood donations by high-risk donors merely to have their blood tested.

The antibody blood test is obviously useful to protect the safety of the blood supply. However, its indiscriminate use can be problematical and even do harm. Appropriate application must take many factors into account, among them the test's capabilities and limitations, as well as the need for absolute confidentiality. To summarize briefly, the test detects antibodies to the AIDS virus. This indicates only that infection has occurred. It does not diagnose for present disease or predict who will develop AIDS or ARC.

Problems related to the test have arisen in several areas. For example, the U.S. military announced that it would use the test to screen recruits. Within several weeks it expanded its plan to include everyone now in service, but specifically promised to take no action against personnel discovered to be homosexuals or IV-drug abusers. Shortly thereafter, it corrected itself and stated that identified homosexuals and drug abusers would be discharged from service.

In another area, some insurance companies and business firms are beginning to use the test to screen out potentially bad insurance risks and undesirable employees. California and some other states have passed regulations that prohibit basing a judgment of insurability or employability on antibody test results.

There is also the issue of confidentiality. Who besides the patient and doctor has the right to such information? Chapters 9, 12, and 15 deal with these issues in greater detail.

FUTURE PUBLIC HEALTH PROSPECTS

It is difficult to imagine what lies ahead. Experience has demonstrated that only a collaborative effort can offer hope of containing and eventually eradicating the disease and mitigating its human costs. Government, organized medicine, the high-risk and general communities, religious groups, the legal profession, and other segments of society must work together, backed by a nationally funded, locally planned and implemented education program.

Certainly, new infectious diseases will threaten humanity in the future, but none is likely to present as broad a challenge as AIDS, with its public health, ethical, social, political, and legal ramifications. If the epidemic of AIDS is not managed wisely, its impact on confidentiality, civil liberties, civil rights, and the legal protections of everyone may come into question. How we as a society deal with this tragic disease will say a great deal about us as individuals.

SUMMARY

Communities across the nation and around the world are facing one of the most complex health problems of the century. Their responses vary widely. San Francisco provides a model for a comprehensive and collaborative approach, dealing not only with health but also social, ethical, legal, and political aspects.

Nationwide, many controversial issues remain: how to prevent the spread of AIDS among IV-drug abusers; the question of isolation of people with AIDS; proper use of the blood test for antibodies; the role of government vis-à-vis such matters as bathhouses; concerns about confidentiality.

Public health officials have played and will continue to play an important role in the control and eventual eradication of AIDS. How best to do this will be debated for years to come.

14   Economic Costs of AIDS

PETER S. ARNO
PHILIP R. LEE

The AIDS epidemic has generated a need for a variety of medical, public health, social, and educational resources in a growing number of communities throughout the country. The financial impact has been felt by individuals stricken with the disease, by families and friends of AIDS patients, by nonprofit community-based health and social service agencies in areas where high-risk groups are concentrated, by hospitals and physicians caring for AIDS patients, by the private insurance industry, by employers, and by authorities at every level of government.

Economic costs are both direct and indirect. The major component of direct costs is the care of patients in and out of the hospital, including physician services, drugs, nursing and home health care, and related expenditures. Indirect costs reflect the economic loss to society, generally measured by lost wages due to sickness and early death. Direct costs are high if hospital and nursing home care looms large in patient treatment. Indirect costs are high if illness and death occur in young people at the peak of their earning power. Both of these circumstances are characteristic of AIDS.

In this chapter, we will report on direct and indirect costs of AIDS experienced in selected U.S. communities. We will consider the organization of services, the means used to pay for the care of AIDS patients, and how these affect total costs.

DIRECT COSTS

The AIDS epidemic raises questions about the cost of health care, particularly in cases of catastrophic illness, and who should pay the bill. Despite the seriousness of the AIDS epidemic and its dramatic spread throughout the nation, information on the costs of treating AIDS patients has been largely fragmentary and of uncertain reliability. Only four cost estimates have been reported in the medical literature. The first (Groopman and Detsky, 1983) estimated the cost at $50,000 to $100,000 per patient but gave no basis and no detailed breakdown. The second (Landesman et al., 1985) estimated the average direct lifetime hospital cost to be $42,000 per patient but was based on only 16 patients.

In a preliminary survey of the first 10,000 AIDS cases in the United States, researchers at the Centers for Disease Control (CDC), estimated the lifetime hospital cost per AIDS patient to be $147,000 (Hardy et al., 1986), obtained from approximate figures for the number of inpatient days per AIDS patient (167 days) and the average cost per day ($878). This amounts to a total cost of almost $1.5 billion for the first 10,000 cases.

The most detailed study to date was directed by Anne Scitovsky of the Palo Alto Medical Foundation and the Institute for Health Policy Studies, University of California, San Francisco (Scitovsky et al., 1985). She reported that the average cost for 445 admissions to San Francisco General Hospital (SFGH) during 1984 was $9,024 per patient ($773 per day for 11.7 days). For 85 of these AIDS patients, who died in 1984 and received all inpatient hospital and professional services at SFGH from diagnosis to death, the average cost was $27,571, and a total of 34.7 days were spent in the hospital. These figures are only about one-fifth the CDC estimate for 10,000 cases. The single largest factor explaining the difference is the total number of days spent in the hospital (167 vs. 34.7 days).

The cost of treatment of AIDS patients reported at SFGH may well represent the low end for hospitalized AIDS patients around the country. There are several reasons for this. First, the figures are drawn from a county hospital where charges are generally lower than those in most private hospitals. More importantly, the average 11.7-day length of stay for AIDS patients at SFGH contrasts with reports of 17.9 days in Los Angeles (McHolland and Weller, 1986), 25.4 days in New York City (Sencer and Botnick, 1985), and 52 days in Trenton, New Jersey (Baxter and Ksell, 1985).

These variations in length of stay may be due in part to differences in patient mix, types of opportunistic infections requiring treatment, medical practices, and availability of community-based social, psychological, and general support services in different parts of the country. For example, AIDS patients whose first diagnosis is Kaposi's sarcoma (KS) are often treated as outpatients and require fewer hospital admissions and shorter hospital stays than those with *Pneumocystis carinii* pneumonia (PCP) or other opportunistic infections. At SFGH, the average length of stay for patients with KS was 7.6 days compared to 18.1 days for those with PCP. Furthermore, KS accounted for 13.3 percent of the total AIDS admissions at SFGH but only 3.5 percent in New York City public hospitals.

Patient mixes also vary substantially and affect the average hospital stay. Two patient groups remain hospitalized longer than others—intravenous (IV)-drug abusers and children with AIDS—and areas with large numbers of such patients can be expected to have higher hospital costs. For instance, 1,707 AIDS cases were reported among IV-drug abusers in New York City through March 1986 (29 percent of the city's total), while only 16 IV-drug-related cases were reported in San Francisco (1.0 percent of that city's total) during the same period. These patients are generally indigent and are more likely to be homeless, have poorer health, more complications, and a higher rate of opportunistic infections than other AIDS patient groups. These factors increase the likelihood of a longer hospital stay and greater direct cost of care. For example, the public hospitals in New York City are overwhelmed with IV-drug-related AIDS cases. Sixty percent of AIDS patients in these facilities are IV-drug abusers, more than twice the proportion of this patient group found citywide.

Also, through March 1986, New York City reported 119 pediatric AIDS cases (children under 13), 47 percent of the nation's total, compared to only 4 in San Francisco. Longer hospital stays for pediatric cases may be due to several factors. Most children with AIDS have parents who are or have been IV-drug abusers (at least one parent in 79 percent of New York City's pediatric cases). Many of these parents are unable to care for their children at home. In addition, alternative facilities for children outside the hospital are lacking, and it is extremely difficult to place children with AIDS in foster care.

The need for intensive care of AIDS patients may also strongly affect total costs. In the SFGH study, the cost for patients who stayed at least one day in an intensive care unit (ICU) was $23,360, more than three times the cost for other AIDS patients ($7,331). Although information on ICU care of AIDS patients is not available from other hospitals, some evidence suggests that ICU use for AIDS patients at SFGH (11 percent of AIDS admissions) may be lower than elsewhere. In part, this may reflect the presence in San Francisco of community-based counselors, who educate patients about the course of their illness and the capabilities of technological life-support systems, possibly resulting in patients' decisions to forgo intensive care in the terminal stages of their ailment (Arno, 1986).

Perhaps the single most important reason for the lower cost of hospital care of AIDS patients in San Francisco is the existence of an integrated system of outpatient and community-based services for AIDS patients. (See Chapter 13.) These services not only provide an important part of the care received by AIDS patients but also significantly reduce costs for the local health-care system since they allow many patients to remain outside the hospital longer and, after admission, to be discharged earlier than similar patients in other cities. The range of available community services includes public health education, outpatient clinics, home-based hospice care, psychosocial counseling, practical support, and housing.

Outpatient clinical services for SFGH's AIDS patients date from September 1981 and were expanded in the fall of 1982 to include a special multidisciplinary clinic (infectious diseases, oncology, psychiatry, psychology, nursing, dermatology, and social work). In the summer of 1983 a special 12-bed inpatient ward was established, which provides a full range of inpatient services plus a close link to the AIDS clinic and community-based services. In August 1984 a special outpatient clinic was opened at the University of California, San Francisco (UCSF). During 1985 the clinics at SFGH and UCSF averaged approximately 1,000 visits per month (SFDPH, 1985). Undoubtedly, these services play an important role in reducing the overall level and costs of hospitalization in San Francisco.

Outpatient and inpatient services at SFGH are integrated with those provided by community-based groups such as the Shanti Project, Hospice of San Francisco, and the AIDS Foundation. Counselors work directly with SFGH AIDS patients and, as part of discharge planning, help them arrange for care outside the hospital, which may make it feasible for them to shorten their stay.

Another influence for holding down hospitalization costs in San Francisco is the provision of permanent housing through the Shanti Project, temporary housing through the AIDS Foundation, and home-based hospice care through Hospice of San Francisco. These organizations offer inexpensive alternatives to inpatient care. Although there have been mixed and somewhat ambiguous reports on attempts to measure the cost-effectiveness of hospice care around the country, the home-based program of Hospice of San Francisco has been unequivocally economical. Costs for the 165 AIDS patients served by Hospice during its fiscal year 1984–85 averaged $94 per day and totaled $4,401 per patient (Arno, 1986). These figures are only about one-eighth the daily and less than one-half the total inpatient costs reported in the Scitovsky study. Obviously, AIDS patients must sometimes be hospitalized, particularly for acute periods of sickness requiring close medical supervision. But other times this may be unnecessary, if patients have another place to live where suitable home health care and support services are available.

Clearly, an estimate of the direct cost of AIDS care nationwide requires accurate details on specific infections, complicating factors such as IV-drug abuse, and the proportion of child patients, as well as all cases newly diagnosed each year. Because the bulk of direct AIDS costs are hospital related, data are also required on the true number of discharges, the costs per day, and the average length of stay. A 1986 Scitovsky and Rice analysis for the CDC estimates direct costs of AIDS in the United States at $837 million during 1985 and projects between $837 million and $3.4 billion by 1990, depending upon the prevalence of AIDS cases at that time.

INDIRECT COSTS TO SOCIETY

Placing a price tag on the direct costs of illness is just the economist's first step in measuring the total financial burden on society, but direct costs are often the only ones cited by hospital administrators, insurance companies, and government officials. There is a significant indirect social cost when large numbers of productive members of society become ill and die. Society is robbed of their potential social contribution. Although the number of AIDS deaths has been relatively small when compared to the nation's leading causes of death, the indirect costs are high because of the relative youthfulness of its victims. According to the CDC, 90 percent of all persons with AIDS in the United States are between the ages of 20 and 49.

The most common method used to calculate the indirect costs of illness is to estimate the wages lost due to disability and premature death (Rice, 1966). The Hardy study for the CDC was the first attempt to measure the substantial indirect economic loss to society caused by AIDS. For the first 10,000 cases it was estimated that 8,387 years of work, valued at $189 million, were lost due to disability, and $4.6 billion in future earnings were lost due to premature death (shorter-than-average life span). The number of premature deaths was obviously the most significant factor. Scitovsky and Rice estimated the indirect costs of AIDS at $3.3 billion during 1985 and projected a range between $3.3 billion and $16.2 billion by 1990, depending on the prevalence of AIDS cases at that time (Scitovsky, Rice, et al., 1986).

FINANCING PATIENT CARE

Financing for hospital and physician care and community-based social services for AIDS patients, like that for care of the rest of the nonelderly population, has been supplied primarily by a mixture of private health insurance, Medicaid, direct out-of-pocket payments by patients, charity, and local government financing.

For many AIDS patients the disease means loss of job, loss of health insurance, catastrophic medical care costs, and social isolation, in addition to the burden of a debilitating and fatal illness. Those who lack private health insurance or have inadequate coverage must personally pay for very expensive care, rely on the charity of physicians, hospitals, and community agencies, or seek public assistance from Medicaid or publicly funded municipal hospitals.

These choices are not unique to AIDS patients but reflect a basic and growing problem in our health-care system, namely a pattern of fragmented financing for acute and long-term care that does not assure access to needed services. Estimates of Americans with no health insurance coverage at all range from 27 to 35 million (Swartz,

1984; Monheit et al., 1984; Davis and Rowland, 1983). The number rises to at least 50 million when those with inadequate coverage are added to the total.

The Role of Private Health Insurance

Private health insurance (including insurance provided through health maintenance organizations) is the primary means of paying for inpatient hospital care for AIDS patients. In California, approximately 90 percent of such care was covered by private insurance (McHolland and Weller, 1986). Unfortunately, complete data are not available for other states. In cities where high-risk groups are concentrated, the proportion of AIDS patients covered by private insurance is much smaller. In San Francisco hospitals, approximately 43 percent of AIDS patient discharges are covered by private insurance, 31 percent by Medi-Cal (California's Medicaid program), 3 percent by Medicare, and 23 percent are self-pay or covered by other sources (West Bay Hospital Conference, 1986). In the New York City municipal hospital system private insurance plays even a smaller role. The payer mix for AIDS patients there is 65 percent Medicaid, 21 percent self-pay, 13 percent commercial insurers, and 1 percent Medicare (Sencer and Botnick, 1985).

Medicaid

The public sector has responded in some states and communities to assure provision of necessary care and to cover the costs for AIDS patients. Notably, New York and California Medicaid programs are more liberal in eligibility requirements and scope of benefits than those in most other states, but it remains to be seen whether the rest of the country will respond as generously as the epidemic continues to spread.

Two programs administered by the Social Security Administration (SSA) can benefit eligible AIDS patients: Social Security Disability Income (SSDI) and Supplementary Security Income (SSI). In April 1983 the SSA ordered that disability benefits be paid to all applicants with AIDS-related infections who were unable to work and (with their employers' contributions) had paid enough payroll taxes (Social Security) to qualify. Initially, there was a time lag of several months between applying for and receiving funds, and many died before their first benefit payments arrived. This flaw in the system took almost two years to correct. In February 1985 the SSA issued interim regulations allowing an AIDS patient who cannot work to qualify for benefits as soon as AIDS is diagnosed, which reduced the waiting time for receiving benefits to just a few weeks.

Individuals who have received SSDI payments for two years are eligible for Medicare but few AIDS patients survive long enough to become eligible. Currently, the U.S. Congress has a proposal under consideration that would extend Medicare eligibility to AIDS patients, but its chances of passing are considered remote.

The SSI program is a means-tested (public assistance) program designed to assist the aged, blind, or disabled who meet the income and asset requirements for public assistance (for example, a poverty-level income and lack of assets such as home ownership). The important point about SSI eligibility for AIDS patients is not the monthly SSI payment, which is small, but the fact that SSI beneficiaries in 34 states are automatically eligible for Medicaid. In 16 other states more stringent eligibility requirements apply for Medicaid (Newcomer, Benjamin, and Sattler, 1985). In California about 12 percent of all AIDS patients' costs are covered by Medicaid (McHolland and Weller, 1986), and, as stated earlier, this figure is closer to 30 percent in San Francisco. Although exact data are not available for New York State, in New York City it is clear that the percentage is higher than in California.

There are no national standards for disability determination that encompass all AIDS-related disabilities, specifically severe AIDS-related complex (ARC). Developing such standards would result in more consistency across states in terms of eligibility of these individuals for SSI, SSDI, and Medicaid. Again, this problem is not unique to AIDS but is common for many severely disabling diseases.

Another problem is that, since there is no known cure, many AIDS patients are treated with experimental drugs. Most private insurance plans and Medicaid programs do not reimburse for hospital care when experimental drugs are used in treatment. The assumption is that a patient is admitted for research purposes, not primarily for necessary inpatient care. Thus, this portion of treatment costs is shifted from public and private third-party payers to individuals or to local government when the care is provided in a local public hospital.

State Public Health Expenditures

Much of the financial burden for dealing with AIDS has fallen on the states. Since the beginning of 1983, in addition to state funds for Medicaid used to pay for inpatient and outpatient hospital care and physician services, approximately $45 million to $50 million in state funds have been spent to support AIDS programs. Thirty-three states and the District of Columbia reported spending a total of between $21 million and $22 million on surveillance, laboratory services, education and information, outreach, antibody testing, and administration; another $21.8 million was allocated to research, and the balance was devoted to social services and treatment. The bulk of these funds earmarked specifically for AIDS-related programs involved only a few states: $27.6 million in California, $8 million in New York, $3.3 million in Massachusetts, $2.0 million in New Jersey, and $576,000 in Florida (Intergovernmental Health Policy Project, 1985).

Local Government Response

The concentration of spending is largely due to the geographical concentration of the AIDS epidemic in a few urban areas. New York City, San Francisco, Los Angeles, Miami, and Newark account for more than half of the nation's total reported cases. This has placed the local health-care systems in these cities under mounting strains. Nowhere has the financial impact been more severe than in New York City and San Francisco, the two cities with the largest numbers of reported AIDS cases in the world. Both cities have poured substantial local resources into contending with the epidemic. Averaging the estimates from New York City's Office of Management and Budget and New York State's Comptroller's Office indicates that AIDS expenditures in New York City for fiscal year 1985–86 are expected to total $137 million, approximately $56 million (41 percent) from city taxes and $81 million (59 percent) from state and federal grants and contributions to the Medicaid program. The bulk of these expenditures are for Medicaid payments to hospitals and physicians. This compares to an estimate of $37 million during fiscal year 1985–86 for San Francisco, which has one-third the AIDS caseload of New York City (Arno and Hughes, 1986). Approximately $9 million of this total (24 percent) is derived from local taxes and $28 million (76 percent) from state, federal, and private sources.

A major difference between the two cities is how local tax monies have been allocated. It is estimated that over 90 percent of local New York City AIDS funds are spent on inpatient hospital care, largely through the city government's 25-percent share of Medicaid expenditures and a direct subsidy to the New York City Health and Hospitals Corporation (the municipal hospital system). This compares to 25 percent of local government funds spent on inpatient care in San Francisco. In part, these figures reflect differences between the cities in Medicaid expenditures, patient mixes, and diagnosed infections, as discussed earlier, but also indicate a different emphasis and level of support for nonhospital care and social services for AIDS patients. For example, during fiscal year 1984–85, the three major community-based groups in San Francisco, the AIDS Foundation, the Shanti Project, and Hospice of San Francisco, received 62 percent of their funding from the city and county of San Francisco as compared to New York City's contribution of 3 percent of the total revenue for the Gay Men's Health Crisis, the major community-based group serving New York City during 1984.

It has been argued that local government support for community-based services by nonprofit agencies not only provides higher quality care for AIDS patients but is also a rational and cost-effective fiscal policy (Arno, 1986). The economic argument rests on two premises: 1) that the availability of community-based services is linked to reductions in the length and expense of hospitalization of AIDS patients, and 2) a hidden subsidy of large quantities of unpaid labor (volunteers) provides more services per dollar expended than if local government supplied the services itself.

Unpaid or donated labor is the backbone of most community-based AIDS organizations in the United States. According to one national survey, nearly 80 percent of services by these groups was performed by volunteers (U.S. Conference of Mayors, 1984). In New York City and San Francisco, the magnitude of donated labor is enormous—conservatively estimated at 100,000 to 150,000 hours per year in each city (Arno and Hughes, 1986). Despite this heavy reliance on a large supply of unpaid labor, community-based groups all depend on substantial financial support from either local government or private sources. This support is used to build and maintain organizational structures with paid staff who recruit, train, supervise, and back up the volunteers. Many other cities have expected volunteers to give these services themselves without a base of financial support, thus weakening the efforts and threatening the long-term viability of the organizations.

Who Will Pay?

The question of who pays, and how the costs will be borne, is of increasing importance as the epidemic grows in magnitude. It is difficult to determine how much public funding goes specifically to AIDS-related programs. The federal government, through continuous prodding by Congress, has allocated increasing amounts of funds primarily for research. These funds have grown dramatically from $5 million in fiscal year 1982 to $234 million in fiscal year 1986. Although federal appropriations have increased substantially, little if any direct appropriations have been made for patient care.

Currently, five sources of federal funds are potentially available to pay for the care of AIDS patients: 1) the federal tax subsidy for the purchase of private health insurance by employers, 2) the federal share of Medicaid funds, 3) the Veterans Administration, 4) to a limited extent, Medicare, and 5) funds at the National Institutes of Health Clinical Center for clinical drug trials. No data are available that identify these five sources of federal financing for hospital care, physicians' services, home care, or nursing home care for AIDS patients. The two largest federal contributions are certainly the federal tax subsidy and the federal share of Medicaid funds used to pay for such care, although only the latter includes a direct expenditure of government funds.

The financing of AIDS care has been hampered by a general lack of government policy in paying for catastrophic illness. This problem is accentuated by current federal and state attempts to slow the growth in health-care expenditures. The five states with the largest numbers of AIDS cases—New York, California, Florida, New Jersey, and Texas—have taken different approaches to cost containment. New York has emphasized regulation to assure access to care for the poor while containing rising health-care costs. Texas and California, on the other hand, have long favored the encouragement of competition to promote greater cost sharing by consumers. Other states, such as Florida, have combined both policy strategies (Lee and Arno, 1986). These vastly different approaches to cost containment, combined with a lack of cohesive federal health-care financing mechanisms, have resulted in a fragmented mix of policies that leaves many individuals afflicted with AIDS without coverage (public or private) for essential services.

SUMMARY

The economic impact of AIDS on our society is already great and can only increase as the epidemic continues to grow. The overriding concern of those who question the prevailing federal strategy is the inadequacy of state and local resources to assume full responsibility for stopping the spread of the epidemic and treating its victims. Underlying the debate over how resources are to be allocated and where the burden should fall is a clear but controversial question about the government's role and responsibility in protecting the public health and providing medical care. AIDS has been viewed as a series of local problems rather than as a national public health disaster.

If the epidemic continues to grow unabated, the expense will soon exceed the limits of contributions by local government, private charity, and unpaid labor. Pressures on local health-care systems will mount, requiring substantial state and federal financial infusions. How we as a society choose to handle AIDS will have a profound influence on the direction of health policy in this country. The tragedy of AIDS mirrors critical weaknesses in our health-care system and points the way to sorely needed reforms.

15 Public Health and the Gay Perspective: Creating a Basis for Trust

JEFFREY LEVI

By the 1988 presidential election, if current trends continue, more Americans will have been diagnosed with AIDS than died in the Vietnam War. The suffering and social dislocation associated with that conflict were extensive. When it is realized that nearly 75 percent of AIDS cases are occurring within only 10 percent of the population—the gay and bisexual male community—the devastation for that community may be better understood.

The impact of AIDS is not felt in a vacuum. The social and political climate for the gay community has made it more difficult to deal with AIDS simply as a public health crisis. This climate has created difficulties for public health and prevention measures, posed obstacles to research, and exacerbated civil liberties and discrimination problems of gays. Ultimately, the success of any strategy adopted to stop the spread of this epidemic will require that society overcome its prejudices and make an affirmative effort to allay the distrust gays have of established institutions.

GAY SOCIAL AND LEGAL STATUS

AIDS has brought into focus the long-standing legal and social vulnerability of gay men and lesbians in American society. Gays and lesbians are a disenfranchised group in the United States. Simply being identified as homosexual risks discrimination and rejection. To date, the courts generally have not extended to gays the same right to equal protection of the laws granted all other citizens. Only Wisconsin and the District of Columbia have passed statewide legislation banning discrimination based on sexual orientation. (About 70 localities have also provided such protections in varying degrees.) This means that in all other jurisdictions it is legal to fire people, deny them housing, and impose other deprivations simply because they are gay. Half the states still have sodomy laws that make homosexual acts a crime, often a felony. This second-class status poses special difficulties for a public health response to AIDS. For example, although homosexual and bisexual men are a risk group for AIDS, admission to being gay as part of a surveillance or research effort is, in half the country, confessing to a crime. This, combined with other vulnerabilities associated with being gay, means that the legal status of gays is in itself a public health problem.

The legal system also does not recognize the family relationships that gays and lesbians form. Gay lovers have no legal standing—whether in seeking spousal benefits or in simpler issues like visitation rights at hospitals. At a time when public health officials are urging gay men to have fewer sexual partners, everything in the social and legal framework of American society discourages the maintenance of stable, long-lasting relationships. Again, the legal status of gays runs counter to public health objectives.

In this instance, as in so many others, the law simply reflects the deep-seated prejudice against homosexuals that exists in the broader society. Gays have long suffered rejection by families and society, a rejection sanctioned by most religions, which have persistently taken Biblical injunctions against homosexuality literally after they long ago reinterpreted other injunctions in their proper historical context.

The vulnerability associated with being gay has increased during the AIDS crisis. AIDS discrimination, even without public health justification, has become a surrogate and cover for antigay discrimination. Individuals and organizations can now hide their homophobia by wrapping themselves in the mantle of AIDS fighters. In jurisdictions where such tabulations are kept, the number of gay-related discrimination complaints has increased during the AIDS crisis—as has the level of antigay violence (see note 1 in References and Sources).

This poses a serious challenge to effective public health work. It threatens to drive underground the target community for prevention and control efforts. Indeed, a distinction must be made between gay-identified individuals and those who are homosexually active; the latter, a far larger group, deliberately chooses *not* to identify openly as gay, in part to avoid the social, legal, and economic penalties society can impose.

Those most directly combating AIDS have a continuing history of tension with the gay community. The medical profession has not welcomed gay practitioners or patients, and it has been only just over a decade since the American Psychiatric Association removed homosexuality from its list of mental disorders. The public health community has done little better. For example, the same Public Health Service that leads the federal government's fight against AIDS also enforces the legislative ban on gays entering the United States under immigration law, a provision of federal law that declares homosexuals to have psychopathic personalities. Indeed, it is no accident that in many communities the first gay institution established is a gay health clinic because the existing medical and public health establishments are not serving the need.

The level of distrust is heightened by the widely held view that federal and local responses to AIDS were delayed because those primarily affected by the disease are homosexuals, and that efforts began in earnest only when officials became afraid that AIDS might spread to the "general community" (see note 2). At the federal level, official reluctance has been evident. With every budget cycle, Congress has had to prod the Reagan Administration to increase funding to combat a disease the Administration itself has labeled the nation's number one health priority (see note 3). Cynical public relations maneuvers have been used to make opposition look like support. In presenting the President's fiscal year 1987 budget proposals, the Administration claimed it was asking for $20 million more in AIDS spending than in 1986. This was true but deceptive; it omitted the fact that $51 million in budget cuts were proposed for fiscal 1986.

Antigay attitudes have had an even greater impact on state and local responses to AIDS. Health officials and the gay community have often had to divert previous resources to fight off New Right attempts to use disease prevention as a cover for increased discrimination against gays and repressive measures against AIDS sufferers. In too many communities, public health officials have hesitated to act for fear they might appear, in the local conservative political climate, too "soft" on gays. Thus, education and services needed to help the sick and prevent the spread of AIDS have been delayed or never provided. Such fear is being paid for in the loss of lives that might have been saved by education to prevent infection. A tragic irony is that officials who fear to educate only compound their problems: The level of hysteria they must then quell in their constituencies is heightened by their failure to disseminate authoritative information.

CONSEQUENCES FOR PUBLIC POLICY

The discriminatory treatment of homosexuals has created a tension between those most affected by AIDS and those in a position to devise a public health policy to combat it. It has been suggested that the civil liberties concerns of the gay community should be set aside during the AIDS crisis, perpetuating the spurious notion of a conflict between civil liberties and sound public health policy. In fact, sound public health policy requires a healthy respect for the rights of those at risk whose cooperation is essential to control the disease. Public health officials must take affirmative steps to gain the confidence destroyed by traditional discrimination. Anything less will drive underground those most needed to be reached—compounding an already difficult public health problem.

There must be recognition at every level of government of the special vulnerabilities of those affected by AIDS. In particular, confidentiality is a constant issue in all dealings with public health officials. It is not good enough for officials to pledge the same protections afforded for other sexually transmitted diseases (STDs). First, despite an almost impeccable record by health departments in protecting confidentiality for STDs in general, the experience of gays with public clinics has not always been positive. This is why so many gay health clinics have been formed around the country. Second, AIDS is not an ordinary STD. Public interest and political pressure are so high where AIDS is concerned that health officials may not be able to protect identities as successfully as they can for other STDs.

Indeed, all state laws allow for court subpoena of STD records. It is not unrealistic to fear that school boards, for example, may go to court to find out who on their staffs have tested positive for antibodies to the virus HTLV-III/LAV or have frank AIDS. Health departments and researchers must therefore provide subpoena-proof assurances when collecting AIDS-related data (see note 4). This willingness to go the extra mile—to withstand the intense public and official interest and to overcome a history of distrust—is a necessary first step toward gaining an effective working relationship between public health officials and those affected by AIDS.

The level of trust accorded public health officials will also depend on their willingness to take strong stands against proposed coercive measures unjustified by medical facts. Quarantine, for example, is perhaps the drastic action most feared by the gay community and most generally associated with misguided attempts to appease public hysteria about AIDS with a false sense of security.

Quarantine is an extreme measure reserved for emergency use with contagious diseases transmitted by air or contaminated water or food, *not* sexually or through blood as with HTLV-III/LAV. Quarantine would be both ineffective and impractical. Who should be quarantined? Only people with AIDS, or the several million whose blood contains antibodies? How do you determine who is infected, by mandatory testing of all Americans? Public health authorities would do better to use less invasive or restrictive alternatives, such as sophisticated counseling programs targeting susceptible individuals, including the few who tend to behave irresponsibly. Emphasis could be more effectively placed on educating individuals to protect themselves regardless of the responsibility or honesty of their sexual partners. If individuals follow risk-reduction guidelines, they can help to avoid and spread infection, whatever the condition of their partners.

Moreover, brandishing quarantine powers before high-risk groups could have a chilling effect on serious efforts at prevention already showing some success. It could result in gay men, for instance, shunning participation in vital research, evading epidemiological surveillance efforts, and perhaps deciding not to seek needed treatment for fear of inviting punitive action. This was recognized, belatedly, by the Texas health commissioner when he withdrew his

184   J. Levi

proposal for quarantine powers, saying that "the effect on the relationship between this department and the gay community would be disastrous and out of all proportion to the value gained." (It is interesting to note that proposals for quarantine have generally come from departments or politicians who have given little, if any, support to less coercive public health measures, like prevention education, as was the case in Texas—see note 5.)

Testing

The HTLV-III/LAV antibody test poses illustrative questions about the unthinking use of a "traditional" public health measure without due consideration of consequences for the person being tested and the likelihood of achieving desired goals. Public health officials may try to impress political superiors and the public by proposing massive screening campaigns. But what, if anything, can mass tests accomplish that cannot be achieved without them? And what risks do they create for those who are tested?

In the absence of effective medical treatment for those who test positive, it is not unreasonable to question the value of mass screening. Also, at present, the only useful prevention advice public health officials can give is to follow safe-sex guidelines—advice appropriate for all in high-risk groups, whether they test positive or negative. (While a confirmed positive test does indicate exposure to the virus and probable infection, a negative test does not preclude recent exposure.) In other words, everyone in a risk group should assume he tests positive, making the test unnecessary to deliver the message, in fact diverting scarce resources from education to testing. It must be recognized, however, that some individuals in risk groups might need a test result to motivate them to follow safe guidelines. To that end, the test should be available on a voluntary basis, with the assurance of absolute confidentiality. For this kind of program, this means anonymity, since no health department can guarantee that results will be subpoena-proof (see note 6).

Why the caution? Because the use of these test results to discriminate is already well documented. Employers have fired staff on the basis of a positive test result, insurance companies are starting to use the test as a basis for insurability, attempts have been made to require a test as a precondition for visitation rights for gay parents, and, of course, the nation's largest employer—the military—is now screening new recruits. This makes possession of a test result a dangerous weapon that can inflict permanent injury, and requires a protective guarantee of anonymity. As long as the only available help is counseling, identifiers are simply not needed for public health purposes.

Another traditional public health practice often associated with the antibody test is the reporting of test results to state health departments and the follow-up tracing of sexual contacts. This only undermines prevention attempts. If a correlation exists between awareness of antibody test results and changes in behavior—it is assumed that the public health goal is changing behavior, not simply data collection—then the first step in making the test useful is convincing susceptible individuals to be tested. If they fear that test information might fall into the wrong hands, they will not consent to the test, and nothing is gained. Again, protections granted other STD testing are not sufficient for AIDS in a period of hysteria.

The value of contact tracing is also questionable on several grounds. No medical help is available for the contact of an antibody-positive individual, other than instruction in safer sex practices. Such education should be taking place generally, without the need for individual intervention. Given the distrust of public health officials in at-risk communities, contact tracing could promote anonymous sexual encounters—exactly what AIDS-prevention educators are trying to discourage. Contacts fearful that their names might later be turned over to health officials are likely to refuse to give right names to partners, thus defeating possible attempts by partners who learn they are infected to informally notify their contacts of exposure. (A voluntary contact notification program would be appropriate. As part of post-test counseling, individuals who test positive should be encouraged to inform previous sexual partners. This is quite different, however, from direct state action.)

Education

At every turn, in contemplating an appropriate public health response, the need for education is central. Until the medical breakthrough that will prevent and treat AIDS, all that can be done is to teach individuals how to prevent exposure to the virus. Education is not a method of disease control with which many public health officials feel comfortable. Testing or coercive methods are more measurable by statisticians, and may mislead the public into feeling that somehow the disease is being contained, especially if the impression is given that it is being confined to only an identifiable segment of the population. But this raises false hopes and delays the day of reckoning. Sound education can stop the spread of the disease, and public health officials have the responsibility to educate everyone.

For the gay community, AIDS control will involve major behavioral changes (some have already begun, as evidenced by rapidly declining STD rates among male homosexuals). But efforts must be based on participation by the gay community. A heterosexual public health official telling gay men how to change their sexual practices—however accurate and valid the message—is not going to get the same hearing as a similar message from within their own community. Health officials must be ready to entrust some of the task to gay community groups, providing funds and the latitude to do the job. This means accepting approaches that might upset some sensibilities. Sanitizing frank language reflects the prudishness about sex that still exists in society, which is magnified when gay sex is involved. Officials are going to have to choose between delivering the message effectively in the vernacular of the gay community and using evasive euphemisms which, while less disturbing to the majority heterosexual population, will not get the job done (see note 7).

Contracting with local gay community groups does not absolve public health officials of their overall responsibility. It should be remembered that many homosexuals at risk for AIDS do not identify with the organized gay community—often because they are afraid to invoke the social and legal consequences of being openly gay. Thus, education efforts by the gay community alone will not be enough. Only general education will reach closeted homosexuals and bisexuals, some married, whose activities place them at risk and whose lifestyles pose the greatest threat of spreading the disease beyond existing risk groups.

One of the unfortunate results of health departments' diverting resources from traditional STD services to AIDS has been a continuing rise in STDs among heterosexuals (compared with the dramatic decline among gay men). At a time when concern about heterosexual transmission of HTLV-III/LAV is growing, this should be alarming. Many heterosexuals will not believe they are at risk for AIDS, but if they can be convinced to adopt sex practices that prevent transmission of other STDs, they will be preventing AIDS as well.

CONCLUSION

What affirmative steps, then, can public health officials take to more effectively cope with the AIDS crisis? The first is to include affected groups in policy making. The government establishment rarely has the intuitive understanding of the affected minority group needed to gain their cooperation in the effective implementation of policy. The gay community has responded to the AIDS crisis in an unprecedented manner. Its local and national institutions were at work long before government even acknowledged the serious problem. Government can now benefit from that experience by reaching out and showing a willingness to surmount the barriers it created itself.

Part of public health policy should be affirmative action to protect gays from discrimination by extending civil rights safeguards and affording the same social and legal recognition to gay relationships as to heterosexual relationships. Existing laws against discrimination based on disability must apply to AIDS-related disability—thus allowing legal measures to be taken against employers, landlords, and others who penalize individuals with AIDS or perceived to be at risk for AIDS. (There is a cruel irony here: Gays have protection only if they can prove discrimination is AIDS-related.) Enforcement must be strong to convince those at risk that their rights will be protected and that they need not go "underground," which would isolate them from public health assistance and attempts to stop the spread of the disease. Finally, public health officials must lead in forestalling the use of AIDS as an excuse to restore antisodomy laws or to revive their active enforcement. Indeed, an appropriate public health response would be decriminalization —to eliminate fears and make those most vulnerable to these laws accessible to public health efforts.

Despite the threats to their rights and the terrible physical and psychological toll resulting from the AIDS crisis, the gay community is ultimately optimistic that it will emerge stronger than ever. New gay organizations and groups have formed in almost every U.S. city, committed to caring for their own, arising from a consensus that gays must depend on each other more than they had ever realized. More individuals who previously kept their sexual orientation secret have joined gay-identified groups out of a general feeling that in times of crisis there can be no hiding, no closets. The AIDS crisis has created a new generation of gay activists who will continue to work to undo injustices in American society after the crisis has ended.

AIDS has also dramatically changed the gay community's relationship to public authorities. Progressing from a basic goal of keeping government out of their lives, gays now seek ways to spur the government into saving lives and providing their share of needed services—while still fending off government intrusion into private affairs. The AIDS crisis has forced many government agencies—federal, state, city, and county—to work with the organized gay/lesbian community for the first time. The gay attitude is that not only do gays need government action, but government needs the gay community's cooperation and support to solve the crisis. With traditional antagonists working together, finally talking to one another, stereotypical thinking and fears are being overcome in a way that should survive the crisis—making for a stronger gay community, politically and socially, and a more effective and evenhanded government response to all its constituents.

AIDS has been a painful experience for the gay community. Through this experience, it can be hoped that society at large will gain a better understanding of the interrelationship between civil liberties and public health—and of the price paid in lives and economic resources when minority groups are not part of the broader society.

16   Legal Aspects of AIDS
ABBY R. RUBENFELD

To fully understand and respond to the AIDS crisis, it is not sufficient to simply consider the medical and social aspects of the disease. As reported cases have multiplied, so too have the variety of legal problems that result from this medical dilemma. In fact, a legal crisis has quickly developed to accompany the devastating medical crisis of AIDS, and both persons with AIDS (PWAs) and practitioners who provide services to PWAs must learn to recognize and react to the multitude of legal problems involved.

The legal ramifications of AIDS are diverse, ranging from potential liability concerns of employers to widespread discrimination against PWAs and those suspected of being at risk for AIDS, from preparing the necessary documents to accommodate the day-to-day needs of persons with the disease to confronting funeral homes that refuse to accept the bodies of those who have died from AIDS. While it is beyond the scope of this chapter to discuss all the legal issues that arise from this disease, it will flag the primary issues of which PWAs and their friends need to be aware.

Those primary issues fall into two general categories: the legal services needs of PWAs, and the pervasive problem of discrimination against those with AIDS or feared to be at risk for AIDS. Issues of confidentiality and obtaining public benefits are discussed in other chapters. Most of the legal issues considered here are covered by state law, and the specifics may vary from state to state. PWAs and service providers should always review applicable state laws and regulations when dealing with these issues. In addition, since only an overview of issues can be presented here, it is advisable, as in all encounters with the legal system, to consult an attorney familiar with the laws of the state involved.

LEGAL SERVICES NEEDS OF PERSONS WITH AIDS (PWAs)

The legal needs of PWAs vary with individual circumstances and may depend on where they live. Many of those needs relate to provision of medical and other services, housing, insurance, and wills.

Provision of Services

The most basic legal needs of PWAs have to do with such services as ambulances; hospital admission, treatment, and discharge; funerals; and access to cemeteries. These areas are all subject to regulation and licensing by state law. Since speed is essential in reacting to problems in these areas, it is wise to be prepared by knowing which local or state administrative agency has jurisdiction and who is the appropriate person to contact. Local AIDS service organizations (see chapter 25) are a good source of such information.

Help with problems in obtaining services may be found by checking whether the state or local health department has a division dealing with the desired service. If there is such a division, it will probably have rules, regulations, and standards with which the hospital, ambulance company, funeral home, or cemetery must comply, and it may provide a means for filing complaints and/or obtaining immediate relief. In addition, hospitals frequently have a staff or volunteer patient representative or advocate who can process and react to problems. If one is not available, the hospital administrator may be contacted for help.

When services are denied or impeded, legal relief may be possible through a lawsuit for damages, but such a suit can usually be filed only after the fact and is subject to the lengthy delays inherent in the civil justice system. Faster action in cases of discrimination may be obtained from a state or local human rights commission, under state and local laws that outlaw discrimination in places of public accommodation. Almost all states have such laws prohibiting discrimination based on disability or handicap, and AIDS is increasingly being included in this category by courts and administrative agencies.

These state laws may be used to obtain not only money damages but also an injunction prohibiting the discriminatory behavior. In addition, the agency that administers the laws may be able to pursue a case with its own attorneys, thus saving the claimant the expense of hiring a private lawyer. An attorney, or the staff at the local human rights commission, should be consulted to determine what legal relief is available, whether the agency can pursue the claim, and whether hospitals, funeral homes, or ambulance companies are covered by the applicable state or local law.

Housing

PWAs, or those perceived to have or be at risk for AIDS, who are denied rental housing may also be able to file complaints under state or local disability discrimination laws. The text of the applicable law must be reviewed to determine whether it generally covers housing, and what, if any, particular types of housing might be exempt (for example, two-family dwellings).

PWAs who live in apartments and have difficulty paying their rent should anticipate that landlords may take action against them. Generally, however, a landlord must give written notice to a tenant before taking such action. Once notice is received, it is advisable to immediately consult an attorney to determine whether proper procedures were followed and what defenses are available. It is also important to consult an attorney or a local housing agency to determine the rules that apply under rent stabilization or rent control laws that exist in many municipalities. These rules can affect such things as the right to sublet or to share an apartment. It is essential to obtain legal advice in order to protect against eviction and to otherwise take advantage of statutory protections.

Insurance

Uninsured people with AIDS or AIDS-related conditions face virtually insurmountable problems in obtaining medical, disability, or life insurance. One possibility is to find employment where a group insurance policy does not require evidence of individual insurability. Another possibility may be to move in with an insured family member who may be able to extend coverage to eligible dependents.

The situation becomes more complicated for healthy individuals considered "at risk" for contracting AIDS. No test exists that can predict who will get AIDS. Blood tests for antibodies to the virus HTLV-III/LAV, associated with AIDS, indicate only previous exposure. Whether insurance applications may ask for the results of antibody tests or require such tests to be made must be determined under the laws of each state. California, Wisconsin, and the District of Columbia have laws that specifically prohibit this use of the antibody test. Other states, such as New York, have administrative policies that restrict the use of the test for insurance purposes. Given the importance of maximum insurance coverage, such legislation is wise public policy.

If insurance companies apply other criteria to reject applicants they consider at risk for AIDS (for example, unmarried males, aged 25 to 45, living in certain metropolitan areas), they may violate state and local human rights laws that prohibit discrimination based on marital status. In addition, if an applicant lives in one of the approximately fifty municipalities and one state (Wisconsin) that have laws that prohibit discrimination based on sexual orientation and is denied insurance because he or she is gay, the denial will probably violate the law.

To maintain existing coverage, PWAs should carefully check the provisions of their policies. Some policies contain provisions that waive premium payments if the insured is disabled, but may require notice to the company and submission of proof of disability. In addition, protection may be available to PWAs whose policies are in danger of lapsing because of missed payments if the insurance company has failed to send an appropriate notice of termination. Information on insurance-related problems may be available from the state insurance department, and it is always advisable to consult an attorney on insurance questions.

Relief may also be available if an insurance company denies benefits to an insured PWA or attempts to rescind a policy, since state law probably regulates both what circumstances will allow rescission and what constitutes a "pre-existing condition" for purposes of denying benefits. Again, the state insurance department and/or an attorney should always be consulted on such problems.

Wills

Will writing and other estate planning for PWAs does not differ much from such planning for anyone else, with two significant distinctions: it must be done promptly, given the swiftness with which AIDS sometimes kills, and it must recognize that a high percentage of PWAs are gay men who must actively take steps to provide for various contingencies that the law automatically presumes for nongay individuals. No jurisdictions in the United States legally recognize gay relationships, and a gay PWA who wants his life partner, or even one of his friends, to have a power of attorney for him or to inherit his estate must take deliberate steps to implement those desires.

While some states accept handwritten, signed wills, it is always preferable to have an attorney prepare it to make sure that it conforms with state law. In addition to routine provisions in the will, such as the inclusion of all assets and consideration of applicable state and federal tax provisions, PWAs must pay particular attention to two possible problems: establishing mental competence and demonstrating absence of undue influence by others.

Given the debilitating nature of AIDS, wills executed by PWAs when they are very sick may be challenged on the grounds that they did not really know what they were signing (that they lacked "testamentary capacity"), or that they were unduly influenced to make their will in a particular way. To help avoid such challenges, PWAs and their attorneys should not delay in preparing the will, should keep careful notes showing that the PWA understands what is happening, should discuss all family members as potential beneficiaries and specifically whether the PWA may want to exclude various individuals, should not involve a lover or other heir in will drafting, and should obtain signatures from independent witnesses to the will signing who will be able and available to testify if the will is challenged.

In addition to executing a valid will, there are various other means by which PWAs can ensure that their assets are distributed according to their desires. They should discuss with their attorneys the various types of joint ownership available for certain kinds of property, such as real estate or bank accounts. Life insurance policies and pension and profit sharing plans should be reviewed to make sure that the desired beneficiaries are properly named. Assets should be reviewed with a tax planner. Certain kinds of trusts may be suggested by an attorney as possible means of avoiding probate court. Powers of attorney can be given in advance to authorize someone trusted by the PWA to make financial and/or medical decisions in the event that the PWA becomes incapacitated. The most important consideration about wills is to acknowledge the need to have one, and to not avoid making one.

DISCRIMINATION

Discrimination is a pervasive problem, frequently experienced in many different contexts by PWAs and those considered at risk for AIDS. As mentioned above, almost all states and many cities have laws that prohibit discrimination based on disability or handicap, and AIDS is increasingly being recognized as a condition that fits within the protections of such laws. Details of these laws vary from state to state, but they usually cover such matters as employment, housing, public accommodations, and/or provision of services. One of the most troublesome areas is discrimination in employment, including problems encountered by individuals who serve in the armed forces.

Employment Discrimination

Traditionally in the American legal system, private employers have been legally free to hire and fire employees as they see fit. During the past twenty-five years, however, federal and state laws have imposed limits on the circumstances in which employers can fire or refuse to hire various individuals. Laws now forbid discrimination in hiring and terms of employment solely because of race, sex, religion, age, national origin, and disability or handicap, on the premise that fairness demands that otherwise qualified individuals should not be denied employment opportunities simply because of those criteria.

AIDS can be regarded as a "disability" or "handicap" within the meaning of these protective laws. Several state human rights agencies, including New York, Florida, and California, have issued opinions that specifically find that AIDS is covered by their state laws. No states have determined that AIDS is excluded from coverage under their disability laws. In addition, since someone can have AIDS but not be continuously incapacitated, and since AIDS is not transmitted by casual contact, PWAs are often physically able to work long after being diagnosed as having the disease. If employment opportunities are denied because of AIDS, a discrimination complaint can be filed under these state and local laws. Furthermore, many of these laws also protect against discrimination based on "perceived handicap," which means that complaints can also be filed for denials of employment opportunities because someone is regarded as at risk for AIDS or suspected of having AIDS.

PWAs and others discriminated against because of AIDS should consult a local attorney or directly contact the state or local human rights agency that administers antidiscrimination laws to find out the procedure for filing a complaint. Under many of these laws, victims of discrimination have an option of filing an administrative complaint with the responsible agency or going directly to court on their own. Filing an administrative complaint usually means that the agency will investigate the claim and try to resolve it between the parties involved. The agency staff may also handle the case, so that the victim of discrimination will not have to hire a private attorney. Directly filing a lawsuit may sometimes result in more immediate relief, such as obtaining an injunction, but usually requires the assistance of a private attorney. It is advisable to consult an attorney and/or the staff of the appropriate human rights agency for advice on the pros and cons of the two approaches.

Some areas, most notably several California cities, have additional protective legislation that specifically prohibits discrimination based on AIDS or suspected AIDS. Again, local attorneys or human rights agencies should be consulted to determine what statutory protections may be available in a particular state or city. Unionized employees may have even further protection under the terms of their collective bargaining agreements, which usually include restrictions on arbitrary dismissal and may protect against discrimination based on handicap.

Federal legislation also prohibits employment discrimination based on handicap by federal contractors and recipients of federal funds. An employer who has federal contracts or receives financial assistance from the federal government may not discriminate on the basis of handicap under the terms of the Vocational Rehabilitation Act of 1973 (29 U.S.C. §701 *et seq.*). However, despite repeated statements from the U.S. Public Health Service that AIDS is not a threat in the workplace, the U.S. Department of Justice has issued an advisory opinion suggesting severe limitations on the application of federal law to AIDS-based discrimination. Although finding that AIDS is a handicap under federal law, the opinion goes on to disregard both overwhelming medical evidence on contagion risks and the intent of the law itself by saying that fear of contagion might justify discrimination in the workplace based on AIDS or suspected AIDS. No courts have accepted this view, and it is clearly inconsistent with current judicial and administrative interpretations of state handicap laws. Legal challenges to the advisory opinion have already been planned.

Complaints of violations by federal contractors can be made to the Office of Federal Contract Compliance Programs (OFCCP), an agency of the U.S. Department of Labor. Complaints against employers who receive financial assistance from the federal government can be made to the Office of Civil Rights of the U.S. Department of Health and Human Services. Both the Office of Civil Rights and OFCCP have regional offices around the country to which complaints can be directed.

Federal, state, and local government employees may also be able to file claims under civil service laws and federal and state constitutional provisions guaranteeing them due process of law. These provisions simply mean that government employees cannot be arbitrarily deprived of jobs merely because of a handicap or other condition, such as race or sex, that does not affect their ability to work. However, these constitutional protections do not generally apply to private employment. Constitutional claims usually must be in the form of a lawsuit rather than an agency complaint, and an attorney should be consulted for advice.

Military

Discrimination problems of PWAs are even worse when they are members of the armed services. The military strongly associates

AIDS with homosexuality, which is viewed as being incompatible with military service, and therefore often treats AIDS as a disciplinary rather than a medical problem. That distinction is important for military PWAs because they will be denied access to the excellent medical care available at military hospitals if they are discharged because of actual, or even suspected, homosexuality.

The means by which a PWA leaves the military is crucial in determining eligibility for medical benefits. Military personnel discovered to be gay or lesbian are usually brought before an Administrative Discharge Board for a hearing to determine the type of discharge they will receive. A less-than-honorable discharge leaves them without a job and quite possibly without benefits. Service personnel who become sick or disabled while on active duty can be retired on disability, if certain criteria are met. Decisions on whether to grant disability retirement are made by a Physical Evaluation Board. With disability retirement comes a pension and, most important to a PWA, access for life to military hospitals.

Obtaining disability retirement and avoiding a discharge based on homosexuality are difficult and require the advice of an attorney or other advisor with expertise in military law. Service personnel do not enjoy the constitutional protections of civilians and cannot base legal arguments dealing with the conditions of their employment on notions of civilian justice. Consequently, those with AIDS-related problems in the military are cautioned to consult attorneys or other advisors familiar with the Code of Military Justice and the specific regulations for the branch of service involved.

SUMMARY

The legal problems generated by AIDS could fill a book by themselves. Only some broad areas of concern have been highlighted here, with suggestions for courses of action to obtain relief. It cannot be emphasized strongly enough that AIDS-related legal problems should always be discussed with an attorney familiar both with the laws and regulations of the particular state involved and with AIDS in general.

More information can be found in the *AIDS Legal Guide,* a publication of Lambda Legal Defense and Education Fund, Inc., 132 West 43rd Street, New York, NY 10036, (212) 944-9488, a national lesbian and gay civil rights organization. Also, in many cities around the country, attorney groups have been formed to provide *pro bono* (free) legal services to PWAs who cannot afford to retain counsel. In New York City, for example, the organization to call is Gay Men's Health Crisis, (212) 206–8640. Lambda Legal Defense and Education Fund will consult with attorneys about AIDS-related legal problems and litigate test cases around the country to set positive precedents on gay rights and/or AIDS issues, but unfortunately does not have the resources to provide routine assistance for day-to-day legal needs of PWAs. American Civil Liberties Union (ACLU) affiliates in most states can also help PWAs with legal problems. Finally, legal assistance may also be obtained through the National Lawyers Guild, which has established an AIDS Network of attorneys around the country—National Lawyers Guild, 211 Gough, Suite 311, San Francisco, CA 94102, (415) 861–8884.

Five   Research on AIDS Cure and Prevention

17

Prospects for AIDS Therapy and Vaccine

LEONARD SCARPINATO
LEONARD H. CALABRESE

AIDS is an especially formidable disease. About half of all reported cases in the western world have already died. Although a truly phenomenal amount has been learned in the relatively few years since the disease was first recognized, patients for the most part can be treated only for symptomatic illnesses, such as pneumonia or cancer, rather than for root causes. However, intensive research is seeking more fundamental therapy, and progress is being made toward a preventive vaccine.

No area of AIDS research has received as much attention in the recent past as the pursuit of a successful treatment against the AIDS virus HTLV-III/LAV. Unfortunately, though many potentially therapeutic agents are under investigation around the world, not a single patient has been cured of the disease. One consequence is that, like all sufferers from as yet incurable illnesses, AIDS patients are particularly vulnerable to fad therapies, and news of promising treatments must be viewed with extreme caution. Even scientifically respectable new treatments may do as much harm as good and must be tested by carefully controlled clinical trials. The attitude that any treatment is better than none is irrational and to be discouraged. Evidence for falsely raised hopes was the premature announcement to the world in the fall of 1985 that the immunosuppressive agent cyclosporin was a cure for AIDS. Shortly following the announcement, several of the allegedly cured patients abruptly died. While this agent may have promise, it will take a long time and many patients to evaluate.

Current knowledge of how the AIDS virus causes disease has produced a general scientific agreement on the fundamentals of a probable blueprint for successful treatment. The virus is known to infect T cells in the body's immune system (see chapter 4), which in susceptible individuals causes failure of the body's defenses against various infections as well as its surveillance mechanisms against the development of certain forms of cancer. As a consequence, progressive viral destruction of the immune system usually causes AIDS patients to succumb to one or more opportunistic infections or to certain cancers (for example, Kaposi's sarcoma and lymphomas) previously known to flourish when the immune system is suppressed by diseases or conditions other than AIDS. Initially, it was hoped that improvements in the management of opportunistic infections and treatment of malignancies would enable AIDS patients to live longer, even indefinitely, if kept free of these complications. This hope was not fulfilled. Moreover, it has become increasingly evident that the AIDS virus also infects other key tissues in the body, in particular the brain and other parts of the central nervous system less accessible to treatment. The wide variety of neurologic complications observed in infected patients can themselves be fatal. It is now clear that restoration of the body's failing immune system is an important part of the overall treatment of AIDS patients but must be combined with treatment to arrest or eliminate the AIDS virus itself. Therapeutic investigations are now proceeding along three lines: preventive vaccine, immunologic restoration, and antiviral medication.

PREVENTIVE VACCINE

The ultimate form of prevention, other than avoidance of exposure to the virus, is a biologic means for warding off infection. Traditionally, this form of prevention has been a vaccine, but it should be appreciated that an effective vaccine benefits only those now *uninfected*. The hope that a vaccine would be developed within a few years once the AIDS virus was identified has been dashed by increased understanding of the complexities of the virus. Despite present awareness of inherent limitations, there are some reasons for cautious optimism.

The acquired ability to cultivate and "clone" the virus is a distinct advantage for the development of a successful vaccine. Unfortunately, the AIDS virus is not stable, and the overall structure of different strains may vary by as much as 20 percent. This results in a moving target against which it is difficult to develop universally protective antibodies. Furthermore, following their legal experience with swine flu vaccine (billions of dollars of outstanding lawsuits), many pharmaceutical companies fear to commit the necessary resources to vaccine development. It is likely to be several years before researchers can adequately predict how long it will take to develop a successful vaccine.

Because of the problematic medical and social ramifications of AIDS, some researchers anticipate serious dilemmas even if an effective vaccine seems imminent. The vaccine must first be tested on humans to establish safety and appropriate dosage. On whom? No vaccine is absolutely safe, and an untested one is even riskier. It is assumed that obvious candidates would be members of high-risk groups, such as homosexuals. Since many homosexuals already carry antibodies to the AIDS virus, indicating previous exposure, they would not be suitable for vaccine trials (vaccines prevent not cure infection). Suitable volunteers must be exceptionally courageous. They may possibly risk social discrimination by revealing a previously hidden sexual orientation while taking the chance of contracting a fatal disease for which no reliable treatment is available. If they are convinced they can avoid the disease by practicing safe sex, why should they take such a chance? Also, if they modify their sexual habits and avoid exposure, they are not good subjects because the vaccine in their blood remains untested.

Although these and other questions remained unanswered, the value of a vaccine is considered self-evident. Research goes on, and it is hoped that logistic questions will find solutions when they are needed.

IMMUNOLOGIC RESTORATION

Immune deficiency in patients with full-blown AIDS is generally progressive and persistent, due to an ever-multiplying infection and elimination of helper T cells by the AIDS virus (as outlined in chapter 4). Even before the virus was discovered, it was recognized that the infections and malignancies of AIDS were symptomatic of an underlying defective immune system, and the earliest treatments to be investigated centered about restoration of the failing immune system, regardless of its underlying cause. Unfortunately, virtually all efforts met with little or no success because of the persistence of the AIDS virus in the tissues of the immune system. These initial studies, though largely unsuccessful, were not without benefit. The hope now is that they may be combined with antiviral therapy to make them more effective. Since even with an effective antiviral therapy, if and when developed, AIDS patients in late stages may be incapable of regenerating their body's defenses despite elimination of the virus, continuing investigation into immunologic restoration is still vital. Such investigations fall into four broad categories:

  replacement of cells of the immune system
  treatment with hormonal products of the immune
      system (biologic response modifiers)
  immunostimulating drugs and agents
  mechanical therapies

Cellular Replacement

In the final stages of AIDS the body is almost totally depleted of its critical population of helper T cells. These cells have been referred to as the maestros of the immune response and are responsible for orchestrating nearly every variety of host defense against bacteria, fungi, parasites, malignant cells, and their toxic products. Efforts to merely replace these cells, or their precursors, have been largely unsuccessful because the virus simply reinfects the replacements.

Clifford Lane and colleagues at the National Institutes of Health (NIH) have transferred bone marrow from genetically identical siblings into AIDS patients, hoping to replace the tissues where most of the cells of the immune system, including the helper T cells, are formed. While achieving minor degrees of reconstitution of the immune system, the transplants were fated to become infected with the virus and destroyed. Plans are now in effect to repeat the procedure, but with the important addition of potent experimental antiviral agents.

Another approach, tried at several research centers, is thymus transplantation. The thymus, located at the base of the neck, is a critical gland responsible for producing the precursors to helper T cells in the developmental stages of the immune system. The principle is to supply donor precursor cells to enable the body to regenerate its own population of helper T cells. Unfortunately, it was quickly found that these grafted tissues (usually placed in the forearm) also became infected and destroyed by the AIDS virus. Thus, thymus transplantation is another therapy with promise for success if an agent can be developed to at least forestall viral infection of the graft.

Lastly, the replacement of helper T cells themselves has been attempted in several research centers. These cells can be harvested by various means from uninfected donors and directly infused into the AIDS patient. However, again the new cells merely became new residences for the AIDS virus.

Biologic Response Modification

The defect in the immune systems of AIDS patients is complex because the helper T cells destroyed by the virus have many functions. They are responsible not only for the initiation of the human immune response but for coordinating virtually all elements of the immune system. That is why AIDS patients suffer not only defects in immune function directly mediated by T cells but also in other dependent functions, such as production of effective antibodies.

Immune responsiveness depends on the physical interaction among immune cells, but also on the secretion and activity of several hormonal products called lymphokines. Development of the ability to produce and purify lymphokines has led to an exciting new area in immunotherapy known as biologic response modifier therapy. Lymphokines of current interest in the treatment of AIDS are interleukin-II (IL-II), interferon, transfer factor, and thymic hormones. Immunostimulating drugs and other agents are also being tested.

Before a therapeutic agent is accepted for human trial, several preliminary steps must be completed. First, experimental evidence, either in the test tube or in animals, must indicate that the agent may successfully combat the target disease. Second, evidence must be accumulated, usually by animal experiments, to indicate that the drug or treatment method is safe for human use. The treatment then advances to what is known as a Phase I trial, which attempts to establish safety and the appropriate dose for human patients. Only then can the drug be subjected to therapeutic trials of effectiveness (Phase II). It is no wonder, in light of these requirements and the relatively recent recognition of AIDS, that experimental trials and therapies have not yet achieved complete success.

Interleukin-II

IL-II, a natural secretion of T cells and hence deficient in AIDS patients, helps to restore the immune system's ability to kill virus-infected cells. It has been used on AIDS patients by a number of investigators, including Clifford Lane and colleagues at NIH. Although no beneficial clinical responses have resulted as yet, varying degrees of immunologic reconstitution have been observed. Also, probably because IL-II is a natural product, toxicity has been relatively mild. IL-II was also used at NIH in 1985 to treat patients with non-AIDS-related forms of cancer, with significant clinical success. Because of favorable effects in the test tube on the lymphocytes of AIDS patients and in clinical trials on non-AIDS-related cancer, IL-II studies are continuing.

Interferon

Interferon is a natural product of a wide variety of cells and has potent immunologic and antiviral properties. At least three types of human interferon have been identified, known as alpha, beta, and gamma. Alpha interferon has been used with some success to treat patients with Kaposi's sarcoma, although the results differed little from those obtained with conventional chemotherapy. Martin Hirsch, at the Harvard Medical School, and others are testing alpha interferon as an immunopotentiating agent in patients with AIDS and AIDS-related illnesses (ARC), but results are not yet available. Beta interferon has no practical therapeutic implications at present. Gamma interferon, a T-cell-derived protein, is the most potent of all interferons in modulating the immune system, and Phase I testing is under way at several research centers. Preliminary reports suggest that gamma interferon alone has little therapeutic value, but it is also being tested in combination with other biologic response modifiers and antiviral agents. Work on interferons for AIDS therapy is continuing.

In June 1986 the Food and Drug Administration approved the use of alpha interferon for hairy cell leukemia, a rare form. Although only a few thousand people in the United States are affected by the disease, this therapy greatly improves their outlook. The possible importance for patients with AIDS or AIDS-related illnesses is that approval of alpha interferon for hairy cell leukemia patients allows private physicians to prescribe it for AIDS patients if it proves to achieve beneficial results.

Thymic Hormones

The thymus gland is instrumental in converting ordinary lymphocytes (cells of the lymphatic system) into T cells, including helper T cells. It secretes a variety of hormones found to restore failing immune systems in certain situations and thus of theoretically possible benefit to AIDS patients who have profound defects in T-cell mediated immunity. One thymic hormone, known as thymic humoral factor (THF), has been administered to several AIDS patients by Natan Trainin and colleagues at the Weizmann Institute of Science in Israel. Preliminary results show periods of improvement in some patients, but the long-term outcome is still unknown. Treatment with THF is appealing because its beneficial effects have already been demonstrated in immunodeficiency diseases other than AIDS.

Transfer Factor

Transfer factor (TF) is an extract of lymphocytes capable of transferring skin test reactivity (immune response) from normal donors to immunologically deficient recipients. It has been used with limited success in some immunodeficiency diseases such as chronic mucocutaneous candidiasis. Treatment with TF is especially attractive because it is generally nontoxic and relatively easy to produce. John Carey and colleagues at Case Western Reserve University and the Cleveland Clinic conducted a trial with eight AIDS patients using TF obtained from a pool of healthy heterosexual donors and from four donors infected with HTLV-III/LAV but without symptoms of AIDS. After weekly injections for four weeks, the patients showed an enhanced immunity (a response to skin tests, previously lost) and an increased capacity of their lymphocytes to be stimulated in the test tube. However, no clinical improvement was observed during the brief trial. Clearly, more studies are needed on the potential therapeutic benefit of TF.

Immunostimulating Agents

Drugs

Among the many compounds tested in clinical trials for their ability to enhance the immune system are isoprinosine, cimetidine, azimexon, indomethacin, and inosine prinobex. Isoprinosine has received the greatest attention, but has not yet clearly demonstrated therapeutic benefits. The drug has not been approved by the Food and Drug Administration (FDA) for public marketing for any medical purpose, but the FDA has permitted investigational tests on a limited number of AIDS and ARC patients. Many patients with AIDS and related diseases have gone to Canada or Mexico to buy isoprinosine for supervised or unsupervised use. Toxic effects are minimal, but include elevation of blood uric acid which may precipitate gouty arthritis, nausea, and vomiting. The manufacturer, Newport Pharmaceuticals, offers several testing plans in which eligible physicians may enter AIDS patients.

To date, many anecdotal reports claim beneficial effects for isoprinosine, particularly when combined with an antiviral drug such as ribavirin. In the test tube, isoprinosine stimulates many lymphocytic functions suppressed in AIDS patients. In limited human trials, it has enhanced the ability of other stimulating drugs to increase the number of lymphocytes, but not to normal levels. No clear clinical benefits have yet been demonstrated with isoprinosine alone or in combination with other agents.

Gamma Globulin

Levels of gamma globulin (the blood's store of antibodies, or immunoglobulins) are actually elevated in patients with AIDS and AIDS-related diseases. Paradoxically, however, AIDS patients are unable to make new antibodies against specific infections. Infants and children with AIDS and AIDS-related diseases, whose immature immune systems have not yet produced an abundant supply of antibodies, may benefit from gamma globulin therapy. For others, gamma globulin offers no apparent advantages since their levels are already normal or higher. Gamma globulin may be useful in certain complications of AIDS patients, such as immune thrombocytopenia (low blood platelets).

Mechanical Treatment—Plasmapheresis

Plasmapheresis ("pheresis" in Greek means "take away") is the removal of the liquid part of the blood (plasma) followed by return of the blood cells (nonliquid part) to the patient. It is relatively safe and has been found useful when certain disease-causing substances travel in the blood circulation. In AIDS, several abnormal substances have been found in the blood, including potentially harmful ones such as immune complexes and acid-labile interferon, and Jeffrey Lawrence and colleagues have identified a soluble immunosuppressive substance in the plasma of most AIDS patients that may contribute to the underlying immune defect. However, plasmapheresis in tests with a number of AIDS patients temporarily raised lymphocyte levels but produced no cure.

Another mechanical process is the passing of plasma over special absorbent columns that help to remove toxic compounds such as immune complexes, and the return of the cleansed plasma to the patient's blood supply. Tests on AIDS patients with Kaposi's sarcoma by Bertram and colleagues at the University of Southern California (USC) and Kiprov and colleagues at the Children's Hospital of San Francisco produced shrinking of tumors in six of seven patients at Children's Hospital and in two of nine patients at USC. Some immunologic reconstitution was also noted. Filterable substances in blood thus seem to be contributing to the disease in AIDS patients, but further studies are necessary.

ANTIVIRAL THERAPY

The general agreement that AIDS is caused by the virus HTLV-III/LAV has been a source of both great encouragement and great frustration. It is remarkable that only four years after AIDS was first described, medical scientists had not only isolated the causative virus but developed methods to grow the virus in the laboratory and to screen for potentially counteractive drugs. While it might seem that an effective treatment should therefore be widely available in a relatively brief time, stubborn obstacles to antiviral therapy must be recognized. Historically, controls over human virus infections have been slow to develop, are usually only partially effective, and require a long and costly process involving several key steps. First, knowledge of the virus' life cycle must be learned to give investigators a hint as to the type of drug they should be searching for. Second, a process must be developed to screen large numbers of drugs for antiviral activity in the test tube. Third, promising drugs must then be tested in humans, first to demonstrate safety and then, in clinical trials, to determine effectiveness.

Samuel Broder at NIH has screened several hundred drugs for anti-AIDS virus potential and is pursuing all promising leads. Several are now being used in human trials, but no satisfactory antiviral agent is yet available. Furthermore, many of the drugs have serious potential adverse effects and may ultimately do more harm than good. This makes careful clinical trials essential. The following is a brief description of available drugs now being tested in humans.

Suramin

Suramin is an antiparasitic drug used to treat African sleeping sickness and River Blindness and was one of the first to show activity against the AIDS virus. In Phase I and early Phase II trials, it has displayed some ability to clear the virus from a patient's blood. However, after the drug is withdrawn, the virus immediately reappears, and no clear-cut clinical successes have been achieved. Furthermore, a great theoretical drawback is suramin's inability to penetrate the brain, now believed to be a major repository for the virus.

Ribavirin

Ribavirin has recently been approved by the FDA for treatment of respiratory syncytial virus infection in children, a relatively common cause of severe pneumonia, but is available over the counter in Mexico. Since it has the dual characteristics of inhibiting replication of the AIDS virus in the test tube and minimal side effects, it is a popular drug for clinical trials. It has also become a popular underground treatment for AIDS patients in doses of 600–1800 mg a day. Clinical trials are now being conducted at several university hospitals across the country, but definitive results are not yet available. Many tests combine ribavirin with isoprinosine.

Azidothymidine

Azidothymidine may be the most promising drug now being studied. It comes in pill form and is able to penetrate the central nervous system, both desirable attributes. Phase I studies are now under way at NIH and several university centers across the country. Thus far, side effects appear minimal at current doses.

HPA-23

HPA-23, originally developed in France by the Rhone Poulenc Company, gained notoriety when doctors at the Pasteur Institute used it to treat Rock Hudson. Isolated cases of limited clinical improvement have been reported, but no long-term cures. Adverse reactions included reduction of blood platelets, bleeding, abdominal pain, and liver damage. This drug is now being studied in several U.S. research centers.

Phosphonoformate

Phosphonoformate was developed in Sweden primarily as an anti-herpes treatment. It effectively inhibits replication of the AIDS virus in the test tube and is undergoing a Phase I trial in a handful of patients in the United States.

Ansamycin

Ansamycin is an experimental treatment for *Mycobacterium avium-intracellulare* infections, frequent in AIDS patients. Its ability to inhibit the AIDS virus in the test tube makes it particularly interesting. Preliminary studies suggest that its use against *Mycobacterium avium-intracellulare* infections also tends to inhibit replication of the AIDS virus.

AL-721

AL-721 is a fat-soluble drug that makes it more difficult for the AIDS virus to bind to its target cells. It can be given orally and appears to be relatively nontoxic. Clinical trials are just getting under way.

Cyclosporin

Cyclosporin is used worldwide as an immunosuppressive agent to prevent transplant organ rejection and to treat a variety of autoimmune diseases. In the fall of 1985, a group of French investigators announced that cyclosporin appeared to be a potential cure for AIDS. Unfortunately, they also announced shortly thereafter that several of the treated patients had died. Cyclosporin may still offer possible benefits in the treatment of AIDS since many investigators believe that an autoimmune process is the ultimate mechanism that kills helper T cells. Cyclosporin must be used guardedly because its suppression of immunity makes it theoretically more toxic than other antiviral drugs for AIDS patients who are already severely immunosuppressed.

Imuthiol

Imuthiol is an immunomodulator that seems to encourage helper T cells to mature without activating them to start an immune response. This promises potential advantages for patients infected with the AIDS virus, with or without symptoms, since it is believed that activation of helper T cells is necessary for destruction of the cells and propagation of the infection. Preliminary investigations at the Hôpital St.-Vincent DePaul in Paris suggest that imuthiol is safe, but its effectiveness in the treatment of AIDS is yet unproven.

GENERAL PRINCIPLES FOR TREATING PATIENTS INFECTED BY THE AIDS VIRUS

More basic than immunotherapy or antiviral therapy for anyone infected with HTLV-III/LAV are principles for maintaining the health of the immune system. The AIDS virus, like many other viruses such as herpes, measles, and cytomegalovirus, causes lifelong infection that the body's immune system constantly tries to keep under control. In AIDS patients, the immune system fails, and the virus ultimately destroys immune system cells themselves and central nervous system tissues. It is critically important for anyone infected with the AIDS virus to do everything possible to bolster the body's immune system.

While no specific measures are known to directly aid the immune system, many things can be done to avoid harming it. Malnutrition is probably the most common worldwide cause of suppressed immunity and can be combated by eating appropriately. A balanced diet, including all major food groups, an adequate number of calories, and no deficiencies in vitamins or trace minerals, is optimum. A well-balanced multivitamin supplement is recommended to insure nutritional adequacy. The addition of amino acids, other types of food supplements, and massive quantities of vitamins and minerals is of no proven value, can be expensive, and should generally be avoided. Infected people should also avoid excessive fatigue and stress and get sufficient sleep.

While the effect on the immune system of various drugs, particularly "poppers," is still in question, it is best to avoid all drugs that may even potentially alter the body's delicate physiologic systems. Perhaps of greatest importance is the avoidance of unnecessary exposure to infections, such as sexually transmitted diseases. Current thinking on how AIDS develops suggests that chronic challenge of the immune system by other infections may be an important cofactor for enabling the AIDS virus to cause overt disease. That is, the constant activation of the immune system in patients continually fighting off other infections seems to favor propagation of the AIDS virus. Those with relatively quiescent immune systems not under severe attack may fare better in the long run. Although these suppositions are not proven, they are supported by some evidence and form a strong basis for cautionary recommendations, for example, to practice safe sex, which protects against sexually transmitted diseases and the risk of chronic immune system stimulation by foreign substances, such as semen, from sexual partners. Such precautions make good sense for everyone, whether infected or not.

LIMITED OPPORTUNITIES FOR EXPERIMENTAL TREATMENT

Persons with AIDS, and others worried by learning of infection with the virus, understandably seek help from any source, such as experimental treatment programs. However, these are not now widely available. While many university centers are doing Phase I and

Phase II trials of a number of drugs, enrollment is strictly limited by test criteria and available openings. Unfortunately for the thousands of people afflicted with full-blown AIDS or lesser symptoms of HTLV-III/LAV infection, enrolling oneself into an experimental treatment program is extremely difficult at present. Anthony Fauci, director of the National Institutes of Allergy and Infectious Disease, has estimated that the programs may accommodate about 3,000 patients by the end of 1986. However, the means for patients to find the nearest experimental treatment program for which they may qualify have yet to be defined. It is recommended that they stay in contact with the local AIDS Task Force (see chapter 25), which actively cooperates with area physicians specializing in AIDS.

SUMMARY

Intensive research is seeking or testing ways to combat AIDS. Drugs, hormones, blood-cleansing mechanisms, and vaccines are being investigated for potential benefits (without undue toxic risks) such as restoration or stimulation of immune system effectiveness destroyed by the AIDS virus, antiviral action, removal of harmful substances from the blood, symptomatic relief, and prevention of infection in those not previously exposed. Although many results have been promising, none can yet be declared successful. Until an effective therapy and preventive vaccine are developed, individuals can help themselves by such means as avoiding exposure to AIDS and other infections (following safe-sex guidelines and shunning the abuse of drugs) and eating a balanced diet. Reputable experimental treatments are available to relatively few patients; fad remedies are unlikely to be useful and may be harmful.

Six   Avoiding or Coping with AIDS

18   Caring for the AIDS Patient

MARY CUFF PLANTE

The health-care needs of individuals with acquired immune deficiency syndrome (AIDS) change during the course of the illness and must often be met in a variety of settings. The care providers also vary and may be the individual patient, professional nurses, home health aides, family, or friends.

Typically, the AIDS patient experiences multiple hospitalizations for treatment of acute opportunistic infections. In the hospital, of course, the primary care provider is a professional nurse. Between acute episodes, the patient may be able to resume normal activities and take responsibility for self-care. In later, debilitating or terminal stages of the disease, family and friends may elect to provide care at home with the help of visiting nurses or home health aides. AIDS presents especially difficult problems for the patient and care givers as indicated in table 1.

Care of the AIDS patient depends on types and severity of infections and malignancies that accompany the disease, and on the extent of physical debilitation brought on by chronic diarrhea, malnutrition, fevers, and complications of therapy. The patient is also likely to have profound emotional needs, not only because of an awareness that the disease may be fatal and possibly transmitted to a loved one but also because victims come largely from socially stigmatized groups. Individual emotional responses to AIDS of course vary with inherent coping abilities, spiritual strengths and

TABLE 1. CARE PROBLEMS FREQUENTLY ENCOUNTERED WITH AIDS PATIENTS

Problem	Related Factors
Respiratory distress Inability to supply oxygen to tissues	*Pneumocystis carinii* pneumonia Respiratory and other opportunistic infections Anxiety
Malnutrition Dehydration	Chronic diarrhea Lesions of the mouth and esophagus Kaposi's sarcoma of the gastro- intestinal tract Nausea and vomiting induced by medications Increased metabolic rate with fevers Depression of chronic illness
Mental changes Sensory or motor impairment Potential for accidental injury	Social and physical isolation Psychological response to catastrophic illness Infections or malignancies of the central nervous system
Social isolation Loss of control/powerlessness Disturbance in self-perception Anxiety/fear	Imposed isolation requirements Community/family/health-care personnel's attitudes Physical dependency Poor prognosis Symptoms of acute infections
Inability to provide proper home care	Lack of community support services Inadequate home-care information Lack of people to assist with care

beliefs, the availability of support from family, friends, and others, and the degree of illness.

The following discussion of the needs of the AIDS patient is divided into acute care in the hospital and home care, with references to chronic problems that require attention throughout the course of the disease.

HOSPITAL CARE

AIDS patients are usually admitted to a hospital for treatment of life-threatening opportunistic infections. These infections are caused by organisms, common in the environment, that have little effect on a healthy person with normal immune defenses, but may produce severe illness when the immune system is deficient, as in AIDS. On admission to the hospital, AIDS patients are often acutely ill, physically debilitated, and apprehensive.

Objectives

The objectives of care for the hospitalized AIDS patient are:

Identification and treatment of infections
Maintaining the function of affected organs
Symptomatic relief
Prevention or early detection of complications related to treatment
Improvement of general well-being
Compassionate mental and emotional support

The first step is an assessment of the patient's physical and emotional condition (see table 2), which includes interviews with appropriate health-care professionals, a physical examination, and various diagnostic procedures and laboratory tests. These may be disturbing to patients who are physically and emotionally exhausted by their illness. Health-care personnel should explain the necessity for the assessment and be especially sensitive to concerns about the confidentiality of divulged information. Assurances should be given that such information will be kept private and shared only when necessary to benefit the patient's treatment.

Care is then planned on the basis of the assessment. The plan focuses first on the most critical problems, which, in most cases, are opportunistic infections and malfunction of infected organs.

Lung Infection

The most common opportunistic infection of AIDS, requiring hospitalization and skilled nursing care, is *Pneumocystis carinii* pneumonia (PCP). Usually symptoms include rapid, labored breathing, a nonproductive cough, and extreme anxiety because of an

TABLE 2. ADMISSION ASSESSMENT OF THE AIDS PATIENT

Patient's description of the nature, onset, and duration of acute symptoms prior to hospitalization, including:

  Respiratory distress, shortness of breath, rapid breathing, or
    nonproductive cough

  Headache, neck stiffness, or sensitivity to light accompanied by
    nausea and vomiting

  Changes in thought processes or behavior noted by family or friends

  Changes in vision, hearing, balance, or mobility

  Loss of appetite, volume and frequency of diarrhea, nausea, vomiting,
    and extent of weight loss

  Fevers or night sweats

  Lesions on skin or in the mouth

  Ability to perform normal daily activities

  Neurologic or psychiatric symptoms

A review of patient's medical history and related events, including:

  Occurrence and onset of prodromal symptoms such as lymph-node
    enlargement, fevers, night sweats, viral-like illnesses

  History of sexually transmitted diseases, parasitic and other types of
    infection requiring treatment

  Recent blood transfusions

  Recent travel, especially outside the country

A discussion of psychological factors that influence the illness or hospitalization, including:

  Sexual orientation

  Recreational drug use

  Response to acute illness, including expectations of hospitalization and
    degree of anxiety and expressed fears

  Availability of emotional support from family or others

  Availability of financial and social support

A physical examination to establish baseline function of major organ systems, with particular attention to systems subject to infection, including:

  Neurological—evaluation of thought processes and sensory or motor
    defects

TABLE 2.   ADMISSION ASSESSMENT OF THE AIDS PATIENT (Continued)

Respiratory—ability of the lungs to exchange oxygen
Skin—lesions related to infection or malignancy
Gastrointestinal—motility of the intestines and the presence of
   malignant growths

Diagnostic and laboratory tests, including:
Complete blood count, including the numbers and types of white
   blood cells
Blood chemistry
Blood gas analysis—oxygen-carbon dioxide balance
Antibody titers—signs of recent exposure to infections
HTLV-III/LAV antibody tests
Chest and abdominal X-rays

Also included may be:
Bronchoscopy—to examine lung tissue for infection or malignancy
Spinal tap—to examine spinal fluid for CNS infections
Endoscopy—to directly examine the gastrointestinal tract
CAT scans of the brain—to detect lesions or infection

inability to draw enough oxygen from the air into the bloodstream. Immediate care consists of relieving respiratory distress, supplementing the oxygen supply to the tissues, and drug therapy to inhibit continued growth of the infecting organism.

Symptoms may be relieved by the administration of high concentrations of oxygen through a face mask. However, some patients with advanced pneumonia may need more intensive support from a respirator machine connected to an endotracheal tube placed in the windpipe. The respirator delivers high concentrations of oxygen directly to the lung and reduces the effort required to breathe. Since the procedure can be frightening to an already anxious patient and also causes some physical discomfort, the care provider should give reassuring explanations of its necessity and benefits. It is also important to explain that the tube prevents speaking, and to provide a pad the patient can write on.

Drug therapy for PCP is usually a combination of trimethoprim and sulfamethoxazole (TMP-SMX), administered intravenously, or intravenous pentamidine. These drugs are not without significant side effects that might require their discontinuation. TMP-SMX may cause kidney problems, nausea, vomiting, severe rashes, and sometimes an impaired ability to produce certain blood cells, such as platelets, necessary for blood clotting, and granulocytes, white blood cells that fight bacterial infections. Pentamidine may impair kidney and liver function, decrease the production of white blood cells, and produce painful abscesses at injection sites. Intravenous infusion of pentamidine may cause a sudden drop in blood pressure and a rapid pulse rate. Drug therapy must be accompanied by close monitoring, including blood tests, pressure measurements, and careful personal observation.

Acute respiratory distress often provokes severe anxiety and fear of dying. Also, the isolation by some hospitals of AIDS patients with PCP intensifies feelings of social ostracism. Relaxation exercises and controlled breathing techniques often help to alleviate some symptoms. Exploring fears with the patient may help to reduce them. Sometimes the most effective therapy is the simplest—the concern and comforting presence of a caring person, which is at least as important as technical monitoring. If the hospital does require patient isolation, the care provider should make sure that all concerned understand the basis for such a precaution.

P. carinii is regarded by most authorities as an inactive parasite present in the lung tissue of more than 90 percent of adults. Only when the immune system is severely compromised is this organism able to multiply and produce a life-threatening lung infection. Pneumonia caused by this organism is virtually nonexistent among healthy adults, and health-care workers and healthy visitors are not at risk of contracting it from a PCP patient. However, in acute-care settings many patients have suppressed immunity for various reasons. It is remotely possible that those caring for a patient with PCP could inhale droplets containing the organism and transmit it to other patients with immune deficiencies. While such transmission is considered unlikely, health-care providers may wear face masks as an added precaution. Visitors who are unlikely to make contact with immunosuppressed patients elsewhere in the hospital usually do not have to wear masks. Additional measures to deal with potential social isolation will be discussed below.

Central Nervous System Infection

The central nervous system (CNS) is the second most common site of acute infections in AIDS patients. The most frequent are cryptococcosis (due to a fungus from weathered pigeon droppings) and toxoplasmosis (due to a parasite excreted by cats). Meningitis (inflammation of membranes of the brain and spinal cord) and encephalitis (inflammation of the brain itself) may be caused by a number of different organisms. Less common are primary CNS lymphoma and a viral syndrome called progressive multifocal leukoencephalopathy (PML). Infections of the brain with the AIDS virus is also a common cause of CNS impairment.

The signs and symptoms of CNS infections are especially distressing to the patient and family. They often include severe headaches, sensitivity to light, neck stiffness, vomiting, fevers, and sometimes seizures and loss of some sensory or motor functions. A loss of vision or the ability to maintain balance increases the dependence of patients on care providers and is a frustrating reminder of their disease. Discomfort may be alleviated by a dark, quiet environment and medication to control vomiting and fevers. Medications to control seizures often make the patient drowsy and distort perception. Seizures or motor defects require precautions to assure patient safety, for example, padded siderails, urging the patient to call for help in walking, and keeping the surroundings free of clutter. However, patients may also find these precautions restrictive.

Occasionally, CNS infections or malignancies cause changes in behavior and mental confusion that are very disturbing to the family and friends of young, previously normal individuals. These dismayed witnesses may need professional assurance that alterations in the patient's personality are uncontrollable consequences of the infection.

Changes in behavior and mental ability may be so great that the AIDS patient can no longer maintain personal hygiene or react properly to prevent injury. This may necessitate 24-hour attendance for an extended period, which can drastically increase the financial burden of treatment. Also, the need for others to help maintain personal hygiene intensifies the patient's feelings of helplessness and dependency. The professionals who must tend to a disabled patient's hygiene can help to lessen these feelings by making sure to give help in private and by encouraging the patient to be as self-sufficient as possible. The exercise by the patient of some control over these tasks can go far to diminish the sense of total powerlessness.

The loss of bowel and bladder control with advanced CNS disease increases the risk of contamination of linens and equipment with body fluids. This requires extra isolation precautions, including the wearing of gowns and gloves by personnel when in the patient's room. It is important to emphasize here that isolation procedures are intended to reduce the risk of exposure to blood or body fluids that may harbor the virus HTLV-III/LAV. CNS infections are not themselves transmitted by person-to-person contact and do not require patient isolation when not associated with AIDS.

Medical treatment for the CNS infection includes potent drugs with potentially toxic effects. Amphoteracin B, used to treat fungal infections such as cryptococcal meningitis, may cause fever and shaking chills, a decrease in blood pressure, an increase in heart rate, chest pain, muscle weakness, and impaired kidney function. Medication for treating toxoplasmosis may decrease the ability of the bone marrow to produce adequate numbers of blood cells, among other possible side effects.

Malnutrition and Dehydration

Malnutrition and dehydration are recurrent problems for the AIDS patient, both in the hospital and at home. One of the most troublesome causes is chronic, persistent diarrhea, which may be due to viral or parasitic infections, malignancies involving the gastrointestinal tract, or unidentified causes. Massive diarrhea, up to 17 liters a day, sometimes occurs with *Cryptosporidium* infections.

Exacerbating the nutritional problems of AIDS patients are loss of appetite, nausea, and vomiting due to treatment with antibiotics or chemotherapy. Lesions in the mouth and esophagus from Kaposi's sarcoma or *Candida* or herpes infections often make swallowing painful and decrease the desire for food. At the same time, fevers may significantly increase the metabolic rate and increase caloric requirements.

The factors that combine to produce malnutrition often result in extreme weight loss, wasting of muscle tissue, and loss of skin tone. Tissue healing and repair are adversely affected by an inadequate protein intake. Malnutrition also impairs the immune system, further suppressing the AIDS patient's ability to withstand infection.

The objectives of care for the malnourished patient are:

Identification of the source of diarrhea or malabsorption, and appropriate treatment
Alleviation of distressing symptoms
An increase in protein and calorie intake
Restoration of fluid balance
A decrease in metabolic caloric demands

Medical treatment for the underlying cause of malnutrition is not always available or effective. Many responsible organisms are difficult to identify. Others, such as *Cryptosporidium*, were rarely seen in man prior to the AIDS epidemic, and effective drug therapy is limited. Treatment, therefore, is frequently limited to symptomatic relief.

Some drugs, such as Kaopectate, that act locally in the intestine to absorb toxic substances and protect the intestinal wall, may be partially effective in controlling chronic diarrhea. More frequently used for the diarrhea of AIDS are systemic drugs, containing narcotics, that slow the movement of food through the intestinal tract and increase the tone of the intestinal wall. However, they often achieve only temporary improvement.

Antiemetics, used to decrease nausea and vomiting, may be helpful when administered before meals or before the giving of medication known to induce vomiting. The control of nausea and a change to small, frequent feedings usually increase food consumption and the absorption of nutrients. Local anesthetic gels applied to mouth sores and the avoidance of hot, cold, or spicy foods can ease the pain of swallowing, improve appetite, and increase food intake.

If malnutrition is not too severe, the patient may be able to gain weight with high calorie-high protein drinks recommended by a nutritionist. However, these high calorie drinks contain concentrated glucose which, in some patients, promotes water absorption into the intestine and consequent watery stools or diarrhea.

More severe malnutrition, especially in patients who are unable to swallow, requires liquid feeding through a tube inserted through the nose and into the stomach. Such liquid feedings may also induce diarrhea, particularly if large volumes of a concentrated glucose-protein solution are administered too quickly. Diluting the solution and feeding by slow and continuous infusion usually eliminate this problem.

Patients unable to absorb nutrients through the gastrointestinal tract may be given concentrated glucose-protein solutions intravenously (hyperalimentation). Intake directly into the bloodstream may exceed 5,000 calories per day and usually produces rapid improvement. Since hyperalimentation requires the insertion of a catheter into a major blood vessel, the major risk is infection, always a special threat to AIDS patients. Not only is the skin penetrated, but highly concentrated glucose solutions are an excellent medium for the growth of bacteria, which then have direct access to the bloodstream through the intravenous catheter. Extreme care must be taken by health-care personnel to prevent infection as well as to monitor the patient's nutritional condition.

A malnourished patient must also be helped to expend less energy to decrease caloric requirements and conserve nutrients for vital functions. For example, a fever increases the metabolic rate approximately 7 percent for each degree above normal temperature, and a prolonged fever can significantly deplete available energy. A feverish patient is given acetaminophen (Tylenol) and temperature is closely monitored as part of nutritional management. If fevers resist control with acetaminophen, or are extremely high, a cooling blanket may be applied to lower body temperature. The rapid breathing and heart rate that accompany fevers, drug reactions, and anxiety also consume calories. Teaching the patient relaxation techniques and controlled breathing exercises is a beneficial adjunct to medical treatment.

Isolation Precautions—Effect on Patient Morale

The AIDS patient has special problems that arise from isolation requirements for a potentially transmissible disease. Both care providers and patients should thoroughly appreciate the reasons for precautions to avoid unnecessary misunderstandings.

Available evidence indicates that AIDS is caused by a virus transmitted by an exchange of body fluids, predominantly through sexual contact or exposure to infected blood or blood products. Although their risk appears to be very small, it is reasonable that care providers take precautions against exposure to AIDS patients' blood and body fluids. AIDS patients admitted to a hospital are placed in a category of isolation known as "Blood and Body Fluid Precautions." These precautions, recommended by the Centers for Disease Control, are discussed in detail in chapter 19.

Secondary infections or complications sometimes require modification of the basic precautions. While the majority of secondary infections seen with AIDS are not transmissible to a healthy individual, other patients in a hospital may have impaired immunity and be more susceptible. Health-care workers are in frequent contact with many of these patients and must take extra precautions against conveying an infection from one patient to another. One example of extra precautions, mentioned earlier, is respiratory isolation and the wearing of face masks for PCP. Face masks are also worn for patients with tuberculosis or other potentially transmissible respiratory infections. It should be emphasized again that it is not necessary to wear masks while caring for an AIDS patient if transmissible respiratory infections are absent. There is no evidence at all that the AIDS virus can be transmitted through the air.

Immunosuppressed patients, including those with AIDS, are especially vulnerable to herpesvirus infections, which may cause painful lesions over large areas of the skin. The fluid in these lesions is highly infectious and often contaminates linen and nearby surfaces. Isolation precautions are more stringent if patients have such extensive infections, to prevent care providers from inadvertently transmitting infectious material to other immunosuppressed patients. Both visitors and health-care workers may develop herpes infections if they come into contact with the fluids from herpes lesions, although such infections will be much less severe. Additional isolation precautions include wearing gowns and gloves at all times, use of a private room, and covering lesions with a moistureproof dressing whenever the patient must leave the room.

Further precautions are necessary if the patient loses bowel or bladder control, or is mentally incapable of complying with cautionary advice. Such precautions were described above in relation to CNS infections.

Modifications discussed thus far have included additions to basic blood and body fluids precautions. If the AIDS patient has no transmissible secondary infections, only the basic precautions are applied. Care providers may enter the patient's room without putting on special gowns or gloves if they do not have to handle blood or be exposed to body fluids. Also, AIDS patients capable of self-care and free of transmissible infection may share a room with other patients.

While care providers must be concerned with appropriate isolation precautions to avoid exposure to the AIDS virus and to prevent transmission of secondary infections to other patients, they should have equal concern to protect the AIDS patient against the adverse effects of isolation. Feelings of being an outcast, loss of control, and diminished self-esteem, frequent in most AIDS patients, are heightened by isolation imposed during hospitalization. Patients may also be depressed if family and friends withdraw because they dread the diagnosis, cannot cope with a debilitating disease, and fear the eventual loss of a loved one. A patient may also create isolation by choosing not to discuss the illness or problems of lifestyle with family, friends, and co-workers.

Unconscious avoidance by health-care personnel and decreased opportunities for casual contact may result from the time-consuming demands of isolation procedures. Care providers, too, may distance themselves to avoid the pain of losing a patient they have become close to. Finally, despite extensive programs to educate health-care workers about the realities of AIDS transmission, a few still avoid AIDS patients for fear of contracting the disease or because of prejudice against members of the high-risk groups.

Psychosocial Support

The responsibility of the professional nurse is to provide a setting with social and environmental stimulation, to help the patient find inner resources and external sources of support, and to educate family, friends, and other health-care workers regarding appropriate isolation practices.

Helping the patient to interact positively with others can include a conscious effort to visit often, even when there are no specific tasks to perform, spending more time with the patient, and not only talking but touching and otherwise communicating acceptance and personal concern. Ambulatory patients who do not require isolation should be encouraged to leave their rooms and use common patient areas. When the patient must be confined to the room, radio, television, and reading materials may increase the feeling of contact with the outside world and provide distraction from immediate concerns.

Support groups for people with AIDS have been established in many metropolitan areas in the United States (see chapter 25 for a list of local referral centers). Patients who do not wish to avail themselves of such support groups should be urged to seek individual counseling or spiritual support to help cope with their disease. (Chapter 20 gives a detailed discussion of support systems and strategies.)

The professional health-care provider must assume the role of educator to promote optimum care for AIDS patients. Fear of AIDS by the public will continue to add to patients' distress until it is established without question that AIDS is not highly transmissible and does not pose a threat to the general population. Professional care providers must not only convey the known facts about AIDS to patients, families, other health-care workers, and the public, but must also confront and correct misinformation to change inappropriate responses to AIDS patients.

HOME CARE

Care may be provided in the home during three phases of AIDS: when the patient is free of serious infection and able to perform normal daily activities; when the patient is debilitated by chronic illness and requires considerable assistance; and the terminal phase of the disease.

Objectives

The objectives of home care vary somewhat with the phase of the disease, but the following are likely to apply at one time or another:

Avoid patient exposure to infectious environmental organisms

Alleviate concerns of patient and those close to the patient regarding transmission of infection or AIDS

Maintain or improve nutritional state

Obtain adequate emotional support for patient and others close to the patient

Assist the terminally ill patient to complete unfinished tasks and achieve a dignified death

Hygiene and General Precautions

A question often asked by AIDS patients is how to decrease the chance of contracting opportunistic infections. Many organisms capable of causing infection in an immunosuppressed person are common in the environment, so exposure cannot be entirely avoided. However, good hygiene can reduce the risk. Since hand-to-mouth transmission of infectious material is extremely common, frequent handwashing with antimicrobial soap is the most basic and effective means of preventing infection, especially after using the bathroom and after handling pets, raw foods, soil, or houseplants. The risk of infection can also be reduced by avoiding places containing decaying vegetation, pigeon or other bird droppings, or accumulations of dust, since these are sites known to harbor fungal and bacterial organisms. Also, the patients should not travel to geographic areas where amebic or protozoal infections are endemic.

Within the home, normal house cleaning is usually adequate, but specific recommendations to inhibit the growth of microorganisms include disinfection of the bathroom with household bleach, frequent cleaning of air-conditioning filters, and periodic cleaning of aerators on water faucets. Food should be properly prepared to avoid or kill infectious organisms. Meats should be well cooked, and uncooked or commercially prepared meats should not be eaten. Raw fruits and vegetables should be peeled or carefully washed before being eaten. No eating utensils or drinking glasses should be shared.

Adequate nutrition at home helps to bolster resistance to infection. Frequent high calorie and protein snacks should be added to the diet. Meals should be balanced, with calories added through the use of such things as cream- or egg-based sauces, cheeses, milk powder, and grains. Fad diets, such as those based on macrobiotics, are frequently unbalanced and have not been demonstrated to be of significant worth.

Because they can catch infections so easily, AIDS patients must avoid very close contact with people known to have infections, viral illnesses, coldlike symptoms, or draining lesions, and should stay away from crowds and crowded rooms. However, remaining totally housebound, without social contact or stimulation, is not advisable since this would only contribute to the sense of isolation that so often accompanies AIDS.

Sexual activity raises a practical, moral, and ethical dilemma for AIDS patients that they must resolve without evading the knowledge that intercourse may not only transmit their disease but also expose them to other serious sexually transmitted infections. If a decision is made to engage in sexual activity, AIDS patients and partners would be well-advised to avoid direct oral or rectal contact and to use a condom.

The AIDS patient at home often has fears about transmitting AIDS to other household members. Friends or family involved in caring for the patient may have ambivalent feelings about their risk of exposure that they are reluctant to express. Professional assistance with home care can provide an opportunity for patient and family to explore these fears in a reassuring environment and to be given information necessary to alleviate inappropriate concerns. For example, in addition to the known facts about how AIDS is transmitted, they should be told that health-care workers involved in the care of AIDS patients incur very little risk of contracting the disease. In numerous studies, nonsexual family contacts have not been infected with the virus from infected family members. Precautions to prevent exposure to the patient's blood and body fluids are similar to those employed in the hospital, as detailed above and in chapter 19.

Home-Care Skills

People in the home often worry about their ability to provide adequate care and comfort to the physically dependent patient. The skills required for home care may include bathing, positioning and turning the patient in bed, helping with walking, feeding, making the patient comfortable, and some specialized skills such as changing dressings. Many of these skills can be demonstrated for home-care providers under professional guidance while the patient is still hospitalized. Visiting nurses and home health aides can provide and demonstrate the skills in the home. Also, in most cities, home-care courses are available through community service agencies, in some cases specifically for the care of AIDS patients. Further information about these courses may be obtained by calling one of the resource groups listed in chapter 25.

Emotional Stress

At home, as in the hospital, the AIDS patient needs emotional support. Family and friends are the patient's major source of emotional support, but participation in a community-based support group can add the needed perspective of a peer group. When group participation is not possible, many AIDS-related organizations will provide counselors who visit the home.

An often neglected aspect of home care is the stress imposed on the care giver. Tending to a sick loved one is a physically and emotionally demanding task. After a time, the most devoted care giver may feel trapped by circumstances, frightened, exhausted, and frustrated or angry with the patient. While these feelings are natural and understandable, they may be difficult to accept and can induce guilt, especially if inappropriately expressed. Family and friends should be encouraged to take time off for themselves and to seek relief either from support groups or from relatives or acquaintances who will occasionally take turns caring for the AIDS patient.

AIDS is still a disease with no known cure. Patients must at some point face the fact that death may not be far off. Many find that planning for the terminal phase of illness alleviates some of the fears and anxiety that surround it. One issue for both the patient and loved one is the extent of medical intervention desired when death appears imminent. Some may prefer to die at home without being subjected to life-prolonging measures and machinery. Others may elect hospitalization and various degrees of care. The wishes of patient and family should be thoroughly discussed in advance with the primary physician so that the limits of desired treatment are understood. Home-care providers may also find themselves assisting the patient to complete unfinished final tasks, such as arranging for the disposal of property and possessions, resolving conflicts with estranged members, and specifying funeral rites. Doing whatever has to be done while there is still time insures that the patient's wishes will be carried out and often provides a degree of comfort in the final days of the illness.

SUMMARY

AIDS patients have many care needs similar to those of other seriously ill persons. However, unique aspects of this disease, such as its transmissibility and association with specific groups in the population, require heightened awareness and sensitivity on the part of care providers. Whether care is provided by skilled professionals in the hospital or by family and friends at home, the common goal is to care about the AIDS patient as an individual and to communicate that caring through their actions.

19 Preventing AIDS

JOHN W. SENSAKOVIC
BENJAMIN GREER

INTRODUCTION

In a dimly lit isolation room in a local medical center, an 18-year-old girl battles for her life against a severe and very unusual pneumonia. She has AIDS, apparently acquired from her 20-year-old boyfriend, an intravenous (IV)-drug abuser who has AIDS. The girl will not survive despite the efforts of a medical team of infection experts. The problem will not end here. The following day, a hospital employee will be suspended for refusing to enter the room in which the girl had been treated. A policeman will be suspended for refusing to escort the boyfriend arrested on a drug charge. The girl's family is distraught, not only over the loss of their daughter, but over their own health and that of their other children. The funeral director expresses worry about preparing the body and is reluctant to have the casket open for viewing.

This sequence of events is not unusual. AIDS inspires fear of contracting the illness not only in people who come near or contact an AIDS patient but in others remote from a patient, such as diners in a restaurant, riders on public transportation, people drinking from a water fountain, non-AIDS patients in a hospital, and blood donors. The dread of contracting such a devastating illness, about which much scientific knowledge remains lacking and to which so much media attention is paid, is not at all surprising. Unfortunately, the fear is too often out of proportion to the risks known from scientific studies of the transmission of AIDS. The known facts indicate realistic precautions that should be taken and unrealistic fears that should not be allowed to misguide behavior and unnecessarily add to suffering.

A rational perspective is based on two important scientific findings. First, the AIDS virus is transmitted effectively only through infected blood or semen, and the production of overt disease by transmitted virus seems to require additional conditions such as a significant level of infection, repeated exposure, and probably even simultaneous infection with another virus or other cause of reduced immunity. For this reason, the AIDS virus spreads in risk groups where these conditions are likely to be present: homosexual and bisexual males, IV-drug abusers, sexual partners of infected individuals, and infants born to infected mothers.

Second, the AIDS virus is easily killed by cleaning agents, such as bleach, alcohol, and detergents, and even by drying. This vulnerability of the virus further assures that transmission is likely only through close sexual contact or transfer of infected blood, and not from casual exposure to the virus in the environment. Also, the virus is quickly killed by all routine methods of disinfection used in the hospital.

PREVENTION FOR HEALTH-CARE PERSONNEL

Health-care professionals, by the nature of their work, are repeatedly exposed to infectious diseases. Although they are aware of the risk from the moment they enter the profession and know they are obliged to face it, they also expect that the scientific community and regulating agencies will protect them, wherever possible, from undue risks. Just as it would be unprofessional and unacceptable for any health-care professional to refuse to care for a patient because of possible risk of infection, so it would be unacceptable for the scientific community and regulating agencies to allow such risk to exceed currently accepted levels. To fulfill this obligation, responsible agencies such as the Centers for Disease Control (CDC) have recommended precautions to minimize the risk to health-care professionals of contracting AIDS.

Transmission routes of AIDS resemble the transmission routes of the hepatitis B virus: blood, blood products, and sexual contact.

Fortunately, the AIDS virus is not transmitted as easily as hepatitis B, and is much more sensitive to adverse conditions. Therefore, taking precautions against AIDS by avoiding contact with infected semen or blood, as is done in caring for hepatitis B patients, actually provides a degree of "over-protection."

Most recommended precautions aim to prevent contact with the blood of known or suspected AIDS patients because health-care workers face the theoretical risk of becoming infected by an accidental stick with a contaminated needle, a cut by a surgical instrument, or the splashing of contaminated blood on an open wound. Despite the enormous number of contacts between health workers and AIDS patients, cases of transmission have been exceedingly rare and accompanied by special circumstances. A study of over 700 needle sticks revealed no documented cases of AIDS in health workers. Nevertheless, all direct contact with possibly infected blood should be avoided. Extraordinary care should be taken to avoid accidental injury from contaminated needles or instruments. This precaution applies especially to physicians, nurses, personnel who draw blood, and laboratory technicians who test it. Gloves should always be worn when handling blood specimens and objects exposed to the blood of AIDS patients. Gowns should be worn when clothing may be soiled with blood, and hands should be washed immediately and thoroughly after contact with possibly contaminated blood. Blood specimens from AIDS patients should always be labeled as such and accidental spills cleaned up promptly with a disinfectant solution such as household bleach. Contaminated articles should be placed in a leakproof bag and labeled before sterilization or incineration. All instruments used on AIDS patients should be properly sterilized before reuse.

Needle stick injuries often result from inadequate attention to the procedure, usually when the protective cover is being replaced over the needle. For this reason, needles should be used with utmost care and undistracted concentration. Gloves should be worn when blood is being drawn, and needles used to draw blood should not be reinserted into the needle cover or broken before disposal but placed directly into a puncture-resistant disposable container. Unlike other needles, which are sometimes broken before disposal to prevent reuse, these needles may cause splashing of infectious blood if broken.

TABLE 1:   PRECAUTIONS FOR HOSPITAL PERSONNEL
TREATING POSSIBLE AIDS PATIENTS

Avoid being stuck or cut by contaminated needles or instruments.
Avoid contact of open wounds with contaminated materials.
Wear gowns and gloves, especially when there is risk of contact with
bodily secretions and excretions.
Wear masks and eye protectors for possible spray of contaminated fluids.
Wash hands thoroughly.
Label contaminated specimens and materials.
Clean spills quickly with bleach.
Do not break needles.

*Adapted from CDC Morbidity & Mortality Weekly Reports 31: 577–579,
1982.*

Since the AIDS virus has been found in AIDS patients' body fluids
other than blood, including semen, saliva, tears, vaginal secretions,
urine, and feces, these are assumed to be potentially infectious,
although extremely less so than blood, if at all, in most cases.
Nevertheless, it is prudent to handle these substances with the same
careful precautions recommended for blood to reduce the risk of
infection as much as possible.

Isolation of AIDS patients is somewhat controversial. If appropriate care is exercised to avoid exposure to body fluids and excretions,
isolation may be unnecessary and may merely depress patient
morale. A private room is probably desirable, if only as a reminder
of the importance of recommended precautions. If the patient is
unable to maintain good hygiene, a private room is mandatory, as are
gowns, gloves, and scrupulous hand washing. Masks are not necessary, unless saliva or sputum may possibly be sprayed into the air, for
example, during suctioning to clear the airways of a patient whose
breathing is being assisted by a mechanical ventilator. Such a risk
also requires the use of protective eye coverings.

Recommended, generally accepted precautions for hospital floor
and laboratory personnel are outlined in tables 1 and 2. If carefully
followed, they will minimize risks to health-care personnel and help
to forestall the use of exaggerated, unrealistic, and unnecessary
procedures that often increase the anxieties of staff and patients, and

TABLE 2:   PRECAUTIONS FOR LABORATORY PERSONNEL
TESTING POSSIBLY CONTAMINATED SPECIMENS

Do not pipet by mouth.
Dispose of needles properly. Do not break, to prevent splashing.
Wear lab coats.
Wear gloves.
Wash hands thoroughly.
Disinfect work area with bleach.

Adapted from CDC Morbidity & Mortality Weekly Reports *31: 577–579, 1982.*

sometimes even interfere with the provision of optimal and much needed medical care.

Because the AIDS virus is easily killed outside of the body, it poses no risk in the environment if routine disinfection is properly applied. The same precautions used for hepatitis B, a much more resistant and infectious virus, are more than adequate against AIDS, whether in surgery, dentistry, the hospital ward, or the mortuary.

PREVENTION FOR RISK GROUPS AND SEXUAL PARTNERS, THE GENERAL PUBLIC, AND HOME CARE OF AIDS PATIENTS

The scientific community has well defined the infection risk and necessary precautions for health-care personnel, but has not adequately conveyed a similar message to the general public. In part, this may be due to less-than-informative sensationalism in the coverage of AIDS by some media representatives, and sometimes to a reluctance by scientists to give the appearance of diminishing the seriousness of the AIDS problem. The hysteria of an inadequately informed public underlies reports of overreactions such as taxi drivers refusing to accept homosexual passengers, homosexual waiters losing their jobs, and blood donors declining in number because of unfounded fears of becoming infected with AIDS at blood banks.

Risk Groups and Sexual Partners

Male homosexuals and bisexuals and intravenous (IV)-drug addicts face by far the greatest risks of AIDS, since the virus is spread

TABLE 3: SEXUAL PRACTICES AND RELATIVE RISK FOR AIDS

Safe	Possibly Safe	Unsafe
Massage, hugging	Wet kissing	Receptive anal intercourse (without condom)
Dry kissing	Vaginal and anal intercourse with condoms	
Voyeurism, fantasy		Vaginal intercourse (without condom)
Mutual masturbation	Sucking—stop before climaxing	
Frottage (body-to-body rubbing)		Rimming (oral-anal contact)
	Cunnilingus (oral-vaginal contact)	Fisting (manual anal intercourse)
		Semen or urine in mouth

primarily by infected semen and blood. Within these groups, the risk is associated with close sexual contact, especially receptive anal intercourse, and injection of drugs with contaminated needles.

Many homosexuals are already infected, over 60 percent in some areas. Many have no symptoms of disease but continue to carry the AIDS virus in their blood and semen and may transmit it to sexual partners. The risk of infection for anyone, homosexual or not, increases with the number of sexual partners and the practice of receptive anal intercourse. The risk can be virtually eliminated by total abstinence from sex and diminished by avoiding unsafe behavior, for example, by limiting the number of partners and choosing partners known to be uninfected. (A negative antibody test is not a certification of freedom from infection, because the test result is occasionally false, and a recent infection may not yet have produced detectable antibodies.)

Practices called "safe sex" offer a reasonable way to reduce the risk of acquiring AIDS. Sexual practices can be divided relatively into categories of safe, possibly safe, and unsafe (table 3). Safe sex practices involve minimal exposure to body fluids and tissue damage. These practices include massages, hugging, dry kissing, voyeurism, fantasy, mutual masturbation, and body-to-body rubbing (frottage). Possibly safe sex incurs a risk that depends on the degree of oral or genital trauma and exchange of body fluids. While the AIDS virus has been isolated from saliva, there have been no documented cases that resulted from kissing. Since the theoretical risk exists, wet kissing may have a small risk factor. Vaginal or anal intercourse with condoms should provide protection. Condoms have been shown to block the transmission of other viruses like cytomegalovirus and herpesvirus. Nevertheless, it is safest to withdraw before climaxing. Sucking may be safe if the partner does not climax prior to stopping the act. The AIDS virus has also been isolated from vaginal secretions, and therefore cunnilingus (oral-vaginal contact) may create a small risk.

Unsafe sex should not be practiced. Receptive anal intercourse (without the use of a condom) results in tearing of the rectum and allows body fluids to be absorbed into the bloodstream. Vaginal intercourse without a condom also is unprotected sex. "Rimming" (oral-anal contact) allows infectious saliva to be absorbed through the anus. Feces are full of bacteria that can cause infections for both partners. "Fisting" (manual-anal intercourse) causes rectal tearing and allows entrance of AIDS-infected body fluids. The swallowing of semen or urine in the mouth is also extremely risky.

IV-drug abusers not already infected with the AIDS virus may be taking a 50:50 gamble of becoming infected when they share needles for injections, since some studies have found over half the group tested to carry the infection. Contaminated needles or syringes can transmit the virus directly into the bloodstream. IV-drug users can reduce their risk only by abstaining totally from injecting drugs or using sterile needles and syringes (not generally legally obtainable).

Members of high-risk groups, whether or not they think they are free of AIDS, should not donate blood, to minimize the risk of unknowingly infecting others.

Heterosexual transmission of AIDS does occur and is causing considerable concern in this era of increased promiscuity. While the heterosexual spread of AIDS is not as common as for herpes and gonorrhea (at least in the United States and Europe), unlike these other venereal diseases, infection with the AIDS virus is often fatal with no cure at hand. Although homosexuals face the greatest risk, AIDS is not just a homosexual disease. Reports of AIDS acquired through heterosexual contact have been increasing. Women can be infected by sexual intercourse with infected men (often bisexual men or IV-drug abusers), and men can be infected by sexual intercourse with infected women, often prostitutes or IV-drug abusers. Here, too, the risk can be reduced by avoiding casual sex with partners not well known or of uncertain background, and by limiting the number of partners. Although it is desirable that the partner be in good health and not promiscuous, apparent good health is no guarantee of protection. AIDS has an incubation period of up to several years, during which time no symptoms may appear but the infection may be contagious to an as yet unknown degree. Even if some symptoms do appear, they may be too few or vague for a physician to diagnose as AIDS. Promiscuous heterosexual activity, though apparently a relatively minor risk factor at present, is likely to become a serious route for the spread of AIDS.

For one risk group, the recipients of blood and blood products, advances in medical knowledge and technology have produced a bright outlook in the prevention of new infections. The blood supply formerly contained contributions from donors infected with the AIDS virus at a time when little was known about the disease. Some recipients of blood transfusions became infected, especially hemophiliacs and patients with sickle-cell disease who received blood products from a large number of donors. The more donors, the greater the chance that one was unknowingly infected. The risk was always small and outweighed by the benefits of essential blood transfusions. Now that donors can be tested for exposure to AIDS, and members of risk groups are advised not to donate blood, screening procedures make the blood supply exceedingly safe. Also, blood products are treated to kill any virus that might enter the blood pool sometimes accumulated from thousands of donors.

Patients who require transfusions of blood or blood products need take no special precautions. Their safest bet is to rely on the standard blood supply. (See chapter 9 for more details.)

The General Public

The general public has sometimes been unnecessarily alarmed by false rumors, for example, that blood donors can get AIDS by giving blood, or that even casual contact with AIDS patients is dangerous. No donor has ever been infected by giving blood. All blood-drawing equipment is either disposable (sterilized at the factory and used only once) or resterilized before being put back into service. No known case of AIDS has ever been attributable to casual contact with someone who has AIDS, even relatively close contact in a household. Although reasonable precautions should be taken against contact with possibly infected body fluids as a matter of principle, AIDS seems remarkably difficult to acquire except by the well-known routes of intimate sex and mingling of blood.

The uninfected public should heed the precautions recommended for risk groups, keep informed about scientifically verified facts available from many sources, such as this book, and act rationally. Although fear of a fatal disease for which no cure is yet available may be understandable, unreasoning fear does more harm than good. Casual association in classrooms or other public places with people who may be infected with AIDS is not only much safer than many other associations that cause no concern but is impossible to avoid since the infected population may already number in the millions.

Some professionals, such as firefighters, first-aid personnel, and police and corrections officers, have questioned the possibility of contracting AIDS on duty, for example, in transporting patients or prisoners, or when administering cardiopulmonary resuscitation (CPR). Casual contact, as in transporting a patient, carries no risk. In CPR, a theoretical risk exists in contact with saliva or blood during mouth-to-mouth resuscitation. Direct mouth-to-mouth contact with known AIDS patients should best be avoided, but CPR should not be withheld from a patient with an unknown history, since transmission of the AIDS virus by this route is actually unlikely.

Police and corrections officers must deal with prisoners, a group known to have a high incidence of drug abuse and homosexuality. Again, casual contact involves little risk, but bite injuries and contact with blood, excretions, or saliva may occur during violent confrontations. These should be avoided when possible, but if exposure does occur, affected parts should receive thorough washing and disinfection. Experience has shown that a three-prong program can alleviate the fears of both prison staff and inmates and ensure a minimal risk. The program involves education of corrections officers and inmates, special instruction of the institutional health service, and screening inmates for AIDS followed by necessary treatment and assignment to separate quarters, if possible.

Home Care of AIDS Patients

Placement of AIDS patients after release from the hospital is one of the most difficult problems in AIDS management. Anxiety among family members can be devastating, as illustrated by a recent instance. Two young sisters were diagnosed as having AIDS acquired by drug usage. Both were hospitalized together for a long and complicated illness. Family members frequently visited the hospital and were obviously concerned, especially when the girls' survival was in doubt. When the girls finally did improve, they were taken home by their family. Two days later, both were brought back to the hospital emergency room and abandoned with only the hospital gowns they had worn when they left the hospital.

Such a reaction is not unusual, due to the fear and lack of understanding of AIDS. The family is concerned for its own safety and ask endless questions. Where should the patient sleep? Wash? Eat? How should soiled clothing be washed? How should used dishes be cleaned? How should the patient's room be treated? The questions are reasonable and need to be answered. Answers can do a great deal to increase understanding and reduce unrealistic fears.

AIDS patients should have a separate room at home. Contact with soiled clothing and objects should be avoided and gloves worn when handling them. Razors, shavers, and toothbrushes should not be shared, as they can become contaminated with minute amounts of blood. Special techniques for washing clothing and dishes and for disinfection should be followed (table 4).

On the other hand, since casual contact carries no risk, there is no reason that the AIDS patient cannot be returned home if proper precautions are taught to the patient and family. The help of an experienced social worker and visiting nurse can be extremely valuable.

The special needs of AIDS patients should be considered. In addition to its devastating physical effects, AIDS exacts a severe psychological toll. Patients must live with the dread of a potentially fatal illness in a climate of great anxiety among family, friends, and

TABLE 4.   PRECAUTIONS FOR AIDS PATIENTS AT HOME

I.   **Necessary Equipment**
Thermometer
Soap
Household bleach solution (1 part bleach to 10 parts
   water), prepared daily
Large and small plastic bags
Garbage receptacles
Gloves
Paper towels

II.   **Precautions**
1. Wear rubber gloves when handling contaminated and soiled
   articles.
2. Wash hands with antimicrobial soap after handling contaminated
   and soiled articles.
3. Seal contaminated articles in a plastic bag and discard in a large
   plastic-lined garbage receptacle to be emptied daily.
4. Wash contaminated surfaces immediately. Wash bathroom sink,
   toilet, and bathtub once daily with bleach solution.
5. Soak *soiled* clothing and linen in bleach solution in bathtub for 1
   hour before washing.
6. Patients should have their own eating utensils, razor or shaver,
   and tooth brush, kept separate in a plastic bag.

others about the risk of spread. Although the hope of an early cure
cannot realistically be held out to them, their feelings should be
understood and sensitively respected.

To prevent the spread of AIDS, patients (as well as members of
high-risk groups) should avoid risk-enhancing sexual activities, and
drug abuse must be stopped completely. Maintenance of proper
hygiene is essential, as well as a balanced diet with a high caloric
intake to prevent or minimize weight loss. In addition, patients
should get adequate rest and avoid exposure to persons with
contagious illnesses that can further challenge an already deficient
immune system.

Until a cure of AIDS is available, recommendations can only help to minimize risks on the basis of available information, combat disproportionate fears with valid facts and reasonable precautions, and allow AIDS patients the maximum possible range of normal activities.

SUMMARY

AIDS is a viral illness transmitted effectively only through infected blood or semen by intimate sexual contact or direct injection, and not by casual contact with intact skin. The virus is highly vulnerable to most cleansing substances and environmental conditions so that survival outside of infected body cells is unlikely. AIDS may be prevented by avoidance of risky sexual practices such as anal intercourse and of injection of drugs with blood-contaminated needles, known to be primary modes of transmission of the virus.

20 Psychological and Social Issues of AIDS and Strategies for Survival

VIRGINIA LEHMAN
NOREEN RUSSELL

The impact of AIDS can be catastrophic for patients, families, and friends. Some of the most troubling aspects are psychological and social. However, resources are available to help those affected through difficult times.

Many of the psychosocial effects of AIDS are like those of other chronic and devastating illnesses. Patients "... usually experience heightened states of anxiety, fear and depression induced by physical pain and psycho-social distress. A number of factors contribute to these emotions: imminent separation from all that is meaningful in life; treatment regimes of chemotherapy; experiences of physical deterioration.... These dysfunctional emotions reduce the ability of patients to cope with their difficult life situations."

PSYCHOLOGICAL AND SOCIAL ISSUES

Fears of Contagion

Although much has been learned in the relatively few years since the first appearance of the disease, AIDS patients still bear the special burdens of having what many regard as a mysterious illness and the fear of contagion. They worry about transmitting AIDS to loved ones, and their associates worry about contracting the disease. Identification of the virus HTLV-III/LAV as the likely cause (possibly with other contributing conditions) has removed much of the mystery, but in the absence of an effective treatment or preventive vaccine public fear of AIDS continues. In larger urban areas, such as New York City and San Francisco, media coverage and intensive efforts to educate high-risk groups, health professionals, and the general public have largely averted an overtly hysterical response. However, an AIDS patient still may encounter discrimination, for example, loss of employment or failure to be hired, abandonment by friends and family, and denial of appropriate medical care. Remaining questions about the possible, although improbable, routes of infection compound public concerns. Guidelines, widely disseminated, for managing AIDS patients during hospitalization and return to their homes have not completely alleviated fears. Some inconsistency in interpreting the guidelines may also contribute to the fears.

Thus, fear is perhaps the most characteristic response to AIDS. An encouraging sign is that many chronic care hospitals and terminal care facilities that formerly did not accept AIDS patients are developing special AIDS units that provide a limited number of beds. However, the National Hospice Organization has issued a policy statement acknowledging the difficulty in meeting the tremendous need (several hospices now do accept AIDS patients) because AIDS patients often do not fit hospice criteria and incur costs, including medication, nursing care, and supplies, that exceed reimbursement rates. Employers and landlords have become alarmed upon learning that an employee or tenant has AIDS. The mother of an AIDS patient was reluctant to keep her stricken daughter in the home for fear of spreading the infection to the daughter's two children. A man threatened to remove his children from the household if his wife's brother, an AIDS patient, came to live with the family.

Contrary to these fears, a recent study published in *The New England Journal of Medicine* concluded that the risk of contracting AIDS even in an intimate household setting is "minimal to nonexistent." The study included 101 individuals living, but not sexually involved, with AIDS patients for an average of two years. They shared eating utensils, toothbrushes, combs, and razors, and 37 shared beds. The majority had exchanged hugs and kisses. Most of

Most of the families had low incomes, lived in crowded conditions, and took relatively few sanitary precautions, all considered generally conducive to the spread of infection. Unfortunately, the results of this study have not eradicated the fear of contagion, and patients' fears of abandonment are sometimes borne out in reality.

Feelings of stigmatization are frequently underscored during hospitalization. AIDS patients may be placed in isolation, and hospital staff and visitors may wear masks, gowns, and gloves. As each day passes, the patient feels more distant from the real world, intensifying a sense of not belonging, being different, being untouchable. Many liken their experience to that of a leper.

AIDS patients continually dread contracting random infections from their surroundings because their defective immune systems make them less able to resist illness. Some shun public places to minimize exposure to germs.

Dependency and Love

Reactions to a diagnosis of AIDS vary. Some panic, others go into shock. They may take weeks to acknowledge the fact. Some retreat into denial and consult one physician after another in hope that the diagnosis was wrong. They feel disbelief, anger, and self-blame.

Coping with a life-threatening illness is extremely stressful. Repeated hospitalizations may be necessary, each longer than the one before. Medical tests and treatment may be painful, and physicians may differ over appropriate treatment. Since the discovery of the HTLV-III/LAV virus, a small number of AIDS patients have been able to participate in experimental studies, but these are very limited. Thus, patients and families may have to choose between treatments espoused by some physicians and discouraged by others. As the illness progresses and becomes more debilitating, they may worry whether they made the right choice. Since no definitive treatment exists, confidence and trust in the doctor are essential.

Horror stories abound of AIDS patients being shunned by hospital staff, left unattended in their beds, evicted from their homes, and fired from jobs. But stories of rejection are far outnumbered by instances of courageous devotion and care by family, friends, and lovers. Many have traveled long distances to be with the sick, often at great sacrifice, leaving their own homes, families, and towns for a strange city and unfamiliar ways.

Because AIDS predominantly affects young adults—in their late twenties, thirties, and forties—caretaking responsibilities are often thrust on elderly parents in their sixties and seventies, reversing the usual role of young adults assisting and caring for elderly parents. This sudden role reversal tends to accentuate stress by adding to the detrimental effects of illness the forced dependence on elderly parents. Old patterns of child-to-parent relationships become revived.

One example is an energetic mother, in her seventies, of a young AIDS patient who resided in another city. Twice, the mother left behind her job and the rest of her family to care for her sick adult son, preparing his favorite meals and doing household chores. Relations were sometimes tense. He felt she was overly protective, constantly "chatting and moving about." She felt he was insensitive and a bully. She was with him until he died, often spending ten hours a day at the hospital. In another example, the laborer father of a young man with AIDS tended his son around the clock, bathing him and changing bedpans with loving devotion during the course of the terminal illness.

Lovers may be equally devoted, and instances of great attentiveness, sensitivity, and love are frequent. The homosexual lover, although sharing membership in a high-risk group, often places loyalty to his ill mate above concern for his personal safety. AIDS patients are often discharged from the hospital to return home where a lover is the main caretaker, providing comfort and attendance until death comes.

Guilt and Shame

Self-condemnation is common among AIDS patients, particularly homosexuals, and close family members. Suppressed conflicts about homosexuality surface. The patient often feels resentful of discrimination, real and imagined. In a once troubled man who has come to accept his homosexuality with a sense of freedom and pride, the diagnosis of AIDS may reawaken earlier ambivalence. He may be anguished by the thought of AIDS as God's punishment. Those not "out of the closet" may be forced by a diagnosis of AIDS to disclose their sexual orientation to family, employers, and even strangers. Revealing homosexuality at a time of one's own choosing may no longer be an option.

Some families are unable to accept the fact that a son or brother is homosexual. Upon learning that a son had AIDS, one family told friends and neighbors he had leukemia. They could talk to each other about his homosexuality, but felt ashamed with others. Another family simply kept the son's illness secret. Some families have withdrawn from friends and neighbors in shame and fear of discrimination, thus denying themselves important sources of emotional support. Parents often agonize over whether they played a role in their son's becoming homosexual and therefore were to blame for his illness. Also, the death of children before their parents seems to violate the natural order of life.

AIDS and Sexuality

AIDS sufferers have a double sexual concern. By engaging in sex, they may infect a lover and, because of their immunodeficiency, may themselves contract other sexually transmitted diseases that would worsen their own health. Some lose interest in sex either because their sickness saps their energy or they are overcome by anxiety. Many abstain out of moral concern about spreading the disease, even if sexual desire persists. If they are used to a very active sex life, especially if they have frequented gay bars and bathhouses for sometimes anonymous sex, abstinence represents the loss of an entire social support network.

Monogamous male couples are confronted with particularly poignant choices. They are beset with anxiety over whether to have sex, which sexual activities are safe, and mutual concern about each other's health. Although sexual transmission of AIDS in the United States and Europe has been predominantly male to male, women with AIDS have borne infected babies and the AIDS virus has been found in vaginal secretions. Many previously unconcerned heterosexuals now fear contracting AIDS, particularly those who are single, divorced, or separated, whose sexual partners may be bisexual or promiscuous. This fear has lead to a shift in sexual practices, including the increasing use of condoms, greater care in selecting sexual partners, and even degrees of abstinence. More concern is expressed that AIDS may spread to the general public.

Dependency

Patients in later stages of AIDS need assistance with everyday activities, but some strongly resist. One would not even allow friends to help with shopping and cleaning. His determination to go to the supermarket and the bank himself and to clean his own apartment represented his mastery over illness. Completion of even one small household task was exhilarating. Others may accept some help from family and friends, but continue struggling in many ways to maintain their independence. At the opposite extreme, some feel they are helpless, at times unrealistically, and expect others to do everything for them.

Basic personality predetermines response to illness. Independent people who grasped opportunities and displayed initiative before becoming ill continue to strive for independence afterward. Habitually dependent people who expected others to care for them remain in that mold. A freelance graphic designer who learned he had AIDS exemplified the independent type. He actively explored treatment options with his physician, kept himself informed at all times, and rarely asked others to do what he could do himself. In contrast, another AIDS patient, who had always felt short-changed by life and not given his due by companions, became extraordinarily demanding of his friends after he became ill. Family and friends relate and respond to sick loved ones much as they did when they were well. Close ties remain close; those with few friends or only transient relationships may find themselves alone.

Anger and guilt affect both the sick and the caretakers. The sick person is angry at the sickness and feels guilty for being a burden. Family and friends feel guilty both for being well and for sometimes resenting having to serve the needs of the one who is ill. It is important for family, friends, and lovers to take periodic breaks from tending the sick. Having time for themselves serves as a safety valve to release tension and helps the sick to feel less guilty about imposing on others.

AIDS may force work and personal aspirations to be put aside in the battle to survive. A conflict often arises between continuing activities at as high a level as possible and slowing down and allowing others to help. Individual circumstances determine an appropriate compromise, if necessary. For example, the manager of an antiques store went to work every day, despite nausea and diarrhea. His great pride in his shop and his love of his work kept him going. Another AIDS sufferer, with a more physically demanding job, found that he was no longer able to work. Despite much frustration and sadness, he yielded to his undeniable disability and accepted "being pampered." He had always been helpful and giving to others; now he necessarily allowed others to be helpful and giving to him.

Children

An increasing number of children have AIDS, estimated at over six hundred early in 1986. Most are under the age of five, but some are almost thirteen. A few appear to have contracted the disease from blood transfusions, but most were born to women who either had AIDS, had sex with an infected partner, or were members of a high-risk group.

Children with AIDS raise many social issues. Discharge from hospital to home may be difficult due to the mother's inability or unwillingness to care for a child with AIDS, and foster homes may not accept such children. A child's stay in the hospital is sometimes extended because alternative placement is not available. Some specially funded programs offer additional support to foster families willing to care for children with AIDS, but the need for more financial, educational, and psychological aid persists.

Children, like adults, are being ostracized, as evidenced by news stories of attempts by parents' groups to prevent AIDS children from attending day-care centers and school classrooms. Through hard-fought advocacy procedures, some parents of AIDS children have forced school boards to reverse decisions denying access, but success has not been universal.

Increasing numbers of families have one or both parents and a child with AIDS. In the future this will present yet another challenge for program development in the treatment of AIDS. One such program is already being offered at Albert Einstein College of Medicine in the Bronx, New York.

More efforts to educate children and school staff are under way in the New York City public school system and are expanding to public schools, private schools, and colleges countrywide. These programs often began only after students or teachers contracted the disease. They include informational meetings for groups of students, training sessions for dormitory advisors, and leaflets about unsafe sexual practices.

AIDS and Minorities

Early publicity about AIDS tended to focus on the white gay community. Recent newspaper articles addressed the fact that AIDS has affected a disproportionate number of black people. Blacks compose about 12.5 percent of the entire U.S. population, but about 25 percent of reported AIDS cases are black. This disproportion is also true of children. Approximately 56 percent of children with AIDS are black. Hispanics are also disproportionately represented among AIDS cases.

There is fear, particularly within the black community, that inadequate education and dissemination of information have led to the misconception among the black poor that this is a "white man's disease." Poor overall health and limited access to appropriate health care may be contributing factors.

In urban areas, such as Philadelphia, black leaders have expressed concern that access of the black AIDS population to existing resources may be inhibited by a tendency to keep to themselves within their own community. The black population, like white heterosexuals, tends to be reluctant to have their members identified with the growing number of AIDS cases.

Media

Whereas articles about AIDS were once relegated either to the back pages of newspapers or to emotionally laden front page headlines, within the last year journalism has trended toward frequent and comprehensive articles about all aspects of AIDS. Articles are now seen in publications ranging from the *Wall Street Journal* to *Vogue*. Television coverage has expanded from straight news stories to a feature-length film adapted for TV, ("Early Frost" aired in November 1985), episodes on medical series, such as "Trapper

John" and "St. Elsewhere," to special cable TV programs devoted solely to issues about AIDS. Two serious plays about AIDS, *As Is*, by William M. Hoffman, and *The Normal Heart*, by Larry Kramer, have had long theater runs in New York City.

The courage displayed by Rock Hudson in revealing his diagnosis of AIDS and his homosexuality brought information about AIDS to a wider public audience. People in the film industry responded to his tragic death with a series of fund-raising events to augment what many people felt was inadequate financial support from governmental agencies.

Blood Testing

A blood test to detect antibodies to the virus, HTLV-III/LAV, has been particularly helpful in screening blood donations to make the blood supply safe for transfusions. However, presence of antibody does not predict the later development of AIDS. It indicates only previous exposure. Many individuals have expressed concern about confidentiality and fear of discrimination. Some organizations and governmental agencies have advocated that everyone in high-risk groups be forced to undergo blood testing. This poses a civil rights issue (discussed in other chapters) since disclosure of positive test results may adversely affect such matters as employment and insurance coverage.

Facing Death

R. Kastenbaum coined the phrase "bereavement overload," referring to the elderly who experience the deaths of many friends within a relatively short time. A similar phenomenon is seen with AIDS: young adults lose many friends within a few months or years. This is particularly devastating and frightening for the homosexual community.

E. Kubler-Ross described death as "...a fearful, frightening happening...even if we think we have mastered it on many levels." Despite this natural fear, many sick or injured people are able to talk about the fact that they are dying and take steps to put their affairs in order, specifying a preferred funeral service, requesting burial or cremation, and, if cremation, where ashes are to be stored or scattered. Many make wills for the first time. Imminent death is often faced with quiet strength and determination. Conflicts with loved ones may be resolved. For example, a man long estranged from his family met with them the day before he died and openly discussed differences. All apologized for hurtful actions and expressed deep love for one another, allowing the dying man a final feeling of equanimity.

Wills

Having a will is very important. A will not only provides for the disposal of your property as you would wish but also protects your heirs. The state receives a disproportionate amount of your money if you die without having a will. A will also insures a more prompt estate settlement. A separate document is advisable to convey your preference for burial or cremation.

A power of attorney may be necessary if you have no suitable next of kin. This can be especially significant if the dying patient is confused and unable to make necessary decisions. Mental confusion is not uncommon in AIDS, especially in later stages. A durable power of attorney is the most comprehensive, since it does not have to be periodically renewed. Assigning a power of attorney to a trusted friend can make sure the patient receives appropriate medical treatment and helps in dealing with many practical details.

Some hospitals do not recognize the partner in homosexual relationships as equivalent to a spouse or relative; possibly contrary to the patient's wish, parents or siblings may be called on to make important decisions. In such cases, even a power of attorney assigned to a lover will have no force if there is a next of kin. The patient should make sure to learn the hospital's policy ahead of time. It is also recommended that the AIDS patient, lover, and family discuss and understand the patient's wishes, to avoid painful and unnecessary conflict.

SURVIVAL STRATEGIES

Although many AIDS patients may ultimately have to accept the fact of terminal illness and will do so with courage and dignity, often helped by compassionate care, they usually want to go on living and fight for survival.

Knowledge of entitlements and community resources can fortify them in their efforts. Eligibility requirements for entitlements vary from state to state. The following list describes entitlement programs and community sources of assistance.

Financial and Other Entitlements

Public Assistance

If you have AIDS, are unable to work, and are without financial assets, you may be eligible for public assistance. Apply at the nearest local or county welfare agency. Needed are documents that establish citizenship or legal alien status (for example, a birth certificate, baptismal record, or alien registration green card) and records of how you maintained yourself financially in the past year (for example, recent receipts, paycheck stubs, income tax return, and telephone, gas, and electric bills sent to your address). You will also need a detailed letter from your physician or local hospital stating that you have an illness that prevents you from working, full or part time, for at least one year. In many states, you must also apply for federal Supplemental Social Security (SSI) at the same time that you seek public assistance (see Social Security below).

Food Stamps

Depending on your financial status, you may be eligible for food stamps. Check with your local social service department.

Disability Programs
State

In many states employers contribute to a disability program. However, if your company has only a few employees, you may not be covered. The company personnel staff can tell you if you are eligible and help you fill out the necessary forms.

Social Security

The Social Security Administration has two disability programs, Social Security Disability (SSD) and Supplemental Social Security (SSI). A diagnosis of AIDS, as defined by the Centers for Disease Control, establishes your disability. If you have been contributing to Social Security (FICA tax on your W-2 income tax form) and have worked the required length of time, you most likely are eligible for

SSD benefits. Benefits are based solely on your prior participation in the system and proof that you have AIDS. Eligibility for SSI is based on disability plus lack of financial resources. For either program, you apply at the nearest Social Security office whose staff is very helpful and will inform you about both programs. You will need documents to prove citizenship or legal alien status and a letter from your doctor or hospital stating that you have AIDS and are unable to work full or part time for at least one year.

Veterans Administration (VA) Benefits
If you served in the armed forces during wartime, were honorably discharged, and can present proof of permanent and total disability, you may be eligible for a VA disability pension. Check with your local VA office for information and forms.

Union Benefits
If you belong to a union, check with your representative about eligibility for disability programs.

Health Insurance

Individual or Group
Whether you are sick or not, check what your policy covers. Some policies are comprehensive, but others are not. You may wish to supplement the coverage of your present policy. Ask your insurance company about your present policy and possibly desirable additional riders. It is a good idea to compare the policies and costs of several companies for supplemental coverage or even a change to a more advantageous plan.

Government
Most states provide some medical coverage for people with limited financial assets and no medical insurance. Proof of citizenship or legal residency and financial documents to show need are necessary to establish eligibility. In many states, the program covers a wide range of services, such as homemaker help and medical equipment. Local hospitals and social service departments can give you information and necessary application forms.

Veterans Administration
If you are a veteran with an honorable discharge, you can obtain medical care at the nearest VA hospital/clinic. Except for medical

emergencies, veterans with service-connected disabilities are given preference.

Community Resources

Hospitals
The medical staff of teaching hospitals, especially in major cities, is more likely to be experienced in treating AIDS patients. Inquire at your local hospital if any members of the staff have special AIDS training. Many hospitals offer crisis intervention services as well as individual, family, and group therapy. Hospitals that receive federal funding have at least one trained social worker knowledgeable about community resources and entitlement programs who will be able to help you.

Psychotherapy/Counseling Services
Crisis intervention involves on-the-spot telephone and in-person counseling, which can be vitally important to AIDS patients and families. This service is available from hospitals, mental health clinics, and special AIDS support programs. Some churches and synagogues also offer counseling services in addition to pastoral care.

Psychotherapy can be appropriate for the individual, the family, and concerned groups. Therapeutic approaches vary with the training of the therapist and the orientation of the clinic. Which psychotherapeutic counseling is best depends on the needs and circumstances of the patient and family. Psychotherapy services are available through hospitals, clinics, specialized agencies, and private practitioners. Before choosing, ask about staff credentials and costs.

Agencies developed in response to AIDS, such as the Gay Men's Health Crisis and the AIDS Resource Center in New York City, and Shanti in San Francisco, can make referrals to experienced practitioners. Groups such as the American Psychiatric Association, the American Psychological Association, the Society of Clinical Social Work Psychotherapists, and gay and lesbian clinical psychotherapy associations may also be good sources for referrals.

Funeral directors can also help families and friends when it becomes a question of coping with emotionally difficult burdens rather than patient survival. It is advisable to obtain advance information about burial and cremation procedures and costs. State funeral directors' associations can supply the information.

Home Health Agencies

Home health agencies provide services in the home. Every state has a visiting nurse service. At the request of a physician, a nurse will assess the patient's health needs and offer skilled nursing care in the home. The service may also provide homemakers, home health attendants, social workers, and physical therapists. Homemakers do shopping and light housekeeping; home health attendants help with bathing, personal care, and household chores. In large cities, both public and private agencies offer in-home health-support services, and some have staff specially trained to assist with AIDS patients.

The American Red Cross of Greater New York offers a training program, "Home Nursing for AIDS Care Givers," for family and friends of AIDS patients. The course covers basic skills and information necessary for the appropriate care of homebound AIDS patients. It also teaches precautions to control the spread of the disease.

Specialized Agencies

Cancer

For AIDS patients who have Kaposi's sarcoma, a form of cancer, agencies such as the American Cancer Society and Cancer Care are a source of special help, ranging from homemaker services to payment of some of the costs of transportation for hospital visits and the purchase of medical equipment. Cancer Care also offers both individual and group counseling.

Gay Men's Health Crisis, New York City

The need for a special group to deal with the AIDS crisis was made clear at a meeting in August 1981 addressed by Dr. Alvin E. Friedman-Kien. Dr. Friedman-Kien had been credited with citing new cases of Kaposi's sarcoma as an unprecedented outbreak of an old disease of older men in a new context—relatively young, gay men. It was proposed at the meeting of about 80 men to form a group to raise money for medical research. The group became known as the Gay Men's Health Crisis (GMHC).

As the need grew, GMHC, a nonprofit organization, expanded its purpose and services and now has 42 full-time and 2 part-time employees and over 1,100 volunteers. Its structure is open and fluid, with no exclusionary rules and no requirements for membership other than a genuine concern about the health of gay men.

In addition to funding medical research projects, GMHC provides a full range of clinical and educational services. All prospective patients who contact GMHC for help are visited within 24 hours by a licensed mental-health professional from the admissions division. After a comprehensive, psychosocial interview, a report is written with recommendations for treatment and referral to one or more GMHC services, which include crisis intervention counseling, buddy support, patient recreation, an AIDS self-help support group, an AIDS therapy group, a care partner therapy group, a women's support group, financial counseling, and individual psychotherapy.

GMHC also disseminates accurate, up-to-date information and advice about AIDS to the general public and to high-risk groups through regularly held public forums and training seminars, an around-the-clock AIDS Hotline, technical assistance to other volunteer organizations, newsletters and brochures, and maintenance of an archive of published information on AIDS. The GMHC telephone number is (212) 807-6655, and its mailing address is Box 274, 132 West 24 Street, New York, NY 10011.

AIDS Resource Center, New York City

The AIDS Resource Center (ARC) was founded in February 1983 by a group of concerned volunteers who had lost friends or lovers to AIDS. It coordinated its activities with GMHC to fill gaps in service, particularly in housing, direct financial assistance, and spiritual support.

ARC developed short- and long-term housing resources for AIDS patients with the goal of establishing hospice-like facilities and is seeking a suitable building and location to be used as a hospice. It gives grants or loans up to $500 to each AIDS patient needing financial help. Recipients sometimes repay in kind, for example, by doing clerical work or manning the telephone at ARC.

The spiritual support rendered by ARC is unique, and includes weekend retreats for patients and close associates in a scenic, secluded area of Connecticut. A holistic plan encompasses Christian worship, nutrition, exercise, and meditation. Participation in programs is voluntary, and scholarships are available for those unable to pay.

Group therapy at ARC differs from that at other agencies in the use of prayer as the primary source of solace. ARC also offers bereavement counseling, in both individual and group sessions.

Formal spiritual counseling embraces all major religious groups, including all Protestant denominations, all three divisions of the Hebrew faith, Muslims, and various sects. ARC is preparing an educational packet about AIDS for distribution to all churches in the metropolitan New York area.

ARC also sponsors a hospital visit program in cooperation with the Volunteer and Social Work Departments at Bellevue Hospital Center, New York City. Bellevue volunteers receive basic training in working with acutely ill patients, addressing spiritual needs, and using community resources. This program supplements the GMHC buddy system. The volunteers visit AIDS patients only in the hospital and cooperate with the hospital social work staff in providing appropriate service.

Shanti Project, San Francisco

The Shanti (Sanskrit for "inner peace") Project, also a nonprofit organization, was founded in 1974 by Dr. Charles Garfield to provide free volunteer counseling services in the San Francisco Bay area to individuals and families facing life-threatening illness and bereavement. Volunteers are carefully screened, receive extensive training and continuing supervision, and attend weekly support group meetings.

Shanti contracted with the San Francisco Department of Public Health to provide supportive services to the community made necessary by the AIDS epidemic. Funding for Shanti's work comes from the City and County of San Francisco, foundations, and individual contributions.

Services of the Shanti Project include:

Individual Counseling—Volunteer counselors work on a one-to-one basis with AIDS patients and their loved ones and are available for short or long terms according to individual needs. A Shanti volunteer will visit home or hospital.

Support Groups—Support groups are open to patients with AIDS or chronic AIDS-like symptoms and their lovers, families, and friends.

Community Volunteer Program—Shanti volunteers help AIDS patients in such practical tasks as running errands, arranging transportation, grocery shopping, preparing meals, and housecleaning.

Residence Programs—Long-term, low-cost housing is provided for AIDS patients with housing problems. Eligibility requirements include three-month previous residence in San Francisco, a medical diagnosis of AIDS, financial need, displacement from previous residence, and the ability and willingness to participate in the housing program. Application for housing involves filling out forms to establish eligibility and an interview with the Residence Director. Placement depends upon available vacancies. Assistance in finding interim housing is given through the Shanti Residence office, the AIDS/KS Foundation, and the City of San Francisco. Since eligibility requirements are subject to change, those interested should contact the Shanti Project directly.

Newsletter—A monthly newsletter is available to AIDS patients. It contains such information as services offered at low or no cost, educational and social meetings and activities, medical updates, and alternative forms of therapy.

Counseling at San Francisco General Hospital—By special contract with the hospital, Shanti counselors serve an inpatient unit and an outpatient clinic and provide both individual counseling and support groups for patients, lovers, families, and friends.

Training and Educational Seminars—Shanti holds seminars for the public and for professionals caring for the ill and the bereaved. Special programs are available to social service agencies, health-care institutions, counselors, clergy, universities, and the general public. Shanti also advises groups that want to establish similar services in their own communities.

Shanti requires direct contact from anyone requesting counseling service unless physical circumstances make it impossible. Its telephone number is (415) 588-9644, and its mailing address is 890 Hayes Street, San Francisco, CA 94117.

SUMMARY

AIDS patients are forced to make many difficult psychological and social adjustments. They are faced with often painful illness and treatment, possible loss of job, income, and independence, and reassessment of social and personal needs. Relationships change— some become strained, others develop greater depth and value. It is essential that patients, families, and friends avail themselves of the psychological and social support of the community. In addition to agencies described here, a comprehensive list of health resources, hotlines, and referral centers is given in chapter 25.

21   AIDS and Mental Health

JAMES W. DILLEY
PETER B. GOLDBLUM

The psychological impact of AIDS (see chapter 20) is far-ranging, affecting those who have the disease, those at risk, and those who care about and for AIDS patients. What happens when the psychological and social stresses of the disease become too much to handle? Where can a person turn for help? What kind of assistance best addresses the special needs of those with AIDS-related problems? These were some of the questions the San Francisco Department of Public Health asked a group of mental health specialists early in the epidemic. From ensuing discussions a new agency, the AIDS Health Project, was born. The project is primarily funded by the health department and is affiliated with the Department of Psychiatry at the University of California at San Francisco.

The purpose of the project is to assure that appropriate mental health services are available to people with AIDS or AIDS-related complex (ARC), and others at risk for the disease. It also serves family, friends, health-care professionals, and others who are concerned. To accomplish this, the project set out four goals: (1) develop an understanding of the complex relationship between AIDS and mental health, (2) develop ways to help people with AIDS-related mental health problems, (3) take steps to apply the acquired knowledge and techniques through existing medical and mental health agencies, and (4) when needed, establish new programs to address unmet mental health needs.

In this chapter we want to share the experience of the AIDS Health

Project, in the hope of giving the reader a better understanding of the relationship between AIDS and mental health problems and an awareness of the various kinds of help that may be available. We also hope this experience will be useful to individuals and agencies interested in developing community programs to address the mental health needs of those affected by AIDS. To be considered are: how AIDS affects mental health, the process of adapting to the changes AIDS brings about, some of the mental health problems that arise, mental health services needed to help manage the problems, and some of the techniques developed by the AIDS Health Project to meet the special needs associated with the AIDS epidemic.

UNDERSTANDING AIDS AND MENTAL HEALTH

Experience has shown that most people are able to adjust adequately to the psychological and social impact of AIDS; with the help of friends and community they manage, after an initial period of shock, to resume their daily lives. In fact, some people have risen to the challenge and grown psychologically from the experience. Others are not so fortunate. For them, the distress of facing AIDS is overwhelming and psychologically devastating. For mental health specialists, the first recourse to combat the emotional upheaval of AIDS is prevention. If we can teach people to recognize the warning signs of mental health problems and provide interpersonal support throughout the community, we can help them avoid the more severe and incapacitating emotional reactions. The next aim is to assist those who do develop problems. By understanding the usual course of the disease, we can recommend an array of mental health services to help with problems such as severe anxiety, depression, difficulties with drug abuse, and neurologic disorders.

Adaptation

Adjusting to events as devastating as AIDS requires calling upon deepest inner resources. Whether someone is able to deal with such demands is determined partly by the nature of the situation, for example, having AIDS oneself or having a loved one diagnosed with AIDS or die from the disease, and partly by personal factors, such as having coped with traumatic events in one's past. Another dimension is important—time. An appreciation that it takes time to adapt to severe life changes, and that certain expected reactions tend to occur, can relieve undue pressure to "hurry up and adjust." Also, such understanding can help to answer the question "How am I doing?" and to determine whether additional help is needed in coping with trying circumstances. Although we will describe how a patient adapts to being diagnosed with AIDS, it should be remembered that parallel processes of adaptation are at work in those who care for people with AIDS and, for that matter, those adjusting to living in a community where AIDS has become epidemic.

Reaction to Diagnosis

Coming to terms with the inescapable knowledge of having AIDS is a shock, especially for those who did not experience an extended earlier period of milder AIDS-related complex (ARC). For those who had previous signs that their immune systems were not functioning properly, but were able to block out the significance of the signs, the diagnosis is the end of being able to avoid the frightening possibility of being ill.

Reactions to diagnosis vary. Some patients are emotionally over-whelmed. They need immediate and compassionate attention to enable them to begin the process of adaptation. Others are like a patient of ours named Paul. A young business executive, Paul took the news stoically and, in fact, refused to discuss the matter further with his physician until he had some time to think things over. Of course, the ability to deny illness depends very much on how ill one feels. Some patients with Kaposi's sarcoma do not feel physically sick when told they have AIDS. Others, for example, those who have *Pneumocystis carinii* pneumonia and require hospitalization and immediate and total care, are undeniably ill. We have observed a somewhat unexpected reaction in some patients who previously suffered long-standing, debilitating symptoms of ARC. They received the news of AIDS with a paradoxical sense of relief, "At least now I *know* what's wrong."

Some understanding of the reactions of AIDS patients can be gained from studies of adaptation to other stressful events. Three phases have been described: stress, adaptation, and integration. With

AIDS, the response to the stress of hearing the diagnosis ranges at first from an intense emotional outcry to a numb absence of feeling, which is followed by a period of adaptation as the news sinks in and thoughts and feelings about the diagnosis become all-absorbing. Professional assistance may be needed to handle the associated anxiety and depression. At this time many AIDS patients begin to express their fears of suffering and death. Most often they alternate between an intense dwelling on their predicament and a denial of its existence. This alternation is natural and should not be combated. Individuals must be allowed to deal with emotional stress at their own rates. Freedom to do so makes them feel a reassuring measure of control. Denial is often a major defense throughout the course of the illness, especially its early stage. Using this defense is likely to be beneficial as long as it does not interfere with self-care. The final phase, integration, or emotional completion, is a state of relative calm. The fact of sickness is not all-consuming. Patients can pay attention to other matters and even discuss their illness without becoming emotionally overwhelmed.

Different individuals go through the phases of adaptation at different rates. Such differences should be expected and respected. No set time is right for everyone.

An understanding of adaptation to the fact of AIDS is incomplete without consideration of the pressure of immediate and practical problems imposed by having a life-threatening disease. Is care covered by health insurance? Can the patient continue to work? Are financial reserves adequate? What kind of social support is available and what are the implications of disclosing the illness to others?

Because AIDS fluctuates between periods of illness and relatively good health, the phases of adaptation may be repeated. Additional bouts of illness may be even more disturbing by enforcing a stronger realization of continuing disease.

Midstage of the Disease

At a midstage, for example, upon hospitalization with a second or third recurrence of *Pneumocystis carinii* pneumonia or other AIDS-related infection, further adaptation is required. An integration achieved earlier may break down, and troublesome thoughts and feelings take over once more. The ability to use healthy denial may crumble, hope be lost, and emotional exhaustion set in. It is important for a patient to feel free to express discouraging emotions when contemplating possible death and mourning the anticipated departure from loved ones. Patients frequently begin to review their lives, sometimes focusing on a particularly difficult relationship or experience, wanting to discuss it and "get it off their chests." Sometimes they want to finish unsettled business with family members and friends. Many AIDS patients seek counseling to help sort out these feelings. It is a confusing time. "How can I think about death, when I'm hoping to live?" one patient asked.

Perhaps the hallmark of the midstage of illness is the development of a personal attitude toward hope. "What can I hope for?" asked another patient. Discussions of the quality of life, and its shortness, lead many patients to decide to live one day at a time. Some vow to fight: "I want to be the one who beats this thing." They follow medical developments closely and volunteer for experimental procedures. Given the extent of medical research being conducted, and the fact that some people have survived with the disease for as long as five years, this line of thinking must be respected. A counselor must help the client balance both the gloomy and hopeful sides. As patients are able to express fears and hopes, a path of action that accommodates both can be arrived at.

The midstage of the disease adds new strains to relationships. At the AIDS Health Project we have developed special groups for couples in which one partner has AIDS. One couple, Bob and Terry, had been together for two years when Bob learned he had AIDS. At first, their relationship deepened. "We were in this thing together." After Bob's second hospitalization, in Terry's words, "He changed, withdrew, became more independent. This hurt a lot. On the one hand, I understood; on the other, I felt like I was losing him prematurely." In discussing this with other couples facing the same situation, they were able to ease the tension in the relationship. Terry was able to develop a supportive relationship with one of the other men in the group whose lover was also sick, so that he was not so dependent on Bob.

This stage of the disease has vague boundaries. When a patient enters it or moves on to the terminal stage depends partly on objective medical status and partly on subjective perception of how fast the disease is progressing.

Terminal Stage

As the disease advances, and more of the patient's vital systems become involved, a shift takes place, which requires additional attention to emotional needs. The patient whose physical condition deteriorates and who becomes increasingly weak must face the loss of independence and control. At some point, the doctor's actions focus primarily on controlling distressing symptoms such as diarrhea, nausea, and pain. Most patients are discharged from the hospital, either to be taken care of at home or to go to hospice centers. As with other stages of adaptation, most patients are able to face death with the support of loved ones and medical and nursing staffs. Practical assistance in such areas as legal matters and household chores can be supplied by a variety of volunteer and service agencies. Programs like Shanti and Hospice, which train volunteers to help patients face imminent death, are enormously helpful.

A mental health professional, especially a psychiatrist, may be called on at this time to assist the patient or the health team to plan treatment that meets both psychological and medical needs. With training in both psychology and medicine, the psychiatrist is best able to assess and differentiate emotional states that have a physical origin from those resulting from a psychological response to awareness of oncoming death. Based on this assessment, appropriate treatment, medical or psychological, can be suggested.

A common fear of patients in the terminal stage of the disease is of spending their last days in excruciating pain and discomfort. This dread sometimes leads to contemplation or even commission of suicide. Although ethical questions about suicide by the terminally ill are complex, modern drugs and humane medication practices can significantly ease final pain. Also, recent efforts have applied non-chemical methods of pain management. Relief from the worst degrees of pain has allowed many patients to pass their final days with dignity and peace.

A growing concern is the number of AIDS patients who develop neurologic disorders as part of their disease. The symptoms of neurologic damage—disorientation, confusion, memory failure, and loss of bodily control—are particularly difficult for care-givers. One lover cried with dismay, "It's like he's not there anymore. I can only vaguely recognize him." Although there are no magical solutions to this heartbreaking aspect of the disease, the psychiatrist can help the care team by suggesting ways to adjust the surroundings to protect the patient and minimize the risks of confused behavior. Psychiatric medications may also be used to help relieve confusion.

During this final stage of disease, additional attention must be paid to those who have cared about and for the AIDS patient throughout the course of the disease. Assisting loved ones and care-givers to adapt to the various stages of illness will later have great benefit when they are grieving for the ones who have died. At times, and for a variety of reasons, some people find it difficult to mourn such a loss. For example, care-givers in areas where AIDS is epidemic may become emotionally saturated by multiple deaths. The grief of others may be held in because of unsettled conflicts in their relationship with the one who has died. Counseling can be of great assistance to these people. In San Francisco we have a variety of services, such as Hospice, where they can get both individual and group support in their bereavement.

MENTAL HEALTH PROBLEMS

Most people have intense emotional reactions to extreme stress. It is natural to have strong feelings when confronted with bad news. In fact, a lack of appropriate emotions may indicate an unwillingness to deal with the situation. At some time during the AIDS crisis everyone involved will feel varying degrees of fear, anxiety, anger, and sadness. In some the anxiety may be exceptionally severe or sadness deepen into depression. The following are the most common problems that cause people concerned with AIDS to seek counseling from a mental health professional, together with guidelines that help to determine if such help is needed.

Anxiety, Fear, and Panic

Perhaps the emotional response that most often motivates people to seek professional counseling is anxiety. Of all emotions, anxiety may be the most subtle and yet pervasive. Rollo May, a psychologist who has written extensively on the subject, suggests that anxiety is the feeling of uncertainty and helplessness in the face of danger. Needless to say, the AIDS epidemic is a ready source for such feelings. Fear, like anxiety, is an emotional reaction resulting from the perception of danger. However, the objects that inspire fear are more specific than those which produce anxiety. For example, some AIDS patients need help to overcome fear of a particular treatment. One *Pneumocystis carinii* pneumonia patient we saw had a debilitating fear of having a chest tube inserted. After being taught relaxation techniques, he was able to tolerate the tube and treatment could resume. Extreme fear can grow into panic, an acute combination of fear and anxiety with dramatic symptoms, such as rapid pulse, dizziness, cold and profuse sweating, and tremors, together with a sense of impending catastrophe, pervasive inhibitions, and an overwhelming desire to flee or get help.

Depression

Depression, while similar to the sadness everyone experiences from time to time, may be considerably more serious, and professional help is advised if it lasts a long time or becomes severe and incapacitating. Depression is a term used by mental health professionals for a cluster of symptoms that may include a persistent sense of dejection ranging from relatively mild discouragement and gloominess to feelings of extreme despondency and despair. In addition, these feelings are accompanied by loss of initiative, listlessness, insomnia, loss of appetite, and difficulty in concentrating and making decisions. Depressed people frequently think of suicide and in some cases actually take their lives. In rare cases they exhibit frightening psychotic symptoms such as auditory hallucinations.

Although AIDS patients may dread the discomfort, pain, and finality of a life-threatening illness, and understandably experience sadness and anger, when these emotions turn into depression, professional assistance is indicated. Depression in AIDS patients is frequently accompanied by self-reproach and feelings of guilt for getting the disease. Unresolved conflicts about homosexuality may arise in some gay patients. A common depressive thought is that AIDS is punishment for past deeds. A sympathetic counselor can often clarify such thinking about the disease and its causes, thus helping to reduce aspects of the depression. Occasionally, depression is so severe that talking things over is not enough. In these cases, antidepressant medications have been extremely useful, but, on rare occasions, AIDS patients have had to be hospitalized for their own protection.

An illustrative example is Luther, a forty-three-year-old gay man who was seen by a psychiatrist at the outpatient AIDS clinic of the county hospital. He came at the encouragement of his lover, Albert. Luther had been diagnosed with Kaposi's sarcoma three months before coming to the clinic and had since "lost all interest in things." According to Albert, Luther sits home all day in his bathrobe with a blank stare on his face, watching TV. He has stopped caring about personal hygiene. Talks with Luther gave the impression of a man who had given up. He had trouble sleeping, frequently waking up early and not being able to get back to sleep. Since he learned of his diagnosis his appetite had fallen off. Although reluctant to talk, he was able to express deep grief and sadness and at times felt so bad he thought of ending his life.

The psychiatrist prescribed Desyrel, an antidepressant, and Luther agreed to start counseling with one of the staff social workers. During counseling, and with the aid of medication, Luther was able to talk more openly about his situation. Albert joined the counseling for several sessions, and eventually both joined one of our couples groups. When he was reevaluated by the psychiatrist six weeks later, Luther's mood had lifted, although he still felt sad and angry a great deal of the time. His sleep had improved greatly, his appetite was better, and he had more energy, helping around the house and once again enjoying his garden and being with his lover.

Drug-Abuse Problems

The problem of drug abuse by AIDS patients and those at risk has, thus far, received far too little attention. AIDS patients who abuse drugs pose several unique problems. Most who have contracted or are at risk for AIDS because they share intravenous needles are not gay and do not come from the same white, middle-class background as the typical AIDS patient. They frequently have difficulty availing themselves of services developed for the gay AIDS patient. Their problems are multiple: they must not only learn to cope with AIDS but, to receive proper medical treatment, must deal with their drug habit at a time when the stress of illness may drive some of them to depend even more on the solace of drugs, which further interferes with their treatment.

At the AIDS Health Project, we established one of the first programs to address the dual problem of AIDS and drug abuse. Specially trained counselors have developed an appreciation for the complex relationship between AIDS and the use of drugs and alcohol. These specialists help drug-abusing AIDS patients to enroll in therapeutic drug programs and also augment drug programs throughout the city with educational seminars for addicts and program staffs on the connection between the two diseases, AIDS and drug abuse. According to Barbara Faltz, director of this program, "The major obstacle in combating both problems is denial. With this group of people, one must be very firm and tell them that they are risking their lives by shooting up. The best help for them is to get into a program and clean up."

Neuropsychiatric Disorders

AIDS patients frequently develop neurologic and neuropsychiatric disorders (neuropsychiatric disorders are those whose predominant symptoms seem to have a psychological origin but actually arise from specific brain dysfunction). Since AIDS destroys the body's resistance to a variety of infections that attack the brain, and the AIDS virus itself can infest and grow in brain cells, the psychological assessment of patients is complicated and should be made by skilled practitioners.

Early symptoms are often indistinguishable from a more common depression. Subjective evidence, such as forgetfulness, poor concentration, loss of interest in usual activities, social withdrawal, and lack of motivation, must be corroborated by formal mental status testing to effectively diagnose a neuropsychiatric problem. Later symptoms include confusion and disorientation (not knowing the day or the place, getting lost, etc.) in addition to physical problems. Severe and debilitating central nervous system infections are frequently the consequence of a protracted illness. In some cases specialized treatment facilities are needed for proper patient care.

Guidelines

Many people have asked us, "How do you know if you need professional help for your problems?" There is no easy and absolute answer. One way is simply to make an appointment with a private counselor or a mental health center and use the first session to determine if further assistance is indicated. Sometimes we find that people who could benefit from counseling postpone making the decision and come in only after months have gone by and the problem has gotten out of hand. We have developed the following guidelines to help assess whether or not counseling is advisable:

1. Are your emotional reactions interfering with your everyday functioning in the home, at school, or on the job? This includes not having the energy to adequately participate in daily activities.
2. Are your emotional reactions becoming excessive and disproportionate to the situation at hand? For example, is fear becoming panic? Anger turning into rage? Sadness being replaced by depression?
3. Are your emotions interfering with your normal sleep patterns for an extended period of time (more than a week)?
4. Is there a consistent change in your eating patterns not related to your medical condition? For example, have you lost weight or have you had a surge in appetite leading to weight gain?
5. Do you have recurring thoughts of extreme actions, such as killing yourself or others? Do you feel out of control?
6. Are you using drugs or alcohol to cope with your emotions? For example, do you drink or use drugs to escape anxiety, depression, or fear?
7. Are you having distorted perceptions, such as hearing voices or seeing things that are not actually there?

If the answer is yes to any of the above, it is well to talk to a trained counselor who can evaluate the situation further.

MENTAL HEALTH SERVICES

When professional help seems advisable, where do you go? Each community handles mental health services somewhat differently. For example, some cities provide all services in one facility, perhaps connected with a large general hospital. In San Francisco, public and mental health services are distributed throughout the city to ease public access. Through the AIDS Health Project, we have placed mental health counselors throughout the system, assigning more to areas serving the highest number of people at risk for AIDS. We have counselors in mental health clinics, youth programs, and clinics for sexually transmitted diseases. We have also sent counselors into prisons to educate inmates about AIDS transmission. We advertise our services widely in gay publications and other media to make sure that those needing our services can readily find them.

Even though other communities may not have the specialized services provided in San Francisco, each metropolitan area in this country has some form of mental health system. In some communities where these services may be difficult to locate lists may be obtainable from physicians or the local health department. Many of the larger cities also have mental health services specifically for gay people, provided for the most part by gay counselors. It is important that those who decide to seek help find a counselor who respects their lifestyle and is knowledgeable about AIDS. It is legitimate to interview prospective counselors to determine if they are sympathetic or not. If not, ask for someone else.

Services usually include two broad categories: crisis intervention and mental health evaluation, and counseling and support services.

Crisis Intervention and Mental Health Evaluation

The first step in seeking help is to call for an appointment. For some this is a time of crisis—things have gotten so bad they are out of control. Others may not wait that long. In either case, the process is the same. With the help of a skilled counselor, the situation is reviewed and the kind of services needed is determined. In the public sector, this is known as an intake interview. Applicants may or may not get to talk with the one who eventually becomes their counselor. Many people seek help from private practitioners, which allows them more control over the choice of counselor. If the problem is complex or ill-defined, several sessions may be needed for clarification. These may sometimes include visiting other mental health professionals, such as a psychiatrist or psychologist, for more in-depth interviewing and perhaps testing.

Counseling and Support Services

Assistance with emotional difficulties should be part of every facet of the AIDS health-care system. Early assistance may prevent more serious problems from developing. Also, providing a place that offers compassionate support and personal caring can forestall a great deal of avoidable emotional distress. Programs like Shanti Project, which provide both individual and group support to people with AIDS, have made a remarkable contribution to enabling people to cope with their illness. They also hold out a helping hand to friends and family of those who are sick. The use of well-trained volunteers not only stretches limited resources, but the informal person-to-person contact is often more effective than more formal professional counseling. It is important, however, for volunteer programs to be backed by capable professional counselors to serve as consultants and to be available for referral of especially difficult cases.

At the AIDS Health Project we have developed group counseling strategies based on teaching patients more about the disease and how to take positive action to enhance their health so that they will be better able to handle their emotional reactions. For example, in guiding patients disabled by anxiety and depression toward an understanding of how they can exert a measure of control over their lives, we have observed that the sense of hopelessness and help-lessness abate. Bringing patients together in a group also helps to break through their feeling of isolation and challenges negative and destructive thinking. We have taken special steps to assure that the assumptions underlying the groups are made clear. Group leaders, who appreciate and value cultural differences and regard gayness as a natural variant of human behavior, see to it that their views are known to everyone in the group. Participants are taught specific techniques to help them manage the stress of AIDS. But most importantly, they are given the opportunity to talk about their feelings and reactions and gain support from others in the same situation.

In San Francisco, a variety of self-help groups have evolved. Others, like the AIDS Health Project, use professional leaders. Still others, like Shanti Project and the Stop AIDS Project, use volunteers. On a city-wide level, we have tried to develop a network of

AIDS and Mental Health 277

support services to ensure their availability to the maximum number of people who need them. The community takes great pride in its responses to this terrible tragedy. This sense of community spirit, in itself, has been important in helping many to overcome a feeling of powerlessness and summon the courage to face the darkness of AIDS.

22 Spiritual and Religious Issues of AIDS

WILLIAM A. DOUBLEDAY

AIDS and its related epidemic, AFRAIDS (Acute Fear Regarding AIDS), have raised a wide range of religious, spiritual, theological, and pastoral issues and responses. The issues are *religious* in the sense that many religious organizations and prominent figures have felt obliged to respond to the crisis in various ways, with pulpit commentary, public statements, social concern, educational efforts, pastoral care, or pointed disinterest and neglect. Serious religious magazines, such as *The Christian Century, Christianity and Crisis, National Catholic Reporter, The Witness,* and a growing number of denominational publications have devoted substantial attention to the implications of the AIDS crisis.

The issues are *spiritual* in that everyone touched by the disease, whether as patient, loved one, friend, caregiver, tends to ponder questions of life and death that transcend purely physical or emotional reactions. Issues of both meaning and longing become coupled with deep human needs for acceptance, forgiveness, hope, reconciliation, and unconditional love. These needs may be addressed in the context of organized religion or the essentially spiritual care offered by family and friends, hospice volunteers, crisis counselors, or low-key religious professionals. Distressing human emotions such as guilt, anger, and fear frequently also have spiritual dimensions.

For many involved in the AIDS crisis, thoughts and expressions emerge in words characteristic of *theology* and *ethics,* often explicit

"God talk" or religious language. AIDS raises classic issues about the meaning of life and death, the character of human sexuality, the moral implications of sexual behavior, such as homosexual practices, of drug abuse, the idea of sin and the relationship between sin and sickness, the complex choices to be made among treatment options, "code status," and other life-and-death decisions in the hospital or at home. Many patients wonder about the experience of death itself and want to discuss concepts of "afterlife."

Religious groups or individuals moved to offer *pastoral care* to the sick, the dying, or the bereaved—or to those who care for them—often have questions such as what form should such care take, by whom is it best given, and what values and attitudes is it provided or inflicted. While some religious groups, pastors, and chaplains have clearly been motivated by a vision of nonjudgmental service, others have been decidedly judgmental, even condemnatory. Still others have refrained from offering any caring support out of a conviction that the sufferers of the disease are somehow "getting what they deserve."

The underlying philosophy of the pastoral care, apart from specific AIDS-related issues, is likely to influence the way it is given by pastor or chaplain. Some, whose training was modeled on essentially psychoanalytic principles, focus on "being" rather than "doing," and tend to emphasize attentive listening and the exploration of feelings. Others, more deacon-like and service-oriented, may play a more forthright role in meeting patients' practical needs or acting as advocate for them in the health-care system. The two approaches are not mutually exclusive. They can reinforce each other when the pastor is able to achieve a genuine, compassionate presence with patients and their loved ones, including insightful listening and appropriate physical touching. Unnecessary protective clothing, such as masks, gowns, and gloves, detract from the quality of pastoral exchanges.

There can be no question that the nature of the initial risk groups for AIDS, homosexual and bisexual men and intravenous (IV)-drug abusers, heavily colored the religious community's response. The Judaeo-Christian tradition has generally deplored homosexual behavior, and in recent decades both the cause of gay civil rights and the issue of ordaining frank homosexuals have sparked heated debate and division within the liberal religious community and outrage in the conservative branches. AIDS among IV-drug abusers did not immediately alter the character of the faith community's response. In part, this was because the community tended to equate drug abuse with moral weakness rather than see it as a symptom of deeply rooted social ills that afflict the psychological, economic, and spiritual lives of many people, particularly the urban poor minorities. Only when confronted with so-called innocent victims (hemophiliacs, transfusion recipients, and infants), AIDS patients who could in no way be held culpable for exposure to the disease, did theological conservatives concede a significant uncertainty about a close link between traditional moral values and sickness or health. Still, even in mid-1986, many TV and radio evangelists and clergy of various religious groupings continued to suggest, or even proclaim, that AIDS was a punishment from God for the "sins of homosexuals and drug abusers."

More positively, recognizing the disproportionate impact of AIDS on minorities, the Council of Churches of the City of New York, under the leadership of the Rev. Dr. Robert Polk and Ms. Suki Ports, initiated a Minority AIDS Task Force in late 1985, and parallel efforts are under way in other cities. Also, a general awareness is growing that particular risk groups require specialized care, attention, and advocacy. For example, women of child-bearing age at risk for AIDS especially need counseling about the danger to as yet unborn or unconceived children.

Some religious groups have taken the position that, though they cannot and must not condone behavior their tradition considers immoral, they are bound by a strong scriptural mandate to carry out works of mercy for the sick, the suffering, and the dying. Sometimes it is not clear whether they perform such works for the sake of caring, as an exercise in pity, or for self-satisfaction.

In many parts of the United States, a long-standing commitment to caring for the sick has characterized the Roman Catholic Church's response. Its hospitals and nursing orders have been in the forefront of medical and pastoral care for AIDS sufferers in many cities. In New York City, for example, St. Vincent's Hospital, and its Hospice headed by Sister Patrice Murphy, are well known for their superior compassionate care for all sorts of people with AIDS, and Cabrini

Medical Center and St. Clare's Hospital also have made a serious commitment to high quality AIDS medical care. Mother Theresa of Calcutta has been involved in organizing a hospice-type facility under the sponsorship of the Roman Catholic Archdiocese of New York, despite the fact that its Archbishop, John Cardinal O'Connor, in collaboration with Orthodox Jewish and Salvation Army leaders, has actively opposed the New York City Gay Rights Bill, seen by many as an important protection for gay people in general and for people with AIDS in particular.

The question remains: What sort of pastoral and medical care will be given by people and institutions whose basic religious and moral attitude is negative, even punitive, toward the behavioral practices of the patient? The answer probably varies with the particular cultural and religious climates of institutions, communities, and regions of the country. In one New York City voluntary hospital, it came to light that a staff chaplain began visits with AIDS patients by saying: "I am Chaplain X. You are very sick because God is punishing you. If you repent, you might get better. Otherwise, you are going to die a miserable death. Would you like me to hear your confession now?" It is important to realize that every religious tradition and denomination has some pastors, counselors, and chaplains who are able to minister with compassion and sensitivity and others almost certain to deliver a message of guilt, judgment, or outright condemnation. Health-care teams are well advised to explore the religious and moral values and pastoral intentions of religious professionals and volunteers before accepting them for AIDS-related service. It is also important to realize that the traditions and moral attitudes of some members of the health-care team also may adversely affect the quality of care given patients and their loved ones. What is clear is that people who are sick, dying, or bereaved should be shielded as much as possible from proselytizing, judgmental attack, and intrusion into their privacy.

From January 1983 to May 1986, I served as a member of the Department of Religious Services at St. Luke's-Roosevelt Hospital Center in New York City, first as Hospice Chaplain and then as Pastoral Care Coordinator for Patients with AIDS. I was involved in varying degrees with the pastoral, psychological, and medical care of several hundred people with AIDS. St. Luke's was founded in the middle of the 19th century by an Episcopal priest and physician,

Dr. William Augustus Muhlenburg, who named the hospital after St. Luke the Evangelist and Physician, the patron saint of healing.

In keeping with Dr. Muhlenburg's vision of what Judaeo-Christian health care was all about, the large and sprawling St. Luke's Hospital at Amsterdam Avenue and 113th Street in Manhattan is centered around a chapel. It is almost impossible to go anywhere in the hospital without passing the chapel. At the foot of the chapel steps one's eyes are drawn toward the altar and the beautiful stained glass window over it. The window portrays the 25th chapter of the Gospel of St. Matthew, beginning at the 31st verse where Jesus describes the final day of judgment. It is in that passage of scripture that Jesus speaks forcefully about the central importance of corporal works of mercy: feeding the hungry; housing the homeless; clothing the naked; visiting the sick and those in prison. Jesus suggests that when such care is offered to the least fortunate of our brothers and sisters it is offered to him.

In my years at St. Luke's-Roosevelt Hospital Center, I have prayed often in the chapel and been deeply moved by the images in the window. I have been struck by the painful parallels between the people to whom I have been called upon to minister in the AIDS crisis and the people to whom Jesus ministered: in Jesus' day—social outcasts, lepers, prostitutes, Samaritans, tax collectors; in our own day—homosexual and bisexual men, IV-drug abusers, prostitutes, prisoners, Haitians, hemophiliacs, and small children with AIDS born in poverty and deprivation. In light of such a scriptural mandate, and with such images and parallels in mind, a growing number of people of faith have felt called to minister compassionately and nonjudgmentally to all of God's children—men and women of all sorts and conditions, and all people with AIDS.

From the perspective of religious groups in dealing with AIDS, it is important to stress that AIDS is not a *gay* disease. It is a human disease that does not discriminate on the basis of race, gender, age, or sexual orientation. It is a disease caused by a cruel virus, not a punishment inflicted by a cruel God. In God's eyes there are no throw-away people, a view clearly expressed in the parable of the lost sheep, the parable of the lost coin, and most powerfully the parable of the prodigal son (Luke 15).

A growing number of religious groups, both Christian and Jewish, have been passing resolutions calling for care and compassion for people with AIDS. A splendid example, passed by the General Convention of the Episcopal Church at its 1985 meeting in Anaheim, California, called upon all Episcopal dioceses and parishes—upon all clergy and laity:

To offer care and compassion to all who suffer with AIDS.
To repudiate condemnation, rejection, and judgment of or upon those who suffer.
To address the need for education, including education for prevention. (This refers to safer forms of sexual behavior, the sterilization of drug paraphernalia, even discussing the facts about sex, drugs, and associated risks of exposure to the AIDS virus with teenagers and young adults.)
To pray for, liturgically remember, and sacramentally serve the sick, the dying, the bereaved, and all who care for them.

Other religious bodies also have responded with various programs and resolutions of concern. Both the Episcopal Church and the National Council of Churches scheduled a National Day of Prayer and Education on the AIDS Crisis for the autumn of 1986.

A recurring concern of many churches, which has elicited statements and comments, has been the possible transmission of AIDS by the "common cup" in the Sacrament of Holy Communion. The Episcopal Bishop of California, the Rt. Rev. William Swing, addressed this subject in a pastoral letter widely quoted in the news media. Some churches have actually eliminated or modified use of the common cup. Others have adopted or reemphasized the practice of intinction (dipping the wafer instead of sipping the wine). The consensus of most medical and religious opinion is that AIDS transmission through the common cup is *exceedingly* unlikely and no cause for worry. Yet, so many people do seem worried about it that education about this specific concern apparently must be a feature of congregational life in the 1980s.

In appraising the religious community's response to the AIDS crisis, the valuable contribution of the gay religious community itself must be acknowledged. Dozens of cities around the United States have congregations belonging to the Fellowship of Metropolitan

Community Churches (commonly referred to as MCC), a predominantly gay and lesbian denomination that has so far been refused membership in the National Council of Churches but is a source of pastoral care and emotional support in many communities for all who suffer from AIDS. Most major Protestant denominations have gay and lesbian caucus groups, for example, Integrity (Episcopalians), Reformation (Lutherans), Presbyterians for Lesbian and Gay Concerns, Affirmation (Mormons), and many gay Jewish congregations. These also are a source of care and support for people affected by AIDS. The group known as Dignity is a worshiping coalition of concerned Roman Catholic clergy, religious, and laity, many gay or lesbian themselves. They have been in the forefront of actions to meet the AIDS crisis in many parts of the country where parochial clergy and institutional chaplains have felt constrained from participating.

Such groups may help when more traditional parts of the religious community fail to serve adequately in pastoral care, hospital visitations, sacramental ministrations, counseling of loved ones, funerals and memorial services, or bereavement care. But it must be recognized that not everyone needing such services will be comfortable receiving them from gay-related or gay-identified religious groups and professionals. This is especially true of some nongay people with AIDS who feel sufficiently stigmatized by having the disease without taking on the appearance of gay affiliation. This reluctance may also apply to many parents and families of AIDS patients who are disturbed by dealings with gays and gay issues.

The religious community is well aware of the existence of *two* epidemics, AIDS and what the magazine *New Republic* has named AFRAIDS (Acute Fear Regarding AIDS). While medical science tells us that AIDS itself is not casually transmitted, AFRAIDS unfortunately is too casually transmitted by gossip, jokes, graffiti, sensationalist news and entertainment media, and some politically, socially, and theologically conservative TV and radio evangelists. While AIDS sufferers usually benefit from pastoral care, the anxieties of AFRAIDS sufferers are often aggravated by misguided religious professionals who could be countering AFRAIDS with pastoral care, education, and the setting of a compassionate example. The task of the religious community in responding to the AFRAIDS crisis is compounded by the fact that, while AIDS is unfortunately almost invariably fatal within a few years, AFRAIDS thrives in closed minds and hearts and may last for an unshortened lifetime. Many more millions are afflicted with AFRAIDS than carry antibodies to the AIDS virus in their blood.

The fears inherent in AFRAIDS are many: fear of the unknown or mysterious; fear of infection or contagion; fear of death; homophobia (fear of homosexuals); and aversion to drug users and their place in society. Deeply rooted distaste and fear are not changed overnight. But persistent education, correction of misinformation, and discussion can sometimes bring enlightenment, change, or at least the enhancement of human compassion or tolerance of people who are different. Many clergy and lay leaders today see their task as challenging the AFRAIDS epidemic through preaching, teaching, pastoral care, public advocacy, and acting as caring and compassionate—even vulnerable—examples.

The Judaeo-Christian tradition regarding homosexuality has been the subject of debate, thoughtful contemplation, and scholarly investigation. Some of the best literature includes: John Boswell's *Christianity, Social Tolerance, and Homosexuality,* John Fortunato's *Embracing the Exile,* John J. McNeill's *The Church and the Homosexual,* Virginia Mollenkott and Letha Scanzoni's *Is the Homosexual My Neighbor?,* Norman Pittenger's *Making Sexuality Human,* and James B. Nelson's *Embodiment.* Dr. Nelson, Professor of Christian Ethics at United Theological Seminary of the Twin Cities, characterized four basic positions in current Christian views on homosexual behavior: rejecting-punitive, rejecting-nonpunitive, qualified acceptance, and full acceptance. (A similar spectrum of views probably exists in the Jewish community.)

The prevailing opinion of the general population is still largely *rejecting-punitive,* but many religious groups and leaders probably now embrace a *rejecting-nonpunitive* position, which regards homosexual behavior as morally flawed but individual homosexuals as humans worthy of concern. In theory, this position "condemns the sin and loves the sinner."

A substantial number of theological and ethical thinkers have gradually come to a position of *qualified acceptance.* This emphasizes pastoral care of the individual and respect for an individual's personal qualities but stops short of categorical acceptance of gay and lesbian lifestyles. Those holding such a position are more likely to support civil rights protection for gays.

The fourth theological position, held by Dr. Nelson himself and this writer, is *full acceptance*. In essence, this considers sexual orientation to be morally neutral. Drawing upon exhaustive exegesis of biblical passages that seem relevant to homosexuality, and incorporating insights from modern psychological and sociological research, an ecumenical array of commentators now share this position. They conclude that homosexuals, bisexuals, and heterosexuals all have the potential to be loving or unloving, creative or destructive, mutually fulfilling or narcissistic. All sexual behavior must take into account the existence of the AIDS health crisis and the ways the deadly virus is spread. But moral and pastoral attention is better directed toward the quality of life and deeds than toward sexual orientation. Long pastoral experience suggests that the vast majority of homosexuals do not simply choose to be gay, but rather are responding to feelings deeply rooted in their hearts, minds, bodies, and sense of themselves. In spite of some claims of changes in homosexual orientation with spiritual or psychiatric assistance, the evidence is largely inconclusive or unconvincing.

Those who are troubled by a liberalization of the religious community's perspective on homosexuality may find a precedent in the change of attitudes toward divorce and remarriage. Until very recently, most religious bodies held a punitive and essentially nonpastoral position on questions of divorce and remarriage. From the Christian vantage point, it can be argued that the scriptural case against divorce is much stronger than the case against homosexuality. Not one word in the four Gospels refers to homosexuality, but Jesus' words clearly condemn divorce. Fundamentalists who cite the Old Testament (Leviticus) injunction against male homosexuality neglect the other issues to which a literal reading of Leviticus might also invite a less than compassionate response. (For example, the chapter that seems to call for stoning homosexuals to death prescribes a similar punishment for adulterers.)

A reasonable conclusion is that the time has come for us to be more humane and compassionate, to regard each person as an individual rather than a member of a labeled group, and to become less judgmental, ostracizing, and rejecting, not only of people who have divorced and remarried, but of those who are gay. More and more pastors, ethicists, and theologians, from various traditions, find such an attitude in keeping with the essential spirit of their faith.

To be effective, the pastoral and spiritual care of people with AIDS and their loved ones must take into account individual religious feelings and beliefs. A helpful guide is suggested by Sister Anne Munley in *The Hospice Alternative*. In evaluating the spiritual care of dying hospice patients, Munley distinguished five basic religious personality types, each of which she felt required care attuned appropriately to personal differences. She designated them:

Atheist/Agnostic
No Religion/Metaphysician
Personal Religion
Personal and Institutional Religion
Institutional Religion.

Though her research did not include people with AIDS, my own pastoral experience with AIDS patients in both hospice and hospital confirms that her categories are informative and relevant.

Atheist/Agnostics are really quite rare, even in the gay community where alienation from organized religions has long been common. Nevertheless, people with strong antireligious views or conscientious believers in a world without God should be protected from proselytizing, attacks on their convictions, and invasion of their privacy. Religious professionals, such as a chaplain, may offer friendship or even a general kind of spiritual solace, but these should be acceptable to and demonstrably meet the needs of the patient. They should not be merely an exercise of a felt duty or a projection of the pastor's own assumptions.

Patients and others in the "No Religion/Metaphysician" category also should have their personal views accepted without challenge. However, they are more likely than Atheists/Agnostics to enter into and even initiate discussions of spiritual matters such as good and evil or the meaning of the universe. They will however tend to shun "God talk" and other religious language.

"Personal Religion" patients and loved ones are likely not to have belonged to an organized religious body for a long time. They nonetheless have a strong sense of an eternal and loving God who is somehow a Ruler of the Universe. More often than not, they derive a sense of comfort from their belief in some kind of caring God. Not only do they pray and probably read the Bible, but often appreciate it when others do so with them.

Patients and others with a "Personal and Institutional Religion" are similar to those with a "Personal Religion" but differ in having a recent or continuing attachment to a local church or synagogue. For them, connections with a particular congregation and its associated sacraments or rituals take on added meaning.

Patients and loved ones characterized by "Institutional Religion" usually have strong ties to a specific tradition or congregation, and often are especially anxious about living, dying, or grieving correctly, "according to the rules." Not only is it important that the particular tradition be followed, but also the rules, regulations, and rituals that go along with it. Somewhat paradoxically, while a "Personal Religion" seems to offer some comfort in a time of crisis or despair, even when the tie to organized religion seems very slight, an "Institutional Religion" can often induce feelings of guilt, inadequacy, failure, and even hopelessness.

Pastoral care, sacramental ministrations, and counseling can often be enhanced by alertness to the personal spiritual feelings and convictions of the patients and their loved ones. Extemporaneous prayer may be suitable for one, selected scripture readings or cherished rites for another. Ecumenical, even interfaith, ministries may often be appropriate, but for many, particularly "Institutional Religion" people, a ministerial representative from the "right" church or faith may be all important.

Inevitably in AIDS care the question arises of the relationship between sin and sickness. The theological background of the subject is extensive. The entire Book of Job wrestles with it and related questions. Rabbi Harold Kushner's splendid book, *When Bad Things Happen to Good People,* is recommended reading. For Christians the 9th chapter of John's Gospel is useful. Jesus was confronted with the case of a man born blind. The question asked was: "Who sinned? The man or his parents?" Jesus answered:

It is not that this man or his parents sinned. He was born blind
so that God's power might be displayed in curing him. While
daylight lasts we must carry on the work of Him who sent Me.

Thus, the Christian focus is on healing and caring for all rather than
on the sources of or reasons for sickness. In the final analysis, people
may choose to offer care or stand in judgment.

As a chaplain I have met many judgmental health-care workers.
They say: "Patients with AIDS don't deserve our care. God is
punishing them. They brought it on themselves." To combat such
punitive attitudes I have sometimes led tours of the nursing units to
survey the sources of patients' ailments. It was evident that only the
rare patient had not in some way, to some degree, contributed to each
sickness. But only in the case of AIDS have I heard health-care
workers claim it is professional and ethical to neglect or stigmatize
patients. Blaming the victim is neither good medical care nor
acceptable pastoral care. Our mandate demands care and compassion
for all, no matter the source of disease, no matter our personal or
religious views and values—no matter how the patient acquired
AIDS.

Nothing in scripture persuades me that God punishes people with
sickness for their sins. Only an unduly anthropomorphic view of God
sees a bearded gentleman on a throne scratching his head and asking:
"Whom shall I zap today for their sinfulness? I know: Let's give lung
cancer to six smokers, liver cancer to four alcoholics, heart attacks to
four cholesterol gluttons, colon cancer to two people who neglected
to eat enough fiber, and, yes, let's give AIDS to eleven homosexual
men but spare all the lesbians."

Speaking from similar points of view, the Rt. Rev. Paul Moore,
Jr., Episcopal Bishop of New York, once observed: "If God is really
punishing people with sickness for their sins don't you think the
perpetrators of war, terrorism, and nuclear destruction would at least
get herpes?"

Many theologians see serious dangers in any religious view
grounded in either self-righteousness or works-righteousness. Most
who follow the Judaeo-Christian tradition have always asserted: "*We
are all sinners.*" Alienation and disruption enter all our lives. At

times we all fail to realize our finest and highest potential. We are all participants in systemic sins, which include racism, poverty, bigotry, inhospitality, homophobia, and indifference. In fact, these are the systemic sins that create the social circumstances in which the AIDS virus thrives.

In the final analysis, some simple theological precepts can guide each of us in our pastoral and religious response to the AIDS crisis:

God loves us.
God embraces us.
God reaches out to us.

As His people we are called to do likewise:
To love unconditionally.
To embrace all patients and their loved ones.
To reach out with care and concern even for those people we may have excluded from consideration in the past.

23   Death, Dying, and AIDS
WILLIAM A. DOUBLEDAY

Our basic views and attitudes about AIDS and about death and dying have a major impact upon the care and experience of people with AIDS and their loved ones and caregivers. The very choice of words and the tone in which they are spoken can either promote insight and comfort or encourage denial or despair.

Clearly, every AIDS patient is confronted with a life-threatening illness, but not everyone with the disease is dying in an active or immediate sense. Some quite appropriately focus on coping, on living life in the present moment and the short-term future to the fullest and richest possible extent. Continually dwelling on AIDS as invariably fatal, and prematurely describing AIDS patients as end-stage or terminal, may in fact deny patients occasions for hope and deter or discourage maximal and effective life-enhancing medical care. Though most experts agree that AIDS as defined by the Centers for Disease Control (CDC) has an overwhelming mortality rate, the survival of a growing number of men and women with AIDS and AIDS-related illnesses has far surpassed both the predictions of their physicians and the odds portrayed in mortality charts. While hospice care and palliative measures are helpful, even essential, for many patients, many others would benefit from programs rooted in positive thinking, staying well, and multidisciplinary support.

HEARING THE DIAGNOSIS

There is little question that the way we communicate with patients colors their response and their experience of the illness. We can speak of hope or we can project utter hopelessness. We can share instances of lives renewed and daily routines resumed, at least for a time: the musician who did return to the concert stage; the young woman who did travel to a long delayed reunion with her family; the patient who did become an effective public policy advocate for people with AIDS; the individual who at least managed to get personal, financial, and legal affairs in order; the man who found time to say "thank you," "good-bye," "I'm sorry" or "I love you" to some of the significant people in his life.

Too often, diagnoses and prognoses are delivered to patients and their loved ones in ways that are less than helpful or timely. Sometimes, infection control procedures, such as cautionary signs, specially colored trash bags, masks, gowns, and gloves, cruelly communicate a diagnosis symbolically long before tests are completed or a physician actually pauses to speak with the patient, family, or friends. Some institutions, in an effort to reduce fears among staff and the general public, avoid clear statements and discussions of an AIDS diagnosis. Others deliver the news briskly and insensitively, sometimes, for example, after 5 P.M. on Friday or at other times when effective sources of emotional and psychological support within the hospital may be very scarce.

Whether the message is impending death, a finding of AIDS, a milder AIDS-related condition, or simply a positive result from a blood test for antibodies to the AIDS virus, thoughtful consideration of time, place, tone, safeguards of confidentiality, and availability of supportive follow-up from health-care personnel is essential. Serious attention should also be given to the appropriate inclusion of lovers, spouses, parents or other family members, concerned and supportive friends, and possibly others who might be able to help the patient.

It is important to remember that patients and loved ones do not always absorb information the first time they hear it. Some may hesitate to ask questions or voice concerns. The health-care provider who actually sits down with the patient, extends a compassionate touch, and invites questions does much to enhance the exchange. Some physicians—particularly house staff who have borne the brunt of much AIDS-related medical care in recent years—have been heard to express frustration at how little they ultimately can do for AIDS patients. Yet often these same physicians—either due to narrow training or busy schedules—are unable or unwilling to take the time to listen to and make genuine contact with AIDS patients in ways that might help them better to come to terms with their illness. It often falls to nurses, social workers, chaplains, and volunteers to fill the role of sympathetic listener as patients and their loved ones say what is in their hearts and minds. Such listening can be stressful, but it represents an important part of psychosocial and spiritual care, and arguably even has therapeutic medical significance.

INFLUENCE OF MEDICAL, CULTURAL, AND SOCIAL ATTITUDES

In some respects, death and dying in the context of AIDS present dilemmas not unlike those of many other serious diseases at a time when advances in medical technology have made the end of life more complex and uncertain than ever before. The vast array of devices and drugs now available offer—even in AIDS care—remarkable and often seemingly endless options for treatment. Informed consent to forgo heroic medical measures and decisions not to prolong suffering are heavily laden with ambiguity and uncertainty for physician, patient, caregivers, and family alike.

One complication is the present tendency of people to take legal action at even slight provocation. Many medical decisions and, even more, institutional policies are affected by a heightened anxiety to avoid lawsuits or even accusations of malpractice or intentional neglect. Whether this serves patient care and quality of life is a debate that has only just begun.

It is also probably fair to suggest that our culture is deeply rooted in the denial of death. When an artificial-heart patient dies, astronauts are killed in a tragic explosion, an AIDS patient succumbs at the age of 27 years, or an elderly nursing home resident just slips away, a part of us resists the whole notion of human mortality in an age of such powerful medical and technological capabilities.

Political and economic forces—not unique to AIDS—also strongly affect the dying experience of patients. Federal, state, and local budget cuts, retrenchment in the insurance industry, the growth of for-profit hospital corporations, a renewed emphasis on home-care alternatives, and the advent of the diagnostic-related-group (DRG) system of reimbursing hospital costs have cast a cloud of fear and uncertainty over many aspects of the health-care field. At a time

when AIDS patients require more care and more staff, there are
fewer dollars. While hospice programs have been helpful for some
patients, many do not accept patients with AIDS. As government,
third-party medical insurance payers, and hospitals themselves are
pressing to discharge patients more quickly to reduce costs, the
community services and alternative sources of care needed by
discharged patients are frequently unprepared, or worse yet, still
unplanned.

The "cure-focused" character of modern medicine has long been
criticized for sometimes failing to meet the medical and emotional
needs of patients who embarrass their doctors by not getting better,
who in fact are going to die. Though the hospice movement has
brought welcome changes, many facilities dispensing acute care do
not necessarily provide for relief of pain and other distressing
symptoms, emotional support for patients and loved ones, or
compassionate amenities that might bring some comfort. The
experiences of many dying AIDS patients suggest that adequate
palliative care, whether in the hospital or at home, may still be
difficult to attain or sustain through the often painful and lonely
ordeal of approaching death.

AIDS also imposes some unique hardships. Other dying patients
have encountered neglect in a "cure-focused" medical system, and
dying may almost inevitably be a lonely journey, but AIDS patients
unquestionably suffer special neglect and feelings of isolation by
virtue of the fact that most come from already socially stigmatized
groups and have a disease regarded by many as mysterious and
fearsome. Attendants' unfounded fears of casual transmission, the
forbidding presence of precaution signs, and excessive protective
garb worn by health-care workers and visitors make patients feel like
lepers, social pariahs, and worse.

The relative youth of most AIDS patients has also affected the care
they have received. While some young health workers identify
sympathetically, many others shrink away. Our society is more ready
to accept those who die politely in old age than to contend with those
who commit the offense of dying too young and making us
uncomfortably aware of the inevitability of mortality and disease.

Also, in view of the newness of AIDS, too new to have been
conquered, and the hope society invests in medical, scientific, and
technological advances, based on past successes, a dying AIDS

patient has a special significance. Physicians and patients alike cling tenaciously not only to life but to expectations of new drugs, new treatment, and new medical insights either being tested or "just around the corner." This is neither evasive denial nor mere wishful thinking, but rather a positive commentary on the state of modern medicine.

FACING DEATH

In the general literature of thanatology, the Swiss psychiatrist Dr. Elizabeth Kubler-Ross wrote what has come to be a classic, *On Death and Dying.* In extensive and highly original interviews with dying patients, Dr. Kubler-Ross identified five stages in their emotional response: *denial, anger, bargaining, depression, accep- tance.* Her own later writings and the commentary of diverse professionals suggest that the word "stages" is deceptive, because the five emotional states seem to represent only points (sometimes recurring) in a continuous spectrum. It must be stressed that the feelings of people faced with life-threatening illness do not neces- sarily follow any particular sequence. The same patient may exhibit five different emotional states to five different caregivers in the course of five hours or five days. Denial, anger, bargaining, depression, and acceptance are all normal and predictable emotional responses, but each is potentially adaptive and helpful or maladaptive and destructive. Always, the attitudes of both loved ones and health- care providers should be sensitive and attuned to the individual patient.

In AIDS, even more than in most other life-threatening illnesses, *denial* can actually be extremely adaptive, especially if it does not keep the patient from receiving appropriate medical care and attending to necessary personal business. A resolute intention to beat the illness against all odds can be distinctly life-enhancing. Con- versely, a refusal to seek prompt treatment of serious opportunistic infections can hasten death. The patient whose denial *or* mental confusion *or* memory loss leads to the resumption of unsafe sexual behavior or drug abuse creates difficult problems for medical care, psychosocial support, and even public policy. Overall, in dealing with denial, the caregiver must ask: Whose need is it to get past denial, the patient's or my own?

Caregivers for people with AIDS should be prepared to be the targets of *anger*. Anger may be directed at the cosmos, at the bigotry and intolerance of the world, at the horror of AIDS, or inwardly at the self for somehow bringing on the disease. Most of such anger against others is not personal, but it is widely displaced. It is probably better that this anger come out freely as long as it does not become abusive or violent. In some instances infection of the central nervous system contributes to uncontrolled rage, and suicide attempts may represent unleashed anger turned inward. Psychiatric help and drug treatment are sometimes essential for patients troubled by intensely angry thoughts and feelings.

Bargaining by a patient can sometimes be seductive to others. Eagerness to respond positively to the patient's requests and promises may tempt the caregiver, whether doctor, chaplain, or other professional, to enter into unrealistic agreements or expectations about prognosis or treatment. For example, the patient may promise to renounce homosexuality, drug use, financial advantages, or even the extension of life beyond a certain date in exchange for certain short-term rewards or gratifications. The danger is that by participating in such "bargains," the caregiver may encourage pathological or ill-conceived expectations. While stopping drug use is certainly desirable, it is unlikely to reverse the course of illness. In the case of guilt-ridden gay patients, promises to give up their previous lifestyle, friends, and social contacts may even accentuate their feelings of isolation and neglect. Bargaining sometimes takes on cosmic or theological overtones that demand the sensitive attention of religious or spiritual counselors. It is important from the point of view of spiritual care that such "bargains" be weighed against the likelihood that they may actually undermine faith, hope, and future coping.

Only the rare AIDS patient does not experience some very intense periods of *depression*. Given the many losses patients may face— work and income, friends and social supports, body image, personal control, life itself—it is not surprising that many are sometimes overwhelmed by a sense of sadness. But it is also essential to realize that AIDS and associated tumors and infections can have a major effect on the brain and the body's chemical balance. Changes in mood, mental abilities, memory, and speech may be warning signs that need serious medical appraisal, not simply a prayer from the chaplain or referral to a social worker. Depressive episodes should be handled sensitively and individually, since the patients have ample reason to be depressed, but the symptoms may also be part of the disease.

Too few professionals stand ready to deal openly and sympathetically with patients who have reached an *acceptance* of, or at least want to talk about, dying. It is the unusual patient who ever totally reaches a point of placid acceptance of death. Most cling to some element of hope almost to the end. But most also have times and moods when they are ready to talk about death-related concerns. Some ask questions about wills, funerals, or autopsies. Some are curious about what the moment of death may feel like. Some want to know about living wills (for example, desired disposal of remains), code status (whether the doctor has ordered resuscitation if breathing or pulse stops), or what treatments they can allow or reject when all others seem to have failed. Some want to discuss spiritual and religious matters, God, heaven and hell, the afterlife, the forgiveness of past sin. Some may seek help in resolving difficult relationships or situations of alienation in their lives.

The experience of dying from AIDS is similar to that of dying from other illnesses but may be more poignant or painful because of social attitudes and association with a high-risk group. For gay and bisexual patients, the illness represents an intensified experience of "coming out," that is, disclosure of both their sexual orientation and their succumbing to a sexually transmitted disease. Needs for long-term care and the making of critical decisions may often create conflicts between gay friends or lovers on the one hand and the family on the other. For the intravenous drug abuser, whose lifestyle was a continual flirtation with death, the experience of AIDS is a prolonged exercise in depression and despair. Hemophiliacs and transfusion-related AIDS patients face equally painful difficulties in coping and adjusting, which often involve spouses and newborn infants who are at risk of infection. Talking with others in the same risk group and making use of existing support services set up by the group can often help with specific needs and concerns.

In general, the dying person should be supported and encouraged in every way possible to participate in decisions about care planning and treatment options, given every opportunity and needed assistance to put personal and financial affairs in order. It is not inappropriate for a physician, nurse, social worker, or chaplain to ask about the patient's wishes concerning wills, estate planning, "living wills," autopsies, and funeral plans. The patient should be allowed to die with some degree of dignity and some measure of control.

BEREAVEMENT OF SURVIVORS

When death does come, it is followed immediately by the difficulties of bereavement. Most of the survivors will already have wrestled with anticipatory grief. The loss of a lover, a near relative, a close friend, or one who has been under your care imposes severe psychological stress. AIDS has brought bereavement home to many who might have expected to postpone their encounter with it. The dying are suddenly no longer the aged, the long-suffering, the distant relatives, and the victims of accidents, but rather the "boy next door," the neighbor across the hall, even the loved one who slept on the other side of the bed. Bereavement exacts a heavy toll, not only on those who have lost a lover or close friend, but on families and on health-care professionals who experience a succession of losses of patients under their care.

The pain and difficulties of the bereaved in the AIDS crisis may be compounded by other considerations. Many may already have AIDS themselves. Even more live one day at a time as the "worried well." This adds to the feelings of loss, anxiety, and disorientation already brought by grief.

Also, some of the bereaved are denied their rightful place in rituals such as funerals or services. Lovers and friends often are not recognized or included when families take charge after a death. This poses serious problems when families are stubbornly ignorant or blatantly hostile toward gay relationships or lifestyles, even if long-standing. Long and costly illness may also have depleted available funds, leaving the griever with the prospect not only of loneliness but of beginning life anew with reduced financial resources.

The bereaved survivor will likely also face radically different social circumstances. Some old friends may stay away out of fear of the disease or uncertainty about what to say or do. Couples may suddenly find it difficult to include a now single bereaved friend. The griever's sadness, depression, and anger may prove unbearable to "fair weather" friends. If the bereaved is gay and still "in the closet," he may even be unable to acknowledge or express his grief in major parts of his daily life, possibly incurring the harmful effects of a sorrow held inside. Sadly, the pain is likely to be worse at certain times of the year, such as anniversaries, birthdays, Christmas, New Year's, Easter, Passover, the date of diagnosis or death, or some other dreaded or cherished date of remembrance.

Religious observances for the bereaved—funerals, memorials, burial rites, and bereavement care—are probably at best of ambivalent value to many survivors. Even as some clergy and religious groups are seeking to reach out to AIDS patients and their families and friends with some measure of love and caring, the "religious right" continues to see the AIDS epidemic as an occasion for judgment and condemnation. The funeral trade, normally eager for business, has often regarded AIDS deaths with hostility, insensitivity, and outright discrimination. Too often, families taking charge of funeral plans turn to clergy who are insensitive to both the lives and the real loved ones of the deceased. Little comfort is then offered to friends and lovers, and sometimes the pain of rejection is added to the sorrow of loss.

Although it may seem somewhat callous to compare grief over the loss of a loved one to AIDS with reactions to less devastating events, it is useful to note similarities to other human experiences of loss: being fired from a job, divorce, moving to another home, death of a pet, amputation of a limb. Researchers since World War II, when work in the field began to blossom, virtually all agree that grieving, like dying, is unique to each individual, so generalizations do not always apply. At best, models have been formed for interpreting human behavior that suggest that some responses are relatively healthy and predictable while others may be destructive and dangerously prolonged, calling for professional help.

One widely used model of grief distinguishes four stages: shock, search, disorganization, reorganization. Shock is the relatively short period during which the bereaved individual feels the sharpness of the loss and is somewhat dazed, as if struck by a blow. Life seems unreal at this stage.

The search stage is marked by emotional conflict between wanting the deceased back and needing to let the deceased go. The mourner has the sensation of wandering in circles and may even watch for the deceased at home or on the street. The deceased may be intensely present in both thoughts and dreams. Anger may arise, directed inward ("What more could or should I have done for the one I lost? Why did he get sick? How could he abandon me?), and outward against doctors and nurses ("They should have given more or better care."), and toward God. Anger may also be general and widely displaced, coloring and corroding usual relationships with others.

The third stage, disorganization, is a time of redefinition of self. Normal habits and daily routine slowly begin to return. At times the bereaved may be overwhelmed by depression, despair, and a sense of detachment from others. Feelings of loneliness can be profound, showing their effects in sleeplessness, diminished appetite, and vulnerability to physical and mental illness. Even at this stage, the impression often persists that the deceased is still alive and present.

The stage of reorganization, if reached, is marked by a more final resolution of the loss and the beginning of a reconnection with friends and the making of new social and vocational attachments. One way or another, the bereaved finds new and renewed meaning in life.

It is important to keep in mind that any "stage" theory is at best only an interpretive tool. People do not simply progress step by step through the stages, as if following a formula, but rather vary over a range of behaviors and moods with time. Different people respond differently, as is borne out by direct experience with many who have lost relatives, friends, or lovers to AIDS.

Some people adapt less well than others to grief. Often, a knowledge of the individual personality and the relationship to the deceased offers clues to concerned friends and professional counselors that help to anticipate special difficulties. Some questions commonly asked by professionals in the field are:

How great is the loss? Was it a major or minor relationship? Was there a bond of love or need?

What is the personality of the bereaved? Has the griever normally coped well with life's ups and downs in previous experiences of loss? Does he or she have a strong self-esteem and sense of identity?

Was the death anticipated? Was anticipatory grief experienced beforehand? Was the mourner prepared for the loss? Was the relationship with the deceased good at the time of death? Was there a lot of unfinished business? Was the death sudden or violent? A suicide? What was the physical appearance of the deceased when last seen? How was the news of death communicated?

What sort of network of support exists for the survivor? Are the friends or family supportive? What is the survivor's financial situation? Does the person live alone? Are religious feelings helpful or destructive at this point? Are mourning customs, funerals, or other observances available and helpful?

The bereaved— even if at no risk for AIDS—has been shown to be at increased risk for other new illnesses, exacerbation of existing illness, and accidents during at least the first year after the death of a loved one. Appropriate support and care during bereavement can often reduce such risks. Help can be provided by social rituals, group support, or individual psychotherapy. Thoughts of suicide must be taken seriously—Romeo and Juliet-style suicide pacts have been widely fantasized in the gay community in the face of the AIDS epidemic. For all the bereaved, prolonged disruption of sleep or reduction of appetite, severe depression. or inability to manage the demands of daily life and work indicate a need for prompt medical, psychological, social service, or pastoral support or intervention.

SUMMARY

The issues faced by patients dying with AIDS bear many similarities to those faced by anyone with a life-threatening illness. However, an understanding of the special sociological and cultural context of the AIDS epidemic can help in understanding and responding to each patient as an individual. There are times when the caregiver and the patient should focus on coping and on maximizing the life experience that remains. There are also many occasions when it is appropriate and desirable for the patient to discuss matters pertaining to death and dying. The approach and tone of the health-care professional or loved one can do much to facilitate communication and insight.

A variety of models are available to interpret the experiences of both the dying and the bereaved, but in the final analysis every person will benefit from individually sensitive expressions of care and concern. Even as the hour of death can rarely be predicted, the time consumed by grief is equally uncertain. The dying, their loved ones, caregivers, and survivors may all benefit from suitable medical attention, steady emotional support, sensitive spiritual care, friendly volunteer visiting, professional counseling, and group support services as may be individually appropriate.

Seven AIDS Information and Resources

24

Questions and Answers about AIDS
VICTOR GONG
DANIEL SHINDLER

WHAT IS AIDS?

AIDS is an impairment of the body's ability to fight disease. It is acquired, meaning that it is not inherited. The disease depresses the body's immune system, lowering the barriers to many opportunistic infections and malignancies. Because many characteristic signs and symptoms define the disorder, AIDS is called a syndrome, that is, a collection of many different symptoms appearing together.

The most common opportunistic infection and malignancy of AIDS patients are *Pneumocystis carinii* pneumonia and Kaposi's sarcoma, although many other infections may appear in sequence or simultaneously over the course of the disease.

There is no definitive test that can confirm a diagnosis of AIDS. However, the Centers for Disease Control (CDC) has proposed certain strict guidelines that most physicians apply in making the diagnosis. According to CDC guidelines AIDS should be suspected in anyone who is under the age of 60, develops opportunistic infections and malignancies, is a member of one of the known risk groups for AIDS, shows laboratory evidence of impaired cellular immunity, and possesses antibodies to HTLV-III/LAV. However, milder forms of AIDS-related illnesses may be overlooked by these guidelines. The full spectrum of AIDS-related illnesses is unknown, but is thought to include the lymphadenopathy syndrome (swollen glands), autoimmune disorders, and the wasting syndrome.

Thus AIDS can be characterized as a syndrome with a broad clinical spectrum ranging from severe infections and death to asymptomatic disease (for example, in carriers and patients who have recovered), including milder forms with perhaps a better outlook for recovery than overt AIDS.

WHO IS AT RISK?

The first cases of AIDS in the United States were gay men. Since then, other population groups found to be at high risk include:

Bisexual or gay men sexually active with many different male partners
Intravenous-drug abusers who share needles
Hemophiliacs and others who require transfusions of large amounts of blood and blood products
Heterosexual partners of AIDS patients
Infants and children of high-risk parents

WHAT ARE THE SYMPTOMS OF AIDS?

Symptoms may be totally nonspecific. No particular symptoms clearly establish the diagnosis of AIDS, since they may also accompany other illnesses. In its mildest forms, AIDS may even go unnoticed. In severe cases, symptoms may develop and progress very rapidly. The most common symptoms include:

Swollen glands, usually in the neck, armpit, or groin, with or without pain
Unexpected weight loss, usually 10–15 pounds or more in 2 months, not due to deliberate dieting
A persistent cough and shortness of breath not related to a "flu" or cigarette smoking
Purple or pink bumps under the skin or in the mouth, nose, and rectum, looking like bruises that don't go away
Persistent fever for over 1–2 weeks
Night sweats—waking at night drenched in perspiration, persisting for several weeks

Persistent diarrhea not explainable by diet or a "stomach virus"
A thick, whitish coating on the tongue and/or the mouth, with or
without a sore throat (oral thrush)
A variety of neurological symptoms that includes headaches,
numbness, weakness of the extremities, problems with balance,
and even psychiatric symptoms such as depression, delusion,
paranoia, hallucinations, etc.

Since AIDS can potentially affect every organ of the body, many
other symptoms may develop.

WHAT IS AN OPPORTUNISTIC INFECTION?

Without normal immune function, the body is vulnerable to assault
by many environmental toxins and pathogens. An opportunistic
infection is one that does not usually arise in a healthy person with a
sound immune system but strikes when the immune system is
defective. For example, our bodies harbor many potentially harmful
viruses, bacteria, yeasts, and possibly cancer cells. They do us no
harm because a normal immune surveillance system keeps them in
check. However, if the body's immune defenses are disabled for any
reason, these pathogens have the opportunity to flourish and create
infection. Thus, a usually local yeast infection can grow and swarm
throughout the body, and the previously rare and nonaggressive
Pneumocystis carinii can cause a severe pneumonia.

WHAT IS *PNEUMOCYSTIS CARINII* PNEUMONIA?

Pneumocystis carinii pneumonia (PCP) is the most common disease
in AIDS. It is due to a parasite and is characterized by fever, a dry
cough, weight loss, drenching night sweats, and shortness of breath.
Before AIDS was recognized, PCP was seen only rarely, in premature infants, debilitated children and adults, and patients whose
immunologic responses are suppressed by chemotherapy to combat
cancer or to prevent rejection of a transplanted organ. With the
advent of AIDS the number of PCP cases has increased dramatically.
Unfortunately, the underlying immune dysfunction hinders recovery,
and PCP is the leading cause of death in AIDS patients.

WHAT IS KAPOSI'S SARCOMA?

After PCP, Kaposi's sarcoma (KS) is the second most common disease associated with AIDS, afflicting over a third of all AIDS patients. KS is a rare malignant skin tumor that, before 1979, primarily affected elderly men of Mediterranean descent. Typically, it was limited to the skin, rarely affected other organs, and responded well to treatment. Patients often lived 8 to 13 years after diagnosis and usually died of other diseases related to old age.

Another variety of KS is found in equatorial Africa, primarily in young men under 35. This is more aggressive, may or may not respond to treatment, and can spread to other organs. Recently, this type of KS is being seen in organ transplant recipients and cancer patients undergoing chemotherapy.

KS in AIDS patients resembles the African type, primarily striking young homosexual men and aggressively spreading to other organs besides the skin, including the lymph nodes, gastrointestinal organs, and the lungs. Its symptoms are painless, nonitching skin lesions, which vary in size from an insect bite to large raised plaques and are colored dark-blue or purple-brown. They may be located anywhere on the skin or mucous membranes, though some patients may have no skin involvement. Often, patients report a history of fevers, night sweats, weight loss, and fatigue.

WHAT CAUSES AIDS?

Scientific evidence points to the human T-lymphotrophic virus (HTLV-III) as the most likely cause. The lymphadenopathy-associated virus (LAV), discovered in France, is thought to be the same or closely similar to HTLV-III. Hence the compromise term HTLV-III/LAV has been used by the scientific community. Its behavior closely parallels the epidemiologic profile of AIDS, that is, it is transmitted by sexual contact, blood transfusion, and shared intravenous needles, preferentially attacks helper T cells, and can cause malignancies. It has also been isolated in AIDS and AIDS-related complex patients, and antibodies to the virus have been detected in AIDS patients.

Other candidates that have been considered include herpesviruses such as cytomegalovirus (CMV) and the Epstein-Barr virus (EBV),

African swine fever and some other animal viruses endemic to Africa, and even possible mutations of old viruses appearing in a new form. It has also been suggested that immunodeficiency may be the result of a long series of immunologic challenges by common viruses, such as CMV and EBV, that produce an immunodepression which is then aggravated by the presence of other infectious agents, a genetic predisposition, sperm, or toxins, and develops into full-blown disease. A weakness of this multifactorial hypothesis is its failure to satisfactorily explain the appearance of AIDS in infants born to AIDS patients and in some recipients of blood transfusions.

WHAT ARE THE DIAGNOSTIC TESTS FOR AIDS?

Presently no single test can diagnose for AIDS. While routine laboratory tests cannot rule out AIDS, they can be useful in indicating the need for more extensive tests of the immune system. Numbers of red blood cells, white blood cells, and platelets are often low in patients with AIDS and AIDS-related conditions.

Also, healthy people respond to skin tests (injection of special substances called antigens under the top layer of skin) with redness and swelling at the injection site. The absence of such a reaction may indicate that the immune system is not working properly.

When immune deficiency is strongly suspected, the diagnosis may be aided by less routine tests such as lymphocyte subpopulation studies, which measure the number of suppressor and helper lymphocytes in the blood. AIDS patients typically have an abnormally high ratio of suppressor to helper lymphocytes in their blood. They have also been found to have elevated immunoglobulin levels. However, these findings, singly or in combination, are not specific for AIDS. Each is also found in patients with other illnesses.

The advent of a blood test capable of detecting antibodies to HTLV-III/LAV allows for the detection of individuals exposed to the AIDS virus. It is not a test for AIDS.

Blood samples may be taken for special treatment (called blood cultures) to promote the growth of microorganisms. Normally, blood is sterile and should contain no bacteria or other microorganisms. With immune deficiency, however, the body often lacks the defenses to prevent pathogens from multiplying in the bloodstream. These foreign organisms constitute an infection which, with appropriate blood cultures, can be identified and treated.

When a patient belongs to a known risk group for AIDS and has symptoms consistent with opportunistic diseases, the course of action is clear. For suspected Kaposi's sarcoma, a skin sample taken from the affected area is examined microscopically (biopsy) for evidence of Kaposi's sarcoma. Similarly, examination of material obtained from the lung establishes the diagnosis of *Pneumocystis carinii* pneumonia (PCP). Specimens are obtained by bronchoscopy, insertion of an illuminated tube down the throat into the airways of the lung, which permits direct inspection of lung surfaces and sampling of tissue for biopsies. If bronchial biopsies do not show PCP, and it is still suspected, open-lung biopsy is performed. This involves piercing the skin of the back or chest under anesthesia to obtain a piece of lung tissue for examination.

WHAT IS THE T-CELL RATIO AND ITS SIGNIFICANCE?

Lymphocytes are a type of white blood cell involved in the immune response. They can be subdivided into two main groups, B cells and T cells. B-cell lymphocytes are called humoral immunity and are responsible for the manufacture of proteins called immunoglobulins. Immunoglobulins circulate in the bloodstream, recognize foreign toxins, and dispose of them. T-cell lymphocytes are called cell-mediated immunity and are effective against intracellular bacteria, viruses, and fungi. T-cell lymphocytes can be further divided into two subclasses, helper T cells and suppressor T cells.

Helper T cells facilitate differentiation and activation of both T and B cells, helping to turn them "on" when needed. We usually have about twice as many helper cells as suppressor cells in our blood. In AIDS, this ratio is reversed, and we have many more suppressor cells than helper cells. The cause of this aberration is not known, but its effect may be lowered resistance against infections such as herpes, yeast, and *Pneumocystis carinii* pneumonia. Its full effect is still not well understood and is under medical investigation.

WHAT IS THE HTLV-III/LAV ANTIBODY TEST?

The HTLV-III/LAV antibody test is *not* a test for AIDS. It indicates only whether a person has been exposed to the virus that can cause

AIDS. It does not indicate whether the person is still infected with the virus or will ever develop AIDS.

The more commonly used antibody test is termed ELISA, an acronym for enzyme-linked immunosorbent assay. It detects antibodies to the AIDS virus, substances produced by white blood cells one to two months after exposure to the virus. (These antibodies are ineffective in destroying the AIDS virus.) The ELISA test has proven to be a reproducible, specific, and sensitive test for antibodies to HTLV-III/LAV, but no test is perfect. Any blood found positive by the ELISA method, and positive again on repetition of the test, is subjected to an additional complex test called the Western blot. Positive results on all three tests are considered confirmation of exposure to the AIDS virus. However, a negative antibody test does not guarantee freedom from the virus. Antibodies may not yet have developed if exposure to the virus was recent.

WHAT DOES A POSITIVE HTLV-III/LAV ANTIBODY TEST RESULT MEAN?

Again, it must be emphasized that this is not a test for AIDS. A positive test means only that antibodies to the AIDS virus have been detected. The presence of such antibodies could mean:

—the person is immune to HTLV-III/LAV
—the person is healthy but is a carrier of the virus
—the person is healthy now but may later develop overt AIDS or one of the HTLV-III/LAV spectrum of diseases
—the person is ill now and may have AIDS or an HTLV-III/LAV illness
—the result is a false positive. The person was not exposed to the AIDS virus but something else in the blood specimen reacted with the test system to cause this result.

WHAT DOES A NEGATIVE HTLV-III/LAV ANTIBODY TEST RESULT MEAN?

A negative test result could mean two things:

—the person has never been exposed to the AIDS virus
—the result is a false negative, that is, the person has been exposed to the AIDS virus but has not yet produced antibodies or has generated an insufficient quantity to be detected by this test.

A small number of AIDS patients have no detected antibodies to the HTLV-III/LAV virus. A negative test is no guarantee that a person will not develop AIDS.

WHAT SHOULD I DO IF MY HTLV-III/LAV ANTIBODY TEST IS CONFIRMED POSITIVE?

A major dilemma for blood banks and physicians is what to tell donors who have antibodies for the AIDS virus. The Centers for Disease Control has published guidelines for administering these tests. They recommend that people who test positive be told that their long-term outlook is unknown at the present time and that they will probably remain infected and can infect others. They are advised to refrain from donating blood, body organs, or semen. Toothbrushes, razors, or other items that could be contaminated with blood should not be shared. Women who test positive for HTLV-III/LAV antibody or women whose sexual partners test positive for the antibody are at increased risk of acquiring AIDS. Their offspring also are at increased risk of acquiring AIDS. These persons are advised to inform their doctors and dentists about their antibody status so that appropriate evaluations and precautions can be taken to prevent spread to others. Finally, testing for HTLV-III/LAV antibodies should be offered to individuals possibly infected by contact with others who test positive for antibodies to the AIDS virus.

HOW DO HEMOPHILIACS GET AIDS?

Hemophilia is a genetically inherited clotting disorder that affects 15,000–20,000 Americans. An absent or diminished blood-clotting Factor VIII is the cause of abnormal bleeding in some hemophiliacs. Without effective clotting, even minor cuts can cause prolonged, dangerous, and even life-threatening bleeding. For hemophiliacs, the development of Factor VIII concentrate was an important medical advance that vastly improved the quality and span of their lives. Factor VIII is extracted and concentrated from pooled blood plasma of thousands of donors. Like other transfused blood products, it has the potential for spreading infectious disease. The plasma concentrate may be contaminated with the AIDS virus.

The Food and Drug Administration has recently instituted a new heat treatment for preparing blood products such as Factor VIII. This procedure has greatly reduced the risk of transmitting infections, including AIDS, through blood products.

CAN AIDS BE CONTRACTED FROM A BLOOD TRANSFUSION?

Transfusion-linked AIDS cases have been reported. However, after more than six years of national AIDS surveillance, the observed incidence of AIDS in blood recipients is very low. Statistically, the ratio of the number of units of blood transfused to the few cases of AIDS possibly acquired by transfusion is probably greater than a million to one.

The U.S. Public Health Service has met with blood bank associations and instituted screening procedures to minimize the transfusion risk. Many safeguards have been employed. Potential donors are made aware of the general criteria before they come to donate. They are told the facts about AIDS, questioned about present health and past diseases, and advised not to donate blood if they belong to any known risk group or have any symptoms consistent with AIDS. Medical personnel question all donors about fevers, night sweats, unexplained weight loss, persistent cough, long-lasting diarrhea, bruise-like spots on the skin, and swollen glands. A medical history may be taken and a physical examination given if indicated. All blood is screened for the presence of antibodies to HTLV-III/LAV. Any containing antibodies to the AIDS virus is eliminated from the transfusion pool and used for research purposes. These measures have virtually eliminated transfusions of blood and blood products as a route for transmitting AIDS.

IS THERE A DANGER OF CONTRACTING AIDS BY DONATING BLOOD?

Absolutely not. Blood donors do not risk exposure to AIDS. All blood collection centers and blood banks use sterile equipment and disposable needles.

IS THERE ANY RISK OF CONTRACTING AIDS FROM THE NEW HEPATITIS VACCINE?

There was some concern at first about the safety of the new hepatitis B vaccine because it is made from plasma taken from carriers of hepatitis B, and carriers are predominantly homosexual men, a high-risk group for AIDS. Many potential vaccine recipients feared that vaccine processing techniques might not inactivate the AIDS agent. However, a review of vaccinated patients has revealed no increased incidence of AIDS.

The vaccine consists of particles of hepatitis virus obtained from the blood of screened, healthy, chronic hepatitis B carriers by a process called plasmapheresis (virus particles are separated from the blood by centrifugation and subjected to a complex sequence of biochemical procedures to inactivate them). The purification process precludes the survival of any viable viruses, bacteria, or fungal agents, including the AIDS virus.

Hepatitis B vaccine is strongly recommended for people, such as homosexual males, intravenous-drug abusers, and certain health-care personnel, at high risk for developing hepatitis.

SHOULD SPECIAL PRECAUTIONS BE TAKEN BY HEALTH-CARE WORKERS IN THE MANAGEMENT OF AIDS PATIENTS?

Health professionals are concerned about their occupational risk of infection as a result of their daily contact with AIDS patients, and from accidental needle sticks or other exposures to an infectious patients' body fluids. To date, there has been no evidence of AIDS transmission to hospital personnel from casual contact with AIDS patients or their laboratory specimens. Nonetheless, prudence should be exercised to minimize the risk of transmission of AIDS to hospital employees while still giving AIDS patients optimal care. Precautions should stress avoidance of direct contact of skin and mucous membranes with blood, body fluids, secretions, excretions, and tissues from patients judged likely to have AIDS (see chapter 19).

The Centers for Disease Control (CDC) combined the results of several studies that investigated the incidence of antibodies to the AIDS virus among health-care workers. Only three of 1,758 health-care workers (none members of a high-risk group) were found to have antibodies to HTLV-III/LAV. The CDC concluded that 2 of the 3 individuals interviewed (the third was an anonymous donor) probably acquired the virus through occupational exposure.

However, it is always difficult to be totally confident that additional risk factors for AIDS were absent (that is, the person may be a homosexual or unknowingly had sex with an infected partner). Also, for conclusive proof that the AIDS infection was due to exposure to AIDS patients, the antibody status would have to have been determined before as well as after exposure. A case has been reported in a nurse from Great Britain who was known to be antibody negative and then became antibody positive following an accidental needle-stick injury with the blood of an AIDS patient.

Regardless, none of these infected health-care workers has developed AIDS; they only have antibodies to the virus. The study confirms that AIDS cannot be transmitted by casual contact, and that the risk of AIDS transmission by an accidental needle stick or other inadvertent contact with AIDS-infected materials is very low. Epidemiologic studies of hospital personnel show that needle-stick injuries and cuts with instruments accounted for over 80 percent of exposures, and that 40 percent of the accidents were potentially preventable if recommended precautions had been followed.

WHEN SHOULD MASKS BE WORN?

Available epidemiologic data indicate that AIDS is not normally transmitted through the air, so masks are not routinely required. Hospital personnel should wear them only when caring for AIDS patients on respirators (mechanical breathing aids) who require frequent suctioning to clear airways, or for patients suspected of having tuberculosis or who cough frequently. Visitors entering such patients' rooms should also wear masks. A mask should cover mouth and nose. A moist mask loses its effectiveness and should be replaced.

WHEN SHOULD PROTECTIVE EYEWEAR BE WORN?

Protect the eyes wherever blood, body fluids, or secretions may be sprayed into the air. For example, a dentist's drill, a cough, or a sneeze can disperse many droplets into the air where they may remain suspended for a long time. Droplets can settle on the surface of the eye and be absorbed into the body.

WHAT IS THE PURPOSE OF GOWNS?

Gowns prevent the contact of clothes with contaminated materials. They need not be sterile, but should be disposed of properly. Hands should be washed after the gowns are discarded.

WHEN SHOULD GLOVES BE WORN?

Gloves are necessary when there is possible contact with an AIDS patient's blood, body fluid, or excretions, or with objects or surfaces contaminated by them.

IS THERE A DANGER OF CONTRACTING AIDS BY GIVING MOUTH-TO-MOUTH RESUSCITATION TO AN AIDS PATIENT?

Although the AIDS virus has been isolated from saliva, it is doubtful whether it can be transmitted by this means. Nevertheless, some concern about mouth-to-mouth resuscitation is warranted since there may be blood in the patient's mouth.

CAN PEOPLE INFECTED WITH HTLV-III/LAV, WHO HAVE NOT DEVELOPED AIDS, INFECT OTHERS?

AIDS researchers estimate that 1 to 2 million Americans are now infected with the AIDS virus. Most have no signs or symptoms and appear healthy. Initial studies predict that about 10 percent will eventually develop full-blown AIDS and another 25 percent will develop AIDS-related complex (ARC).

However, those persons infected with the AIDS virus can potentially infect others by known modes of transmission such as sexual activity and needle sharing, and may be infectious for five years during the incubation period from initial infection to development of the disease. Those found to have antibodies to the AIDS virus should practice the same precautions advised for AIDS patients. They should also have periodic medical evaluations.

IS AIDS IN THIRD-WORLD COUNTRIES DIFFERENT FROM THAT IN AMERICA OR EUROPE?

AIDS has been reported in 80 countries on 5 continents. In some places the incidence of AIDS is as high as in some major U.S. cities. In third-world countries, especially in Central Africa, AIDS has different characteristics than in America or Europe. In the early 1980s European physicians began seeing in Central African patients an unexplained immune deficiency syndrome resembling cases reported in the United States. Because of the difficulties in reporting and surveillance in these areas, concrete data are lacking. But current evidence indicates that AIDS emerged in central Africa sometime in the late 1970s and early 1980s about the same time it appeared in the United States.

In the third-world countries, AIDS is associated with different risk factors, occurs in different groups of people, and has different clinical features than its North American or European counterparts. For example, the epidemiology of African AIDS offers striking contrasts. The two most important differences are the sex distribution and the risk factors. In Africa, men and women are afflicted with the syndrome in equal numbers, which suggests that transmission of AIDS occurs both from male to female and from female to male. In one study, reported in *Lancet* (1984), most African males with AIDS were promiscuous heterosexuals, and some of the females were prostitutes. Most recent studies confirm the association between infection with HTLV-III/LAV and heterosexual promiscuity and female prostitution in central Africa. None of the African AIDS cases admitted to homosexuality, intravenous-drug abuse, or blood transfusions. However, religious rituals and poor hygiene during medical procedures (using the same syringe on many patients) may play an important role in transmitting AIDS through blood. Further evidence of heterosexual transmission of AIDS in Africa comes from the unpublished cases of two separate clusters of AIDS involving males and females with frequent heterosexual contacts.

Another example is the clinical presentation of AIDS. In Africa, AIDS appears typically as a wasting syndrome of diarrhea, severe weight loss, fever, skin rashes, and oral thrush. It is referred to locally as "Slim" disease. African AIDS is often associated with venereal disease, suggesting that sexual activity may disrupt the outer genital skin and expose it to the AIDS virus. The disease in Africa is also associated with sexual promiscuity, the use of unsterilized needles for injection of drugs, and blood transfusions.

ARE HETEROSEXUALS AT RISK FOR AIDS?

The proportion of cases not belonging to one of the established groups has shown a minimal increase, mostly due to blood product transfusions and a smaller number to sexual contact. However, a small but growing number of cases seem to involve sexually active heterosexual men and women. Heterosexual transmission of AIDS has been reported in both the United States and in Africa. However, the number of such cases in the United States remains small, less than two percent of all reported AIDS cases. When heterosexual transmission has occurred, it has been mainly from male intra-venous-drug abusers to their female sexual partners. Some preliminary reports (small studies) hint that sexual promiscuity may play an even greater role than intravenous-drug abuse in the spread of AIDS among heterosexuals.

The growing concern that AIDS may be expanding its target group was spurred by findings about AIDS in several African countries. The reason for the dramatic epidemiologic difference between Africa and the United States is unclear and may involve many risk factors not widely prevalent in American heterosexuals. For example, differences in genetic susceptibility, sexual practices, coinfection with other pathogens, and other factors that may alter the immune status (such as drugs, malnutrition) may influence susceptibility to AIDS. Heterosexuals in the United States are not exposed to the same chronic immunosuppressive environment as homosexuals with multiple sexually transmitted diseases or intravenous-drug abusers who share contaminated needles. Hence, their susceptibility to HTLV-III/LAV infection and the subsequent development of AIDS is considerably less.

Also, if lessons learned from other sexually transmitted diseases (for example, gonorrhea) are considered, then female-to-male trans-mission of the AIDS virus may be a "less efficient" mode of transmission. Finally, the proportion of women among infected persons in the United States is relatively small, about 7 percent of all reported cases.

In the United States, the Centers for Disease Control reports that about 5 percent of all reported AIDS cases belong to the category "noncharacteristic patients." These patients could not be classified into a group otherwise known to be at increased risk for AIDS. Some of the men claimed to have frequent sexual contact with prostitutes. The exact role of female prostitutes in the heterosexual transmission of AIDS in the United States has not been clearly established. Many of these prostitutes are intravenous-drug abusers and could acquire the AIDS virus by this route. Some investigators have studied the incidence of HTLV-III/LAV infection in female prostitutes from several American cities. Of 92 prostitutes tested in Seattle, 5 percent had antibodies to the AIDS virus. In Miami, 40 percent of prostitutes attending an AIDS screening clinic had HTLV-III/LAV antibodies. There is little evidence of prostitutes infecting their customers or of a woman becoming infected from her sexual partner who was exposed to a prostitute. A study of patients of New York sexually-transmitted-disease clinics showed no evidence of contagion from prostitutes.

Certainly, the public anxiety that heterosexuals harboring the AIDS virus will propagate a new pandemic of AIDS in America is out of proportion to the scientific facts so far amassed about this disease. AIDS is still difficult to acquire. Many other factors besides exposure to the virus are needed before the full-blown syndrome develops in a person with a normal immune system.

DO CHILDREN WITH AIDS POSE A RISK TO OTHER CHILDREN IN THE CLASSROOM?

The start of the 1985 school year brought heated debates and controversy about the classroom acceptance of children afflicted with AIDS. Public concern was raised about the safety of other children as well as of the AIDS children themselves who are exquisitely susceptible to any infections, even, for example, the common cold or measles. Uncertainties about contagion and transmission of AIDS fueled fears that an epidemic would develop in the American educational system. The unwarranted hysteria was exemplified in Queens, New York City, where a massive boycott of classes occurred when school officials decided to allow a young AIDS child to attend class. In Kokomo, Indiana, a 13-year-old hemophiliac with AIDS was barred from his seventh-grade classroom and now receives instruction at home via telephone.

As of June 30, 1986, 310 cases of AIDS have been reported among children below the age of 18. This number is expected to double in the next year. It does not include the potentially greater number of children infected by the virus but without overt AIDS. The majority of the children acquire AIDS virus before or during birth from their infected mother. One child was reported to be infected from sucking the milk of the mother diagnosed with AIDS. Children may also be infected by transfusion of blood and blood products.

There is no evidence that AIDS has ever been transmitted in a school, day care center, or foster care setting, or through other casual contact. None of the family members of the over 14,000 AIDS patients have been found to have AIDS, except for the sexual partners and infants of these patients. Everyday casual person-to-person contact, such as holding or playing with a child or sharing food, poses no threat of contracting AIDS. For most infected school-aged children the risks of transmitting AIDS are nonexistent.

ARE THERE ANY SPECIAL PRECAUTIONS NEEDED IN THE CLASSROOM WITH CHILDREN AFFLICTED WITH AIDS?

The CDC advises excluding from ordinary classrooms only children with AIDS who are likely to bite other children, those who are unable to control their body secretions because of a handicap, and children with uncoverable, oozing wounds or sores. In fact, the threat of infection poses a greater risk for AIDS children, whose disease-fighting abilities are impaired and who are at risk for contagious diseases from other children in a classroom setting. They are also at greater risk of suffering severe complications from such common infections as chickenpox, measles, herpes, and other viruses. The CDC also recommended that each case be decided on an individual basis, taking into consideration the child's behavioral and neurological development, physical condition, and the particular institution of attendance. Such decisions are best made by an expert team. In New Jersey, for example, the panel includes a physician with expertise on AIDS, a pediatrician, a child psychologist, and a health department physician. In New York City, a similar panel consists of medical experts, a parent, and an educator. Once the panel has decided that an AIDS child may attend classes, only the school principal and nurse will be notified that the child has the disease. Issues of confidentiality and rights of privacy are very important because of the atmosphere of fear and the potential for social isolation if the child's condition becomes known to others in the school.

ARE WOMEN AT INCREASED RISK FOR CONTRACTING AIDS?

AIDS afflicts both males and females. Of all U.S. reported cases, about 7 percent are women. More than half these women are intravenous-drug abusers, another 9 percent contracted the disease from blood transfusions, some 20 percent through heterosexual contact, and 18 percent from unknown sources.

Who are the women at increased risk for developing AIDS? Women who use intravenous drugs acquire the disease from unsterilized, shared needles. Women who are sexual partners of IV-drug abusers are also at great risk. Women whose sexual partners are hemophiliacs, bisexual or homosexual men, or promiscuous males are also at increased risk. Women who have donor insemination for pregnancy may also be at risk if the sperm donors have not been screened for antibodies to the AIDS virus. Three women in Australia were reported to have developed HTLV-III/LAV antibodies after having artificial insemination from an infected donor. And women may also acquire AIDS through blood and blood product transfusions.

Some scientists are cautiously studying the increasing incidence of AIDS among women. Much of the anxiety about the spread of AIDS to the heterosexual community stems from the rising number of women AIDS patients. At the International Conference on AIDS in Paris (1986), two disturbing reports conjured even more anxiety among the public. Dr. Warren Johnson of New York Hospital-Cornell Medical Center described his finding that in 1983 the risk groups for AIDS in Haiti were similar to those in the United States (IV-drug

322   V. Gong and D. Shindler

abusers, homosexuals, bisexuals, etc.), but in 1985 the majority of AIDS cases in Haiti were not in these risk groups but in other categories. Also, in 1985, 40 percent of the AIDS patients were women, compared to only 14 percent two years before.

At the same meeting, Col. Donald Burke of the Walter Reed Army Institute of Research reported that among nearly 300,000 army enlistees, 1.5 per 1,000 showed evidence of exposure to the AIDS virus, and the ratio of men to women who tested positive was 2.5 to 1. This contrasts with the 13-to-1 ratio of men to women in total AIDS cases in the United States. However, the army study could not absolutely exclude individuals who may be homosexuals or IV-drug abusers.

DOES AIDS PRESENT SPECIAL PROBLEMS FOR PREGNANT WOMEN?

AIDS not only threatens the mother but also the newborn. The AIDS virus is transmitted to the fetus while in the mother's womb or at birth, which accounts for most cases of AIDS in children. However, a mother has been reported to have acquired AIDS following a blood transfusion and transmitted it to her offspring through breast feedings. How frequently is the virus transmitted to the babies of infected mothers? Scientists are not exactly sure, but some studies indicate that the rate of transmission may be as high as 65 percent.

AIDS poses special risks to pregnant women. Pregnancy in normal healthy women is associated with some suppression of the immune system and may place a previously asymptomatic HTLV-III/ LAV-infected woman at risk for developing full-blown AIDS or ARC.

The CDC advises all women at increased risk for AIDS to be tested for HTLV-III/LAV antibodies. Women who test positive should delay pregnancy until more is known about AIDS and pregnancy and the effects on children. Uninfected women should be counseled on methods of avoiding infection. Infected women who are already pregnant should be counseled on the risks to their fetuses, the management of their pregnancies, and follow-up care for their infants.

25 Health Resources, Hotlines, and Referral Centers
VICTOR GONG

The following is a list of organizations and institutions in the major U.S. cities involved in the AIDS crisis. Their number is growing and their character is constantly changing. Some offer counseling, support groups, and crisis intervention, while others give medical evaluations, including diagnostic testing, screening, and patient care. All provide instructive and useful information. These resources are open to everyone, regardless of race, sex, or sexual orientation.

Inclusion in this list does not constitute an endorsement of the services rendered. It is intended only as a guide to sources of further information and assistance.

AIDS ORGANIZATIONS AT THE NATIONAL LEVEL

AIDS Action Council of the
Federation of AIDS-Related
Organizations
1115 ½ Independence Avenue, SE
Washington, DC 20003
(202) 547-3101

American Association of
Physicians for Human Rights
P.O. Box 14366
San Francisco, CA 94114
(415) 558-9353

American Hospital Association
840 North Lake Shore Drive
Chicago, IL 60611
(312) 280-6000

Gay Rights National Lobby
750 Seventh Street, SE
Washington, DC 20013
(202) 546-1801

KS Research and Education
Foundation
54 Tenth Street
San Francisco, CA 94103
(415) 864-4376

Lambda Legal Defense and
Education Fund
132 West 43rd Street
New York, NY 10036
(212) 944-9488

National Coalition of Gay STD
Services
P.O. Box 239
Milwaukee, WI 53201
(414) 277-7671

National Gay Rights Advocates
540 Castro Street
San Francisco, CA 94114
(415) 863-3624

National Gay Task Force
80 Fifth Avenue—Suite 1601
New York, NY 10011
(212) 741-5800
Crisisline: (800) 221-7044
(212) 807-6016 (New York,
Alaska, Hawaii)

National Hemophilia Association
19 West 34th Street, Suite 1204
New York, NY 10001
(212) 563-0211

National Lesbian and Gay Health
Foundation
P.O. Box 65472
Washington, DC 20035

Public Health Service
Department of Health and Human
Services
Washington, DC 20201
(202) 245-6867

FEDERAL AGENCIES INVOLVED WITH AIDS

Blood and Blood Products Division
U.S. Food and Drug
Administration
Room 220, NIH Building 29
Bethesda, MD 21235
(301) 496-4396

Centers for Disease Control (CDC)
AIDS Activity
Building 6, Room 292
1600 Clifton Road
Atlanta, GA 30333
(401) 329-3479

Health Care Financing
Administration
Hubert H. Humphrey Building
Washington, DC 21235
(202) 245-6726

National Cancer Institute
Building 31, National Institutes of
Health
900 Rockville Turnpike
Bethesda, MD 20205
(301) 496-5615

National Heart, Lung, and Blood
Institute
Building 31, National Institutes of
Health
900 Rockville Turnpike
Bethesda, MD 20205
(301) 496-5166

National Institute of Allergy and
Infectious Disease
Building 31, National Institutes of
Health
900 Rockville Turnpike
Bethesda, MD 20205
(301) 496-2263

National Institutes of Health
Building 1
900 Rockville Turnpike
Bethesda, MD 20205

Public Health Service
Hubert H. Humphrey Building
Washington, DC 21235
Hotline (800) 342-2437

U.S. Department of Health and
Human Services
200 Independence Avenue, SW
Washington, DC 20201
(202) 245-6296

U.S. Social Security
Administration
900 Altmeyer Building
Baltimore, MD 21235
(301) 594-3120

AIDS RESOURCES AT THE STATE LEVEL

Alabama

Alabama Department of Health
Room #900
State Office Building
Montgomery, AL 36130
(205) 261-5131

Alaska

Alaska Department of Health
3601 C Street, Pouch 6333
Anchorage, AK 99502
(907) 561-4233

Anchorage S.T.D. Clinic
825 L Street
Anchorage, AK 99506
(907) 964-4611

Arizona

Arizona AIDS Fund Trust
c/o Robert Hegyi
5150 North 7th Street
Phoenix, AZ 85014
(602) 277-1929

Lee Dominguez
Department of Health
State Epidemiologist and AIDS
Coordinator
Ramada Hall
431 North 24th Street
Phoenix, AZ 85008

Metropolitan Community Church
(MCC)
560 South Stone Avenue
Tucson, AZ 85701
(602) 622-4536

Arkansas

Arkansas Department of Health
4801 West Markham
Little Rock, AR
(501) 661-2395

Gay Counseling Service
Psychotherapy Center
409 Walnut Street
Little Rock, AR 72205
(501) 663-6455

California

Statewide Toll-Free Hotlines
Northern—(800) 367-2437
M–F 9:00 A.M.–9:00 P.M.
S/S 11:00 A.M.–5:00 P.M.
Southern—(800) 922-2437
7 Days 8:00 A.M.–11:00 P.M.

Fresno
Gay United Services of Fresno
606 East Belmont
Fresno, CA 93794
(209) 264-2436
Hotline (209) 264-2437

Los Angeles
AIDS Project
Long Beach Health Department
2655 Pine Avenue
Long Beach, CA 90806

City of Hope Medical Center
1500 East Duarte Road
Duarte, CA 91010
(818) 359-8111, ext. 2202, 2201

Gay and Lesbian Community
Services Center
1213 North Highland Avenue
Hollywood, CA 90038
(213) 464-7276, ext. 267

KS Foundation/Los Angeles
Gay/Lesbian Community Center
1213 North Highland Avenue
Los Angeles, CA 90038
(213) 461-1333

L.A. City/County AIDS Task
Force
313 North Figuroa Street
Room 924
Los Angeles, CA 90012
(213) 517-3228

L.A. Sex Information Hotline
8405 Beverly Boulevard
Los Angeles, CA 90048
(213) 871-1284

L.A. Shanti Foundation
8568 Santa Monica Boulevard
West Hollywood, CA 90069
(213) 874-2030

Social Security AIDS Community
Liaison
Shirley Burkhardt
6730 Sunset Boulevard
P.O. Box 1391
Hollywood, CA 90078
(213) 468-3188

Southern California Physicians for
Human Rights
Suite 109, #165
7985 Santa Monica Boulevard
Los Angeles, CA 90046
(213) 464-7666

Sacramento
AIDS & KS Foundation/
Sacramento
2115 J Street - Suite #3
Sacramento, CA 95816
(916) 448-2437

Social Security AIDS Community
Liaison
Nancy Vise
Area Director's Office
P.O. Box 214008
Sacramento, CA 95821
(916) 484-4788

San Diego
Mayor's Task Force on AIDS
San Diego Health Department
1700 Pacific Highway
San Diego, CA 92101
(619) 236-2705

Owen Clinic
University of California
San Diego Medical Center
235 Dickinson Street
San Diego, CA 92103
(619) 294-3995

San Diego AIDS Project
4304 Third Avenue
San Diego, CA 92103
(619) 294-2437

San Diego Community Clinic
3705 Mission Blvd.
San Diego, CA 92109
(619) 488-0644

San Francisco
AIDS Activity Office
Room #323
101 Grove Street
San Francisco, CA 94102
(415) 558-2381

AIDS Fund/San Francisco
1547 California Street
San Francisco, CA 94109
(415) 441-6407

AIDS Health Project
333 Valencia Street, 4th floor
San Francisco, CA 94103
(415) 626-6637

American Association of
Physicians for Human Rights
P.O. Box 14366
San Francisco, CA 94114
(415) 673-3189

Bay Area Physicians for Human
Rights
P.O. Box 14546
San Francisco, CA 94114
(415) 558-9353 (Administration)
(415) 372-7321 (Medical inquiries)

Berkeley Gay Men's Clinic
2339 Durrant Avenue
Berkeley, CA 94704
(415) 644-0425

Kaposi's Sarcoma Clinic
University of California
400 Parnassus
Room A-328
San Francisco, CA 94143
(415) 476-1363

KS Research and Education
Foundation
54 Tenth Street
San Francisco, CA 94103
(415) 864-4376

Outpatient AIDS Clinic
San Francisco General Hospital
Ward 86
995 Potrero
San Francisco, CA 94110
(415) 821-8830

Shanti Project
890 Hayes Street
San Francisco, CA 94117
(415) 558-9644

Social Security AIDS Community
Liaison
Patti Bittenbender
Area Director's Office
200 Center Street—Room 308
Berkeley, CA 94704

Social Security AIDS Regional
Coordinator
Tom Parent
100 Van Ness Avenue, 2nd Floor
San Francisco, CA 94102
(415) 556-7029

San Jose
AIDS Project
Department of Public Health
2220 Moorpark Avenue
San Jose, CA 94128
(408) 299-5858

Social Security AIDS Community
Liaison
David Janott
Area Director's Office, Suite 4070
280 South First Street
San Jose, CA 95113
(408) 291-7431

Santa Barbara
Four County AIDS Task Force
300 San Antonio Road
Third Floor, Building B
Santa Barbara, CA 93110
(805) 967-2311

Santa Barbara Health Department
Health Care Services
300 North San Antonio Road
Santa Barbara, CA 93110
(805) 967-2311, ext. 455
Hotline (805) 963-3636

Colorado

Colorado AIDS Project
1615 Ogden
Denver, CO 80218
(303) 837-0166

El Paso County Health Department
Clinic
601 North Foote Street
Colorado Springs, CO 80909
(303) 578-3148

Gay and Lesbian Health Alliance
P.O. Box 6101
Denver, CO 80206
(303) 777-9530

University of Colorado Health
Clinic
Section B—Outpatient Section
University of Colorado Health
Services Center
7200 East 9th Street & Colorado
Boulevard
Boulder, CO 80302
(303) 394-8879

Connecticut

AIDS Project-New Haven
P.O. Box 636
New Haven, CT 06503
(203) 624-2437

Hartford Gay Health Collective
281 Collins Street
Hartford, CT 06120
(203) 724-5194

Medical Clinic
Yale-New Haven Hospital
20 York Street
New Haven, CT 06511
(203) 785-4629

Yale Self-Care Network
17 Hillhouse Avenue
New Haven, CT 06520

Delaware

Delaware Lesbian and Gay Health
Advocates
608 West 28th Street
Wilmington, DE 19802
(302) 764-2208

G.L.A.D.
P.O. Box 9218
Wilmington, DE 19809
(800) 342-4012
(302) 652-3310

**District of Columbia
Washington, DC**

George Washington University
Hospital
901 23d Street NW
Washington, DC 20037

Washington Hospital Center
Section of Disease Information
Room 2A-7
110 Irving Street NW
Washington, DC 20010
(202) 541-0500

Whitman-Walker Clinic
2335 18th Street, NW
Washington, DC 20009
(202) 332-5295
Hotline (202) 833-3234

Florida

Key West

AIDS Action Committee
Florida Keys Memorial Hospital
P.O. Box 4073
Key West, FL 33041

AIDS Education Programs
(in affiliation with Florida Keys
Memorial Hospital)
5900 Junior College Road
Key West, FL 33040
(305) 294-5531

Florida Keys Memorial Hospital
Clinic
5900 Junior College Road
Key West, FL 33040
(305) 294-5537

Monroe County Health Department
Public Service Building
Junior College Road
Key West, FL 33040
(305) 294-1021

Miami

AIDS Project-University of Miami
Medical School
Department of Medicine
R-60
1611 Northwest 12th Avenue
Miami, FL 33136
(305) 549-7092

AIDS Support Group
c/o MCC Church
23d St. & NE 2nd Street
Miami, FL
(305) 573-4156

Health Crisis Network
c/o KIPP
P.O. Box 521546
Miami, FL 33152
(305) 634-4636 until 9:00 P.M.
Hotline (305) 358-HELP

Jackson Memorial Hospital
AIDS Center
1611 Northwest 12th Avenue
Miami, FL 33136
(305) 547-6231

Orlando

Orange County Health Department
P.O. Box 3187
Orlando, FL 32802
(305) 420-3347

Tallahassee

Department of Health and
Rehabilitative Services
Florida Health Program Office
Building 1, Room 115
1317 Winewood Boulevard
Tallahassee, FL 32301
(904) 488-2905

Tampa

U.S. Veterans Administration Hospital & University of South
Florida-College of Medicine
13000 North 30th Street
Tampa, FL 33612
(813) 974-4096

University of South Florida
Main Lab, Medical Clinic S.
12901 North 30th Street
Tampa, FL 33612
(813) 974-4214

Georgia

AID Atlanta
811 Cyprus Street, NW
Atlanta, GA 30309
(404) 872-0600

Centers for Disease Control
AIDS Activity
Building 3, Room 5B-1
1600 Clifton Road
Atlanta, GA 30333
(404) 329-3472

Georgia Association of Physicians
for Human Rights
1175 Cumberland Road, NE
Atlanta, GA 30306
(404) 876-8587

Hawaii

Hawaii Department of Health
P.O. Box 3378
Honolulu, III 96801
(808) 548-5986

Sexual Identity Center
2139 Kuhio Avenue
Suite 213
Honolulu, HI 96801
(808) 926-1000

Idaho

Idaho Department of Health
Bureau of Preventive Medicine
Health & Welfare Building
450 West State Street
Boise, ID 83720
(208) 334-4303

Illinois

Chicago Department of Health
50 West Washington
Chicago, IL 60602
(312) 744-7573

Cook County Hospital/Scheer-
Sable Clinic
1835 West Harrison Street
Chicago, IL 60612
(312) 633-7810

Howard Brown Memorial Clinic
AIDS Action
2676 N. Halstead Street
Chicago, IL 60614
(312) 871-5777 (Office/Medical)
(312) 871-5776 (Hotline)

Indiana

Indiana AIDS Task Force
c/o Community Hospital
1500 North Ritter
Indianapolis, IN 46219
(317) 353-5858
Hotline (317) 543-6200

Indiana State Board of Health
Chronic & Communicable Disease
Control
1330 West Michigan Street
Indianapolis, IN 46206
(317) 633-8414

Iowa

Scott County Health Department
Communicable Diseases
428 Western Avenue
Davenport, IA 52801
(319) 326-8618

Louisiana

Crescent City Coalition
c/o St. Louis Community Center
1022 Barracks Street
New Orleans, LA 70116
(504) 568-9619

Health Department of the City of
New Orleans Clinic
320 South Claiborne Street
New Orleans, LA 70112
(504) 586-4668
Hotline (504) 525-1251

New Orleans AIDS Task Force
1014 Dumaine
New Orleans, LA 70116
(504) 899-0482

Maine

Bangor Health Department/S.T.D.
Clinic
103 Texas Avenue
Bangor, ME 04401
(207) 947-0700

Maryland

AIDS Project of the Cancer Center
University of Maryland
22 South Green Street
Baltimore, MD 21201
(301) 528-7394

Gay Community Center Clinic
241 W. Chase Street
Baltimore, MD 21201
(301) 837-2050

Health Education and Resource
Organization
(H.E.R.O)
101 West Read, Suite 819
Baltimore, MD 21201
(301) 947-2437

Johns Hopkins Hospital
Blalock III
600 North Wolfe
Baltimore, MD 21205
(301) 955-3150
(301) 955-7090 Clinic

Mayor's AIDS Study Group
111 North Calvert
Baltimore, MD 21201
(301) 396-3851

Massachusetts

Boston City Hospital
HOB 320
818 Harrison Street
Boston, MA 02118
(617) 424-5000

Boston Department of Health
AIDS Hotline
(617) 424-5916

Fenway Community Health Center
or AIDS Action Committee
16 Haviland Street
Boston, MA 02215
(617) 267-7573

Massachusetts General Hospital
c/o Infectious Disease Clinic
Fruit Street
Boston, MA 02114
(617) 726-3812
(617) 726-2000 (switchboard)

Mayor's Ad Hoc Committee on
AIDS
c/o Boston City Hall, Room 608
Boston, MA 02201
(617) 725-4849

Michigan

Henry Ford Hospital
2799 Grand Boulevard West
Detroit, MI 48202
(313) 876-2563

Minnesota

AIDS Support Group
c/o 2309 Girard Avenue, South
Minneapolis, MN 55405

Minnesota AIDS Project
1010 Park Avenue
Minneapolis, MN 55408
(612) 371-0180

Minnesota AIDS Project
c/o Lesbian & Gay Community
Services
124 W. Lake Street, Suite E
Minneapolis, MN 55408

Mississippi

Mississippi Department of Health
P.O. Box 1700
Jackson, MS 39201
(205) 261-5131

Mississippi Gay Alliance
P.O. Box 8342
Jackson, MS 39204
(601) 353-7611
Hotline (601) 353-7611

Missouri

Gay and Lesbian Health Clinic
P.O. Box 2696
Kansas City, MO 64142
(816) 931-4470

Metropolitan St. Louis Task Force
on AIDS
P.O. Box 2905
St. Louis, MO 63130
(314) 768-8100, ext. 2437

Montana

Judith Gedrofe, RN
State Epidemiologist
Health Services and Medical
Facilities Division
Department of Health
Cogswell Building
Helena, MT 59620
(406) 444-4740

Nebraska

Dr. Paul A. Stoesz
Office of Disease Control
State Department of Health
P.O. Box 95007
Lincoln, NE 68509
(402) 471-2937

Nevada

Nevada Division of Human
Services
Communicative Disease Office
505 East King Street Room 200
Carson City, NV 89701
(702) 885-4800

New Hampshire

John Hedderick
VD Program Public Health
Advisor
Bureau of Communicable Disease
Control
Public Health Service
Health and Welfare Building
Hazen Drive
Concord, NH 03301
(603) 271-4490

New Hampshire Feminist Health
Center
232 Court Street
Portsmouth, NH 03801
(603) 436-6171

New Jersey

**New Jersey AIDS Helpline
(201) 596-0767**

AIDS Health Center
Newark Beth Israel Center
201 Lyons Avenue
Newark, NJ 07112
(201) 926-8025

Mid-State Prison
(609) 723-4221, ext. 228

New Jersey Lesbian and Gay AIDS
Awareness
c/o St. Michaels Medical Center
268 High Street
Newark, NJ 07102
(201) 596-0767

New Jersey State Department of
Health
Communicable Disease Service
Room 702 CN 360
Trenton, NJ
(609) 292-7300

New Jersey State Department of
Health
Northern Regional Office
(201) 266-1910

St. Francis Hospital
601 Hamilton
Trenton, NJ 08629
(609) 599-5000

St. Michael's Hospital
306 Martin Luther King Blvd.
Newark, NJ 07102
(201) 877-5525
Hotline (201) 596-0767

University Hospital
100 Bergen Street
Newark, NJ 07103
(201) 456-6000

New Mexico

New Mexico AIDS Task Force
Department of Health and
Environment
State of New Mexico
P.O. Box 968
Santa Fe, NM 87504
Hotline (505) 827-3201

New Mexico Physicians for Human
Rights
P. O. Box 1361
Espanda, NM 87532
(505) 753-2779

New York
Statewide Toll-Free Hotline
(800) 462-1884

Albany
AIDS Council of Northeastern
New York
332 Hudson Avenue
Albany, NY 12210
(518) 434-4686
Hotline (518) 445-2437

Albany Medical Center
New Scotland Avenue
Albany, NY 12208
(518) 445-3125

New York State AIDS Institute
New York State Department of
Health
Albany, NY 12237
(518) 473-0641
Hotline (518) 473-0641

Binghamton
Southern Tier
56 Whitney Avenue
Binghamton, NY 13901
(607) 772-2803

Buffalo
Western New York AIDS Program
647 West Delavan
Buffalo, New York 14222
(716) 881-1275
Hotline (716) 881-2347

New York City
AIDS Medical Foundation
Suite 1266
230 Park Avenue
New York, NY 10169
(212) 949-7410

AIDS Resource Center
235 West 18th Street
New York, NY 10011
(212) 206-1414

AIDS Unit
New York City Human Rights
Commission
52 Duane Street
New York, NY 10007
(212) 566-1826, 566-5446

Bellevue Hospital
New York University Medical
Center
First Avenue & 27th Street
New York, NY 10016
(212) 561-5151

Beth Israel Medical Center
10 Nathan Place
New York, NY 10003
(212) 420-2650

Gay Men's Health Crisis
P.O. Box 274
132 W. 24th Street
New York, NY 10011
(212) 807-7035
(212) 807-6655

Gay Men's Health Project
74 Grove Street, #21
New York, NY 10014
(212) 691-6969

Memorial/Sloan-Kettering Hospital
1275 York Avenue
New York, NY 10021
(212) 794-7722

New York City Department of
Health
Office of Gay and Lesbian Health
Concerns
125 Worth Street, #806
New York, NY 10013
(212) 566-6110

People with AIDS
Box G-27
444 Hudson Street
New York, NY 10014
(212) 929-5741

Roosevelt Hospital and AIDS
Clinic
St. Luke's-Roosevelt Hospital
Center
428 West 59th Street
New York, NY 10019
(212) 554-7221

St. Mark's Clinic
88 University Place
New York, NY 10003
(212) 691-8282

Social Security AIDS Community
Liaison
Gary Goodman
26 Federal Plaza
New York, NY 10278
(212) 264-9420

Social Security AIDS Regional
Coordinator
Camille Mahr
26 Federal Plaza, Room 743
New York, NY 10278
(212) 264-7299

Rochester
AIDS-Rochester/Rochester AIDS
Task Force
153 Liberty Pole Way
Rochester, NY 14604
(716) 232-7181
Hotline (716) 244-8640

Stonybrook
Long Island AIDS Project
LIAP-SAHP-HSC
SUNY at Stonybrook
Stonybrook, NY 11794
(516) 444-2437

Syracuse
Central New York AIDS Task
Force
Room 407
306 S. Salina Street
Syracuse, NY 13202
(315) 475-2430
Hotline (315) 475-2437

Ohio
Statewide Toll-Free Hotline
(800) 322-2437

Akron
Akron City AIDS Task Force
Akron Health Department
177 South Broadway
Akron, OH 44308
(216) 375-2960

Cincinnati
Ambrose Clenent Health Clinic
STD Clinic
3101 Burnet Avenue
Cincinnati, OH 45229
(513) 352-3143

Cincinnati AIDS Task Force
U.C. College of Medicine
231 Bethesda Avenue
Cincinnati, OH 45267
(513) 352-3143
Hotline (513) 352-3138

Cleveland
Cleveland Clinic Foundation
9500 Euclid Avenue
Cleveland, OH 44106
(216) 444-5258

Cleveland/Cuyahoga AIDS Task
Force
Cleveland Health Department
1925 South Clair Avenue
Cleveland, OH 44114
(216) 664-2525

Cleveland Health Issues
11800 Edgewater Street, #206
Lakewood, OH 44107
(216) 822-7285 (Daytime)
(216) 266-6507 (After 6 P.M.)

Free Medical Clinic of Greater
Cleveland
12201 Euclid Avenue
Cleveland, OH 44106
(216) 721-4010

Gay Education and Awareness
Resources
2100 Fulton Road
Cleveland, OH 44102
(216) 651-1999
Hotline (800) 332-2437

Health Issues Task Force
P.O. Box 14925 Public Square
Cleveland, OH 44114
(216) 266-6507

University Hospital AIDS Referral
Center
2065 Adelbert Road
Cleveland, OH 44106
(216) 844-3227

Oklahoma

Healthguard Foundation
2135 NW 39th
Oklahoma City, OK 73112
(405) 525-9333

Oklahoma Blood Institute
1001 Lincoln Boulevard
Oklahoma City, OK
(405) 239-2437

Oklahoma City Memorial Hospital
University of Oklahoma School of
Medicine
P.O. Box 26307
Oklahoma City, OK 73126
(405) 271-4700

Oklahoma for Human Rights
P.O. Box 52729
Tulsa, Oklahoma 74152
(918) 587-4297
Hotline (918) 587-GAYS

Oregon

Community Health Support
Services
c/o Phoenix Rising/Cascade AIDS
Project
408 Southwest 2d Avenue,
Room 403
Portland, OR 97204
(503) 233-8299

Oregon AIDS Task Force
c/o Dr. Mark Loveless
10535 NE Glisan
Portland, OR 97220
(503) 254-8812
Hotline (503) 254-8812

Oregon State Health Division
1400 SW Fifth Avenue
Portland, OR 97201
(503) 229-5792

Pennsylvania
Statewide Toll-Free Hotline
(800) 692-7254

Graduate School of Public Health
University of Pittsburgh
A-417 Crabtree Hall
Pittsburgh, PA 15261
(412) 624-3928

MCC-Pittsburgh
4401 5th Avenue
Oakland, PA 15217
(412) 681-0765

Philadelphia AIDS Task Force
1129 Spruce Street
Philadelphia, PA 19101
(215) 232-8055
Hotline (215) 232-8055

Pittsburgh Community Health
Services
121 South Highland Ave.
2nd Floor-Highland Bldg.
Pittsburgh, PA 15206
(412) 624-5046

State AIDS Task Force
Pennsylvania Department of Health
Health and Welfare Blvd.
Harrisburg, PA 17120
(717) 787-3350
Hotline (800) 692-7254

Rhode Island

Rhode Island Department of Health
Division of Disease Control
75 Davis Street
Providence, RI 02908
(401) 277-2362

South Carolina

State Department of Health and
Environmental Control
Bureau of Communicable Diseases
2600 Bull Street
Columbia, SC 29201
(803) 758-5621

South Dakota

Kenneth A. Senger
State Epidemiologist
Department of Health
523 East Capitol
Pierre, SD 57501
(605) 773-3364

Tennessee

Lifestyle Health Services
17270 Church Street
Nashville, TN 37203
(615) 329-1478

University of Tennessee Center for
Health Science
956 Court Ave., Room 3B09
Coleman Building
Memphis, TN 38163
(901) 528-5932

Texas

AIDS Project
Oak Lawn Counseling Center
5811 Nawsh
Dallas, TX 75235
(214) 351-1502
Hotline (214) 351-4335

Baylor University Hospital
3500 Gaston Avenue
Dallas, TX 75246
(214) 820-0111

KS/AIDS Foundation of Houston
3317 Montrose Boulevard
Houston, TX 77006
(713) 524-2437

Mayor's Task Force on AIDS
City of Houston
P.O. Box 1562
Houston, TX 77521
(713) 342-0100, ext. 117

Memorial City Hospital
920 Frostwood
Houston, TX 77024
(713) 932-3000

Parkland Hospital
5201 Perry Hines Blvd.
Dallas, TX 75235
(214) 637-8000

Safeweek AIDS Project
1627 West Rosewood
Box 5481
San Antonio, TX 78201
(512) 736-5216
Hotline (517) 733-7300

The Montrose Clinic
104 Westheimer
Houston, TX 77006
(713) 528-5531
(713) 528-5535

University of Texas System Cancer
Center
M.D. Anderson Hospital and
Tumor Institute
Texas Medical Center
Houston, TX 77030
(713) 792-2666/3020

Utah

Utah Community Services Center
and Clinic
525 South 500 East
Salt Lake City, UT 84102
(801) 533-6056
Hotline (801) 533-0927

Utah State Health Department
P.O. Box 45500
Salt Lake City, UT 84145
(801) 533-6191

Vermont

Vermont Department of Health
60 Main Street
Burlington, VT 05401
(802) 863-7240

Virginia

Richmond AIDS Information
Network
Fan Free Clinic
1721 Hanover Avenue
Richmond, VA 23220
(804) 355-4428
Hotline (804) 358-6343

Virginia Department of Health
101 Governor Street, Room 701
Richmond, VA 23219
(804) 786-6029

Washington

Gay Men's Health Group
P.O. Box 1768
Seattle, WA 98111
(206) 322-7043

Harbor View Medical Center
STD Clinic
324 9th, ZA-85
Seattle, WA 98104
(206) 223-3000

Northwest AIDS Foundation
P.O. Box 3499
Seattle, WA 98114
(206) 329-3927

Shanti-Seattle
P.O. Box 20698
Seattle, WA 98102
(206) 324-7920

West Virginia

Preventive Health Services
State Department of Health
151 Eleventh Avenue
South Charleston, WV 25303

Wisconsin

Brady East STD Clinic
1240 East Brady Street
Milwaukee, WI 53202
(414) 964-0965
Hotline (414) 271-3123

Governor's Council on Gay and
Lesbian Issues
State Capitol
Madison, WI 53707
(608) 267-8739

National Coalition of Gay
Sexuality
Transmitted Disease Services
(NCGSTDS)
P.O. Box 239
Milwaukee, WI 53201

Wyoming

Wyoming Department of Health
Hathaway Building, 4th Floor
Cheyenne, WY 82002
(307) 777-7953

Glossary

Acyclovir: A new antiviral agent

AIDS: Acquired immune deficiency syndrome

Aids-related complex (ARC): A heterogeneous group of clinical disorders in high-risk individuals, related to but not necessarily prodromal for AIDS, including diffuse lymphadenopathy, fever, profound fatigue, weight loss, and diarrhea. ARC is usually accompanied by depressed cell-mediated immunity similar to but less severe than that found in AIDS.

Anemia: A condition in which the number of red blood cells is reduced

Antibody: A protein made by the immune system to inactivate antigens and help fight infections

Antigen: A foreign substance that activates the immune system

Autoimmune disease: A condition in which the body's immune system attacks its own tissues

Antibiotic: A drug used to fight bacterial infection

Bacterium: A one-celled microscopic organism

Biopsy: Removal of a tissue sample for examination to establish a diagnosis

Blood count: A laboratory test to determine the number of red cells, white cells, and platelets in the blood

Bone marrow: A soft material in the center of bones where blood cells are manufactured

Bone marrow transplant: Removal of bone marrow from a donor and transfusion of the marrow into a recipient

Cancer: A group of diseases characterized by an uncontrolled growth of abnormal cells that can destroy surrounding tissues and spread to other organs of the body

Candidiasis: A yeast infection that typically affects the tongue, mouth, and esophagus (oral thrush), appearing as white, curdlike patches

Chemotherapy: Administration of anticancer drugs

Cryptosporidiosis: An infection due to a protozoan, commonly seen in cattle and cattle handlers, that usually causes a self-limiting diarrhea but, in AIDS, results in severe diarrhea that can lead to dehydration and malnutrition

Cytomegalovirus: A virus of the herpes family that can cause illnesses that range from flu-like infections to hepatitis, pneumonia, and brain infections

Encephalitis: A serious infection of brain tissue

Endemic: Present in the community at all times (usually referring to a disease)

Epidemic: A disease that affects many people in a particular area at the same time

Epidemiology: The study of the relationships of various factors to the incidence and distribution of a disease

Epstein-Barr virus: A virus that lives in the nose and throat and causes mononucleosis. It has been directly linked with Burkitt's lymphoma.

Etiology: The cause(s) or origin(s) of diseases

Fungus: A member of the plant family that includes yeast, molds, mildew, and mushrooms

Gastrointestinal: Pertaining to organs of the digestive system

Helper-suppressor T-cell ratio: Ratio of the number of helper T cells to the number of suppressor T cells. Normally 2 to 1 in a healthy person, but reversed in AIDS.

Hemophilia: A hereditary blood-clotting disorder that almost exclusively affects males

Hepatitis: Inflammation of the liver, causing jaundice, vomiting, malaise, fevers, and abdominal pain

Herpes simplex I: A herpesvirus that commonly causes cold sores on the mouth and face

Herpes simplex II: A sexually transmitted herpesvirus that causes painful sores around the anus or genitals

Herpes varicella-zoster: The virus responsible for chickenpox in children and shingles in adults

HTLV-III/LAV: Human T-cell lymphotropic virus type III and lymphadenopathy-associated virus are both the same virus or closely similar. Members of the retrovirus family, they are considered a primary cause of AIDS.

Iatrogenic: Resulting from the activities of a physician

Idiopathic (or Immune) thrombocytopenic purpura (ITP): An autoimmune disorder involving a low platelet count that can result in symptoms from easy bruising to bleeding

Immunity: The body's ability to resist disease by a system of defense mechanisms, including the action of antibodies, various white blood cells, and other agents

Immunodeficient: Having an impaired or nonfunctioning immune system

Immunomodulation: Attempts to change the body's immune responses (e.g., to restore an AIDS-impaired immune system back to normal)

Immunotherapy: A treatment of cancer and other diseases with substances that enhance the body's own natural defenses

Incidence: Number of cases of a disease occurring during a given period

Incubation period: The lapse of time from the entry of a germ into the body to the appearance of disease symptoms

Interferon/Interleukin: White blood cell products, called lymphokines, found at abnormal levels in AIDS patients. Interferon is a protein made by the lymphocyte that prevents viruses from infecting other cells.

Intravenous: Into the vein

Lymphadenopathy: Also known as swollen glands. The lymph nodes are swollen, may be tender and firm, and can be the result of many causes besides AIDS.

Lymph nodes: Glands that fight infection by filtering out germs and producing antibodies, and that usually becomes swollen when infection, cancer, drug reactions, or other disease conditions exist in the body

Lymphatic system: A circulatory system of vessels, spaces, and lymph nodes that fight infection

Lymphocytes: White blood cells, called B cells (bursa-dependent) or T cells (thymus-dependent), that are an important part of the immune system

Lymphomas: Cancers of the lymphatic system

Malignant: Cancerous

Meningitis: A serious infection of the membranes surrounding the brain

Metastasis: Spread of cancer from one part of the body to another to form new tumors

Morbidity: Condition of being diseased

Mycobacterium avium-intracellulare **(MAI):** An unusual form of bacteria, similar to tuberculosis, that lives in the airways of our lungs. It rarely causes illness in healthy people, but in AIDS patients can cause disease in many different organs.

Natural killer cells: T cells important in the body's destruction of tumor cells

Neoplasm: An abnormal growth of tissue, either benign or malignant

Opportunistic infection: Infection by a microorganism that may be common in the environment but causes disease only in a host with a poorly functioning immune system

Parasite: An organism that depends on food from a host for survival

Plasmapheresis: A sophisticated form of filtration that separates cells and other products from blood

Platelet: A component of blood that helps in clotting and wound healing

Prevalence: Number of cases of a disease existing at a given time

Prodrome: A collection of signs and symptoms that may precede the onset of overt disease

Protozoa: One-celled microscopic animals

Radiation therapy: Treatment of cancer with high-energy radiation such as X-rays

Red blood cells: Disc-shaped blood components that carry oxygen to body tissues

Reticuloendothelial system: A part of the immune system involved with phagocytosis (engulfing and destroying) of antigens

References and Sources

Chapter 1. Facts and Fallacies: An AIDS Overview

Abrams DI, Mess TP, and Volberding, PA. *Lymphadenopathy: Update of a 40-month prospective study.* Read before the International Conference on Acquired Immunodeficiency Syndrome, Atlanta, GA, 1985

Centers for Disease Control. *Pneumocystis* pneumonia in Los Angeles. *Morb Mortal Wkly Rep* 1981; 30:250–252

———. Persistent generalized lymphadenopathy among homosexual males. *Morb Mortal Wkly Rep* 1982; 31:249–251

———. Acquired immunodeficiency syndrome update. *Morb Mortal Wkly Rep* 1983; 32:465–467

———. Update: Acquired immunodeficiency syndrome (AIDS)—United States. *Morb Mortal Wkly Rep* 1984; 32:688–691

———. Prospective evaluations of health-care workers exposed via parenteral or mucous-membrane routes to blood and bodily fluids of patients with acquired immunodeficiency syndrome. *Morb Mortal Wkly Rep* 1984; 33:181–182

———. Revision of the case definition of acquired immunodeficiency syndrome for national reporting—United States. *Morb Mortal Wkly Rep* Acquired Immunodeficiency Syndrome, Atlanta, GA, 1985

———. Heterosexual transmission of human T-lymphotrophic virus type III/lymphadenopathy-associated virus. *Morb Mortal Wkly Rep* 1985; 34:561–563

———. Update: Evaluation of human T-lymphotropic virus type III/lymphadenopathy associated virus in health-care personnel-United States. *Morb Mortal Wkly Rep* 1985; 34:575–579

———. Update-acquired immunodeficiency syndrome—United States. *Morb Mortal Wkly Rep* 1986; 35:17–21

Chamberland ME, Castro KG, Haverkos HW, Miller BI, Thomas PA, et al. Acquired immunodeficiency syndrome in the United States: An analysis of cases outside high-incidence groups. *Ann Intern Med* 1984; 101:617–623

Fauci A et al. Acquired immunodeficiency syndrome: Epidemiologic, clinical, immunologic, and therapeutic considerations. *Ann Intern Med* 1984; 100:92–106

Fauci AS, Masur H, Gelmann EP, et al. The acquired immunodeficiency syndrome: An update. *Ann Intern Med* 1985; 102:800–813

Friedman-Kien AE, Laubenstein LJ, Rubinstein P, Buimovici-Kien E, et al. Disseminated Kaposi's sarcoma in homosexual men. *Ann Intern Med* 1982; 96 (Part 1):693–700

Gong V. Acquired immunodeficiency syndrome. *Am J Emergency Room Med* 1984; 2(4):336–346

Gong V, Kelen G, and Sivertson K. AIDS update. *Maryland Med J* 1986; 35:361–371

Harris C, Small CB, Klein RS, et al. Immunodeficiency in female sexual partners of men with the acquired immunodeficiency syndrome. *N Engl J Med* 1983; 308:1181–1184

Haverkos HW and Curran JW. The current outbreaks of Kaposi's sarcoma and opportunistic infections. *Cancer J Clin* 1982; 32(6)

Ioachim HL, Lerner CW, and Tapper ML. Lymphadenopathies in homosexual men. *J Am Med Assoc* 1983; 250:1306–1309

Kornfield H, Vande Stouwe RA, Lange M, et al. T-lymphocyte subpopulations in homosexual men. *N Engl J Med* 1982; 307:729–731

Landesman SH, Ginzburg HM, and Weiss SH. The AIDS epidemic. *N Engl J Med* 1985; 312:521–525

Masur H. The acquired immunodeficiency syndrome. *DM* 1983; 30(1): 5–48

Masur H, Michelis MA, Grene JB, et al. An outbreak of community-acquired *Pneumocystis carinii* pneumonia: Initial manifestations of a cellular immune dysfunction. *N Engl J Med* 1981; 305:1431–1438

Metroka C, Cunningham-Rundles S, Pollack M, et al. Generalized lymphadenopathy in homosexual men. *Ann Intern Med* 1983; 99:585–591

Morris L, Distenfeld A, Amorosi E, and Karpatkin S. Autoimmune thrombocytopenic purpura in homosexual men. *Ann Intern Med* 1982; 96:705–713

Rabkin C, Lekatsas A, Walker J, O'Donnell R, Garcia N, and Thomas P. *Acquired Immunodeficiency Syndrome in Heterosexual Males Associated with Sexual Contacts.* Read before the International Conference on Acquired Immunodeficiency Syndrome, Atlanta, Georgia, 1985

Redfield RR, Markham PD, Salahuddin SZ, et al. *Heterosexual Promiscuity: An Emerging Risk Factor for HTLV-III Disease?* Read before the International Conference on Acquired Immunodeficiency Syndrome, Atlanta, Georgia, 1985

Salahuddin SZ, Groopman JE, Mardham PD, et al. HTLV-III in symptom free seronegative persons. *Lancet* 1984; 2:1418–1420

Sarngadharan MG, Popovic M, Bruch L, Schupbach J, and Gallo RC. Antibodies reactive with human T-lymphotropic retroviruses (HTLV-III) in the serum of patients with AIDS. *Science* 1984; 224:506–508

Scott GB, Buck BE, Letterman JG, Bloom FL, and Parks WP. Acquired immunodeficiency syndrome in infants. *N Engl J Med* 1984; 310:76–81

Weiss SH, Saxinger C, Rechtman D, et al. HTLV-III infection among health-care workers: Association with needle-stick injuries. *J Am Med Assoc* 1985; 254:2089–2093

Chapter 2.   Assembling the AIDS Puzzle: Epidemiology

Brun-Vezinet F, Rodouzioux C, Montagnier L, et al. Prevalence of antibodies to lymphadenopathy-associated retrovirus in African patients with AIDS. *Science* 1985; 226:453–456

Centers for Disease Control. *Pneumocystis* Pneumonia—Los Angeles. *Morb Mortal Wkly Rep* 1981; 30:250–252

————. Kaposi's sarcoma and *Pneumocystis* pneumonia among homosexual men—New York City and California. *Morb Mortal Wkly Rep* 1981; 30:305–308

————. Persistent, generalized lymphadenopathy among homosexual males. *Morb Mortal Wkly Rep* 1981; 30:249–251

————. Diffuse, undifferentiated non-Hodgkin's lymphoma among homosexual males—United States. *Morb Mortal Wkly Rep* 1982; 31:277–279

————. Update on Kaposi's sarcoma and opportunistic infections in previously healthy persons—United States. *Morb Mortal Wkly Rep* 1982; 31:291–301

————. Update on Kaposi's sarcoma among Haitians in the United States. *Morb Mortal Wkly Rep* 1982; 31:353–361

————. A cluster of Kaposi's sarcoma and *Pneumocystis carinii* pneumonia among homosexual male residents of Los Angeles and Orange counties, California. *Morb Mortal Wkly Rep* 1982; 31:305–307

————. *Pneumocystis carinii* pneumonia among persons with hemophilia A. *Morb Mortal Wkly Rep* 1982; 31:355–357

————. Update on acquired immunodeficiency syndrome (AIDS) among patients with hemophilia A. *Morb Mortal Wkly Rep* 1982; 31:644–652

_____. Possible transfusion-associated acquired immunodeficiency syndrome (AIDS)—California. *Morb Mortal Wkly Rep* 1982; 31:652–654

_____. Antibodies to a retrovirus etiologically associated with acquired immunodeficiency syndrome (AIDS) in populations with increased incidences of the syndrome. *Morb Mortal Wkly Rep* 1984; 33:377–378

_____. Heterosexual transmission of human T-lymphotropic virus type III/lymphadenopathy-associated virus. *Morb Mortal Wkly Rep* 1985; 34:561–563

_____. Update: Acquired immunodeficiency syndrome—Europe. *Morb Mortal Wkly Rep* 1985; 583–589

_____. Task Force on Kaposi's Sarcoma and Opportunistic Infections. Special Report: Epidemiologic aspects of the current outbreak of Kaposi's sarcoma and opportunistic infections. *N Engl J Med* 1982; 306:248–252

Clumeck N, Carael M, and Rouvroy D. Heterosexual promiscuity among African patients with AIDS. *N Engl J Med* 1985; 313:182

Clumeck N, Sennet S, Taelman H, et al. Acquired immunodeficiency syndrome in African patients. *N Engl J Med* 1984; 310:492–497

Curran JW, Morgan WM, Hardy AM, Jaffe HW, Darrow W, et al. The epidemiology of AIDS: Current status and future prospects. *Science* 1985; 229:1352–1357

Frank E, Weiss SH, Compass JC, Bienstock J, Weber J, et al. AIDS in Haitian-Americans: A reassessment. *Cancer Research* 1985; 45:4619s–4620s

Gottlieb MS, Schroff R, Schanker HM, et al. *Pneumocystis carinii* pneumonia and mucosal candidiasis in previously healthy homosexual men; evidence of a new acquired cellular immunodeficiency. *N Engl J Med* 1981; 305:1425–1431

Groopman JE and Volberding PA. The AIDS epidemic: Continental drift. *Nature* 1984; 307(19)·211–212

Marx JL. Acquired immune deficiency syndrome abroad. *Science* 1983; 222:998–999

Piot P, Quinn TC, Taelman H, et al. Acquired immunodeficiency syndrome in a heterosexual population in Zaire. *Lancet* 1984; 65–68

Van de Perre V, Rouvroy D, Lepage P, et al. Acquired immunodeficiency syndrome in Rwanda. *Lancet* 1984; 62–64

Chapter 3. Causes of AIDS: Etiology

Aledort LM. AIDS: An update. *Hospital Practice* September 1983

Barre-Senoussi F, Chermann JC, Rey F, et al. Isolation of a T-lymphotropic retrovirus from a patient at risk of acquired immunodeficiency syndrome. *Science* 1983; 220:868–871

Curran JW. AIDS—Two years later. Editorial, *N Engl J Med* 1983; 309:609–611

Daniel MD, Letvin NL, King NW, et al. Isolation of T-cell lymphotropic HTLV-III-like retrovirus from macaques. *Science* 1985; 228:1202–1204

Goedert JJ et al. Amyl nitrite may alter T-lymphocytes in homosexual men. *Lancet* 1982; i:215–218

Kanki PJ, Barin F, Souleyman M, et al. New human T-lymphotropic retrovirus related to simian T-lymphotropic virus type III (STLV-III AGM). *Science* 1985; 232:238–243

Kanki PJ, Kurth R, Becker W, et al. High prevalence of antibodies to simian T-lymphotropic virus type III in African green monkeys and recognition of STLV-III viral protein by AIDS and related sera. *Lancet* 1985; i:330–332

Levy JA and Ziegler JL. Acquired immunodeficiency syndrome is an opportunistic infection and Kaposi's sarcoma results from secondary immune stimulation. *Lancet* 1983; ii:78–91

London WT et al. Experimental transmission of simian acquired immunodeficiency syndrome and Kaposi-like skin lesions. *Lancet* 1983; ii:869–873

Popovic M, Sarngadharan MG, Read E, et al. Detection, isolation, and continuous production of cytopathic retroviruses (HTLV-3) from patients with AIDS and pre-AIDS. *Science* 1984; 224:497–500

Shearer GM and Hurtenbach U. Is sperm immunosuppressive in male homosexuals and vasectomized men? *Immunology Today* 1982; 3:153–154

Sonnabend J, Witkin SS, and Purtilo DT. Acquired immunodeficiency syndrome, opportunistic infections, and malignancies in male homosexuals. *J Am Med Assoc* 1983; 249:2370–2374

Chapter 4.   Immunology of AIDS

Ammann AJ, Abrams D, Conant M, et al. Acquired immune dysfunction in homosexual men: Immunological profiles. *Clin Immunol and Immunopath* 1983; 27:315–325

Hokama Y and Nakamura RM. *Immunology and Immunopathology. Basic Concepts.* Little, Brown, Boston, 1982

Reuben JM, Hersh EM, Mansell P, et al. Immunological characterization of homosexual males. *Cancer Research* 1983; 43:897–904

Rogers MF, Morens DM, Stewart JA, et al., and the Task Force on Acquired Immune Deficiency Syndrome. National case-control study of Kaposi's sarcoma and *Pneumocystis carinii* pneumonia in homosexual men: Part 2,

Laboratory Results. *Ann Intern Med* 1983; 99:151–158

Rose NR, Migrom F, and van Oss C. *Principles of Immunology,* Second Edition. MacMillan, New York, 1979

Rubinstein A, Sicklick M, Gupta A, et al. Acquired immunodeficiency with reversed T_4/T_8 ratios in infants born to promiscuous and drug-addicted mothers. *J Am Med Assoc* 1983; 249:2350–2356

Small CB, Klein RS, Friedland GH, et al. Community-acquired opportunistic infections and defective cellular immunity in heterosexual drug abusers and homosexual men. *Am J Med* 1983; 74:433–441

Stahl RE, Friedman-Kien AE, Dubin R, et al. Immunologic abnormalities in homosexual men. Relationship to Kaposi's sarcoma. *Am J Med* 1982; 73:171–178

Chapter 5.   Signs and Symptoms of AIDS

Britton CB, Marquardt MD, Koppel B, Garvey G, and Miller JR. Neurological complications of the gay immunosuppressed syndrome: Clinical and pathological features. (Abstract). *Ann Neurology* 1982; 12(1):80

Buimovici-Kien E et al. Disseminated Kaposi's sarcoma in homosexual men. *Ann Intern Med* 1982; 96(Part 1):693–700

Centers for Disease Control. Acquired immune deficiency syndrome (AIDS): Precautions for clinical and laboratory staffs. *Morb Mortal Wkly Rep* 1982; 31(43):577–580

———. An evaluation of the acquired immunodeficiency syndrome (AIDS) reported in health-care personnel—United States. *Morb Mortal Wkly Rep* 1983; 32(27):358–360

———. Cryptosporidiosis: Assessment of chemotherapy of males with acquired immunodeficiency syndrome. *Morb Mortal Wkly Rep* 1982; 31:589–592

———. Task Force on Kaposi's Sarcoma and Opportunistic Infections. Epidemiological aspects of the current outbreak of Kaposi's sarcoma and opportunistic infections. *N Engl J Med* 1982; 306:248–252

Follansbee SE, Busch DF, Wofsy CB, et al. An outbreak of *Pneumocystis* pneumonia in homosexual men. *Ann Intern Med* 1982; 96:539–546

Friedman-Kien AE, Laubenstein L, Marmor M, et al. Kaposi's sarcoma and *Pneumocystis* pneumonia among homosexual men—New York and California. *Morb Mortal Wkly Rep* 1981; 30:305–308

Gopinathan G, Laubenstein LJ, Mondale B, and Krigel RL. Central nervous system manifestations of the acquired immune deficiency syndrome in homosexual men. (Abstract). *Neurology* 1983; 33(Suppl 2):105

Gottlieb MS, Schroff R, Schanker HM, et al. *Pneumocystis carinii* pneumonia and mucosal candidiasis in previously healthy homosexual men:

Evidence of a new acquired cellular immunodeficiency. *N Engl J Med* 1981; 305:1425–1431

Greene JB, Sidu GS, Leein S, et al. *Mycobacterium avium-intracellulare.* A cause of disseminated life-threatening infection in homosexuals and drug abusers. *Ann Intern Med* 1982; 97:539–546

Herman P. Neurologic complications of acquired immunologic deficiency syndrome. (Abstract). *Neurology* 1983; 33(Suppl 2):105

Klein RS, Harris CA, Small CB, Moll B, Lesser M, and Friedland GH. Oral Candidiasis in high-risk patients as the initial manifestations of the acquired immunodeficiency syndrome. *N Engl J Med* 1984; 311:354–364

Levy RM, Bredesen DE, and Rosenblum ML. Neurological manifestations of the acquired immunodeficiency syndrome (AIDS): Experience at UCSF and review of the literature. *J Neurosurg* 1985; 62:475–492

Masur H, Michelis MA, Grene JB, et al. An outbreak of community-acquired *Pneumocystis carinii* pneumonia: Initial manifestations of a cellular immune dysfunction. *N Engl J Med* 1981; 305:1431–1438

Mildvan D, Mathur U, Enlow R, et al. Opportunistic infections and immune deficiency in homosexual men. *Ann Intern Med* 1982; 96(Part I):700–704

Miller JR, Barrett RE, Britton CB, et al. Progressive multifocal leukoencephalopathy in a male with T-cell immune deficiency. *N Engl J Med* 1983; 307:1436–1437

Morris L, Distenfeld A, Amorosi E, and Karpatkin S. Autoimmune thrombocytopenic purpura in homosexual men. *Ann Intern Med* 1982; 96:714–717

Moskowitz JB, Hensley GT, Chan JC, Gregorios J, and Conleyt FK. The neuropathology of acquired immune deficiency syndrome. *Arch Pathol Lab Med* 1984; 108:867–872

Palacios E, Gorelick PB, Gonzales CF, and Fine M. Malignant lymphoma of the nervous system. *Comput Assist Tomogr* 1982; 6:689–701

Pitchenik AE, Fischi MA, Dickinson GM, et al. Opportunistic infections and Kaposi's sarcoma among Haitians: Evidence of a new acquired immunodeficiency state. *Ann Intern Med* 1983; 98:277–284

Post MH, Chan JC, Hensley GT, Hoffman TA, Moskowitz LB, and Lippman S. *Toxoplasma* encephalitis in Haitian adults with acquired immunodeficiency syndrome: A clinical-pathologic CT correlation. *Am J Roentgenology* 1983; 140:861–868

Shaw GM, Harper ME, Hahn BH, et al. HTLV-III infections in brains of children and adults with AIDS encephalopathy. *Science* 1985; 227:177–182

Snider WD, Simpson DM, Aronyk KE, and Nielson SL. Primary lymphoma of the nervous system associated with acquired immune deficiency syndrome. *N Engl J Med* 1983; 308:45

Snider WD, Simpson DM, Nielsen S, et al. Neurological complications of acquired immune deficiency syndrome: Analysis of 50 patients. *Ann Neurology* 1983; 14(4):403–418

Spivack JL, Bender BS, and Quinn TC. Hematologic abnormalities in the acquired immune deficiency syndrome. *Am J Med* 1984; 77:224–228

Chapter 6.   Infections of AIDS

6A.   Viral Infections

Barre-Senoussi F, Chermann JC, Rey F, et al. Isolation of a T-lymphocyte retrovirus from a patient at risk of acquired immunodeficiency syndrome. *Science* 1983; 220:868–870

Cawson RA, McCracken AW, and Marcus PB. *Pathologic Mechanisms and Human Disease.* C V Mosby, St. Louis, 1982

Essex M, McLane MF, and Lee TH: Antibodies to cell membrane antigens associated with human T-cell leukemia virus in patients with A.I.D.S. *Science* 1983; 220:859–862

Gallo RC. The virus-cancer story. *Hospital Practice,* June 1983

Gallo RC, Sarin PS, and Gelman EP. Isolation of human T-cell leukemia virus in acquired immune deficiency syndrome. *Science* 1983; 220:865–867

Gelman EP, Popovic M, Blayney D, Masur H, et al. Proviral DNA of a retrovirus, human T-cell leukemia virus in patients with A.I.D.S. *Science* 1983; 220:862–865

Lennette EH and Schmidt NJ. *Diagnostic Procedures for Viral, Rickettsial and Chlamydial Infections,* Fifth Edition. American Public Health Association, Washington, DC, 1979

Lipscomb H, Tatsumi E, Harada S, et al. Epstein-Barr virus and chronic lymphadenomegaly in male homosexuals with acquired immunodeficiency syndrome (AIDS). *AIDS Research* 1983; 1(1):59–82

Peter JB and Wolde-Mariam W. AIDS: Putting the pieces together. *Diagn Med,* Feb 1984, pp. 56–65

Sonnabend J, Witkin SS, and Purtilo DT. Acquired immunodeficiency syndrome, opportunistic infections and malignancies in male homosexuals. *J Am Med Assoc* 1983; 249:2370–2374

6B.   Parasitic Infections

Baker RW and Peppercorn MA. Enteric disease of homosexual men. *Pharmacotherapy* 1982; 2(1):21–32

———. Gastrointestinal ailments of homosexual men. *Medicine* 1982; 61(6):390–405

Centers for Disease Control. Cryptosporidiosis: Assessment of chemotherapy of males with acquired immune deficiency syndrome (AIDS). *Morb Mortal Wkly Rep* 1982; 31:589–592

————. Task Force on Kaposi's Sarcoma and Opportunistic Infections. Epidemiological aspects of the current outbreak of Kaposi's sarcoma and opportunistic infections. *N Engl J Med* 1982; 306:248–252

Chandra RK. Immune responses in parasitic diseases. Part B: Mechanisms. *Rev Infect Dis* 1983; 4(4):756

Cruickshank JK and Mackensie C. Immunodiagnosis in parasitic disease. *Brit Med J* 1981; 283:1349–1350

Hakes T and Armstrong D. Toxoplasmosis: Problems in diagnosis and treatment. *Cancer* 1983; 20:1535–1540

Huges WT, Feldman S, et al. Comparison of pentamidine isethionate and trimethoprim-sulfamethoxazole in the treatment of *Pneumocystis carinii* pneumonia. *J Pediatr* 1978; 92:285–291

Kean BH. Clinical amebiasis in New York City: Symptoms, signs and treatment. *Bull NY Acad Med* 1981; 57:207

Keusch GT. Immune responses in parasitic diseases. Part A. General concepts. *Rev Infect Dis* 1983; 4(4):751–755

Krogstad DJ, Spencer HC Jr, and Healy GR. Current concepts in parasitology: Amebiasis. *N Engl J Med* 1978; 298:262–265

Landesman SH and Vieira J. Acquired immune deficiency syndrome (AIDS)—A review. *Arch Intern Med* 1983; 143:2307–2309

Portnoy D, Whiteside ME, Buckley E, et al. Treatment of intestinal cryptosporidiosis with spiramycin. *Ann Intern Med* 1984; 101:202–204

Salfelder K and Schwarz V. Pneumocystosis. *Am J Dis Child* 1967; 114:693–699

Smith JW and Wolfe MS. Giardiasis. *Ann Rev Med* 1980; 31:373–383

Tzipori S. Cryptosporidiosis in animals and humans. *Microbiol Rev* 1983; 47:84–96

Walzer PD, Perl DP, et al. *Pneumocystis carinii* pneumonia in the United States. Epidemiologic, diagnostic and clinical features. *Ann Intern Med* 1974; 80:83–93

Wong B. Parasitic diseases in immunocompromised hosts. *Am J Med* 1983; 76:479–485

6C.   Bacterial and Fungal Infections

Centers for Disease Control Task Force on Kaposi's Sarcoma and Opportunistic Infections. Epidemiological aspects of the current outbreak of Kaposi's sarcoma and opportunistic infections. *N Engl J Med* 1982; 306:248–252

Dutt AK and Stead W. Long-term results of medical treatment in *Mycobac-*

terium intracellulare infection. *Am J Med* 1979; 67:449–453

Gottlieb M et al. The acquired immunodeficiency syndrome—UCLA conference. *Ann Intern Med* 1983; 99:208–220

Greene JB, Sidhu GS, Lewin S, et al. *Mycobacterium avium-intracellulare:* A cause of disseminated life-threatening infection in homosexuals and drug abusers. *Ann Intern Med* 1982; 97(4):539–546

Kaufman CA, Israel KS, Smith JW, et al. Histoplasmosis in immunosuppressed patients. *Am J Med* 1978; 64:923

Krick JR and Remington JS. Resistance to infection with *Nocardia asteroides*. *J Infect Dis* 1975; 142:432

Lane HC, Masur H, Edgar LC, et al. Abnormalities of B-cell activation and immunoregulation in patients with the acquired immunodeficiency syndrome. *N Engl J Med* 1983; 309(8):453–458

Louria DB. Bacterial and fungal infections in AIDS. In *The AIDS Epidemic*, ed. K Cahill. St. Martin's, New York, 1983

Mildvan D, Mathur U, Enlow R, et al. Opportunistic infections and immune deficiency in homosexual men. *Ann Intern Med* 1982; 96(Part I):700–704

Pitchenik AE, Fischi MA, Dickinson GM, et al. Opportunistic infections and Kaposi's sarcoma among Haitians: Evidence of a new acquired immunodeficiency state. *Ann Intern Med* 1983; 98:277–284

Rosenzweig D. Pulmonary mycobacterial infections due to *Mycobacterium intracellulare-avium* complex. *Chest* 1979; 75(2):115–119

Wolinsky E. Nontuberculous mycobacteria and associated disease. *Am Rev Resp Dis* 1979; 119:107–159

Yeager H and Raleigh J. Pulmonary diseases due to *Mycobacterium intracellulare*. *Am Rev Resp Dis* 1973; 108:547–552

Zakowiski P, Fligiel S, et al. Disseminated *Mycobacterium avium-intracellulare* infection in homosexual men dying of acquired immunodeficiency. *J Am Med Assoc* 1982; 248(22):2980–2982

Chapter 7.   Cancers and Blood Disorders of AIDS

Abrams DI, Chinn EK, Lew BJ, et al. Hematologic manifestations in homosexual men with Kaposi's sarcoma. *Am J Clin Pathol* 1984; 81(1):13

Centers for Disease Control. Opportunistic infections and Kaposi's sarcoma among Haitians in the United States. *Morb Mortal Wkly Rep* 1982; 31:353, 360

————. Persistent, generalized lymphadenopathy among homosexual males. *Morb Mortal Wkly Rep* 1982; 31:249

————. Task Force on Kaposi's Sarcoma and Opportunistic Infections. Epidemiological aspects of the current outbreak of Kaposi's sarcoma and opportunistic infections. *N Engl J Med* 1982; 306:248

Chaganti RSK, Jhanwar SC, Koziner B, et al. Specific translocations characterize Burkitt's-like lymphoma of homosexual men with the acquired immunodeficiency syndrome. *Blood* 1983; 61:1269–1272

Ciobanu N, Andreeff M, Safai B, et al. Lymphoblastic neoplasia in a homosexual patient with Kaposi's sarcoma. *Ann Intern Med* 1983; 98:151

Conant MA, Volberding P, Fletcher V, et al. Squamous cell carcinoma in sexual partners of Kaposi's sarcoma patient. *Lancet* 1982; i:286

Cooper HS, Patchefsky AS, and Marks G. Cloacogenic carcinoma of the anorectum in homosexual men: An observation of four cases. *Dis Col and Rec* 1979; 557–558

Dancis A, Odajnyk C, Kriegel RL, et al. Association of Hodgkin's and non-Hodgkin's lymphomas with the acquired immunodeficiency syndrome (AIDS). *Pro Am Soc Clin Oncol* 1984; 3:61a (CC236)

Davies JNP and Loethe F. Kaposi's sarcoma in African children. *Acta Un Int Cancer* 1962; 18:394

DiGiovanna JJ and Safai B. Kaposi's sarcoma. Retrospective study of 90 cases with particular emphasis on the familial occurrence, ethnic background and prevalence of other diseases. *Am J Med* 1981; 71:779–783

Doll DC and List AF. Burkitt's lymphoma in a homosexual. *Lancet* 1982; i:1026–1027

Drew WL, Conant MA, Miner RC, et al. Cytomegalovirus and Kaposi's sarcoma in young homosexual men. *Lancet* 1982; 2:125

Drew WL, Mintz L, Miner RC, et al. Prevalence of cytomegalovirus infection in homosexual men. *J Infect Dis* 1981; 143:188

Fauci AS, Macher AM, Longo DL, et al. Acquired immunodeficiency syndrome. Epidemiologic, clinical, immunologic, and therapeutic considerations. *Ann Intern Med* 1984; 100:92

Fenoglio CM and McDougall JK. The relationship of cytomegalovirus to Kaposi's sarcoma. In *AIDS: The Epidemic of Kaposi's Sarcoma and Opportunistic Infections,* ed. Friedman-Kien AE and Laubenstein LJ, p. 329. New York, Masson Publishing USA, 1984

Friedman-Kien AE. Disseminated Kaposi-like sarcoma syndrome in young homosexual men. *J Am Acad Dermatol* 1981; 5:468

————. Kaposi's sarcoma: An opportunistic neoplasm. *J Invest Derm* 1984; 82:446

Friedman-Kien AE, Laubenstein L, Marmor M, et al. Kaposi's sarcoma and *Pneumocystis* pneumonia among homosexual men—New York and California. *Morb Mortal Wkly Rep* 1981; 30:250

Friedman-Kien AE, Laubenstein LJ, Rubinstein P, et al. Disseminated Kaposi's sarcoma in homosexual men. *Am J Med* 1982; 96 (Part I):693–700

Friedman-Kien AE and Ostreicher R. Overview of classical and epidemic Kaposi's sarcoma. In *AIDS: The Epidemic of Kaposi's Sarcoma and Opportunistic Infections,* ed. Friedman-Kien AE and Laubenstein LJ. New York, Masson Publishing USA, 1984

Gallo RC, Salahuddin SZ, and Popovic M. Frequent detection and isolation of cytopathic retroviruses (HTLV-III) from patients with AIDS and at risk for AIDS. *Science* 1984; 224 (4648):500–503

Gallo RC, Sarin PS, Gelmann EP, et al. Isolation of human T-cell leukemia virus in acquired immune deficiency syndrome (AIDS). *Science* 1983; 220:865

Gatti RA and Good RA. Occurrence of malignancy in immunodeficiency diseases. A literature review. *Cancer* 1971; 38:89

Giraldo G, Beth E, and Huang E-S. Kaposi's sarcoma and its relationship to human cytomegalovirus (CMV). III. CMV DNA and CMV early antigens in Kaposi's sarcoma. *Int J Cancer* 1980; 26:23

Gottlieb MS, Schroff R, Schanker HM, et al. *Pneumocystis carinii* pneumonia and mucosal candidiasis in previously healthy homosexual men: Evidence of a new acquired cellular immunodeficiency. *N Engl J Med* 1981; 305:1425

Harwood AR, Osoba D, Hofstader SL, et al. Kaposi's sarcoma in recipients of renal transplants. *Am J Med* 1979; 67:759

Haverkos HW and Curran JW. The current outbreak of Kaposi's sarcoma and opportunistic infections. *Cancer* 1982; 32:330–339

Hochberg FH, Miller G. Schooley RT, et al. Central nervous system lymphoma related to Epstein-Barr virus. *N Engl J Med* 1983; 309:745

Holecek MJ and Jarwood AR. Radiotherapy and Kaposi's sarcoma. *Cancer* 1978; 41:1733

Hymes K, Cheung T, Greene JB, et al. Kaposi's sarcoma in homosexual men. *Lancet* 1981; 2:598

Ioachim HL, Lerner CW, and Tapper MI, Lymphadenopathies in homosexual men: Relationships with the acquired immune deficiency syndrome. *J Am Med Assoc* 1983; 250:1306

Israel AM, Koziner B, and Straus DJ. Plasmacytoma in a patient with acquired immunodeficiency syndrome. *Ann Intern Med* 1983; 99:635

Jaffe HW, Choi K, Thomas PA, et al. National case-control study of Kaposi's sarcoma and *Pneumocystis carinii* pneumonia in homosexual men. Part I, Epidemiologic results. *Ann Intern Med* 1983; 99:145

Kaposi M. Idiopathiches multiples pigment sarcom der Haut. *Arch Dermatol* 1872; 4:465

Kaposi M. Classics in oncology: Idiopathic multiple pigmented sarcoma of the skin. (Translated and reprinted) *Cancer* 1982; 32:342

Klepp O, Dahl O, and Stenwig JT. Association of Kaposi's sarcoma and prior immunosuppressive therapy. *Cancer* 1978; 42:2626

Kondlaponoodi P. Anorectal cancer and homosexuality. *J Am Med Assoc* 1982; 248:2114–2115

Koziner B, Urmacher C, Chaganti RSK, et al. Acquired immunodeficiency syndrome in the development of lymphoma. In *UT M.D. Anderson Clinical Conference on Cancer*, ed. Ford RJ, Fuller LM, and Hagemeister FB, Vol 27, p. 227. New York, Raven Press, 1984

Krown SE, Real FX, Cunningham-Rundles S, et al. Preliminary observations on the effects of recombinant leukocyte α interferon in homosexual men with Kaposi's sarcoma. *N Engl J Med* 1983; 308:1071–1076

Laubenstein LJ, Hymes K, and Krigel R. Phase II trial of VP-16-213 in disseminated Kaposi's sarcoma. *Proc Am Soc Clin Oncol* 1982; (C-680):174

Laubenstein LJ, Krigel RL, Hymes KB, et al. Treatment of epidemic Kaposi's sarcoma with VP-16-213 (etoposide) and a combination of doxorubicin, bleomycin and vinblastine (ABV). *Proc Am Soc Clin Oncol* 1983; 2:228

Leach RD and Ellis H. Carcinoma of the rectum in male homosexuals. *J Roy Soc Med* 1981; 74:490–491

Levine AS. The epidemic of acquired immune dysfunction in homosexual men and its sequelae—opportunistic infections, Kaposi's sarcoma and other malignancies: An update and interpretation. *Cancer Treat Rep* 1982; 66:1391–1395

Lotze M, Robb R, Frana L, et al. Systemic administration of interleukin-2 in patients with cancer and AIDS: Initial results of a Phase I trial (abstract). *Proc Am Soc Clin Oncol* 1984; 3:51

Lozada F, Silverman S, and Conant M. New outbreak of oral tumors, malignancies and infectious diseases strikes young male homosexuals. *Calif Dent J* 1982; 10:39

Marmor M, Friedman-Kien AE, Zolla-Pazner S, et al. Kaposi's sarcoma in homosexual men: A seroepidemiologic case-control study. *Ann Intern Med* 1984; 100:809

Metroka CE, Cunningham-Rundles S, Pollack MS, et al. Generalized lymphadenopathy in homosexual men. *Ann Intern Med* 1983; 99:585

Mitsuyasu RT and Groopman JE. Biology and therapy of Kaposi's sarcoma. *Seminars Oncol* 1984; 11:53–59

Morris L, Distenfeld A, and Amorosi E. Autoimmune thrombocytopenic purpura in homosexual men. *Ann Intern Med* 1982; 96:714–717

Nydegger VE, ed. *Immunochemotherapy: A Guide to Immunoglobulin Prophylaxia and Therapy*. Academic Press, New York, 1981

Olweny CLM. Epidemiology and clinical features of Kaposi's sarcoma in tropical Africa. In *AIDS: The Epidemic of Kaposi's Sarcoma and Opportunistic Infections*, ed. Friedman-Kien AE and Laubenstein LJ, p. 35. New York, Masson Publishing USA, 1984

Olweny CLM, Kaddumukasa AA, Atine I, et al. Childhood Kaposi's sarcoma: Clinical features and therapy. *Br J Cancer* 1976; 33:555

Penn I. Depressed immunity and the development of cancer. *Clin Exp Immunol* 1981; 46:459

────. Kaposi's sarcoma in organ transplant recipients. *Transplantation* 1979; 27:8

Pitchenik AE, Fischl MA, Dickinson GM, et al. Opportunistic infections and Kaposi's sarcoma among Haitians: Evidence of a new acquired immunodeficiency state. *Ann Intern Med* 1983; 98:277

Poiesz B, Tomar R, Ehrlich G, et al. Association of HTLV with AIDS. *Proc Am Soc Clin Oncol* 1984; 3:13 (Abstract C-52)

Real FX, Krown SE, Krim M, et al. Treatment of Kaposi's sarcoma with recombinant leukocyte α interferon (abstract). *Proc Am Soc Clin Oncol* 1984; 3:55

Safai B and Good RA. Kaposi's sarcoma: A review and recent developments. *Cancer* 1981; 31:2–12

Safai B, Mike V, Giraldo G, et al. Association of Kaposi's sarcoma with secondary primary malignancies. Possible etiopathogenic implications. *Cancer* 1980; 45:1472

Salan AJ, Greenwald ED, and Silvay O. Long-term complete remission of Kaposi's sarcoma with vinblastine therapy. *Cancer* 1981; 47:637

Schoeppel SL, Hoppe RT, Dorfman RF, et al. Hodgkin's disease in homosexual men at risk for AIDS. *Proc Am Soc Clin Oncol* 1984; 3:64 (Abstract C-250)

Stribling J, Wertzner S, and Smith GV: Kaposi's sarcoma in renal allograft recipients *Cancer* 1978; 42:442

Volberding PA. Therapy of Kaposi's sarcoma in AIDS. *Seminars Oncol* 1984; 11:60–67

Ziegler JL, Beckstead JA, Volberding PA, et al. Non-Hodgkin's lymphoma in 90 homosexual men. *N Engl J Med* 1984; 311:565

Ziegler JL, Miner RC, Rosenbaum E, et al. Outbreak of Burkitt's-like lymphoma in homosexual men. *Lancet* 1982; 2:631

Ziegler JL, Templeton AC, and Vogel CL: Kaposi's sarcoma: A comparison of classical, endemic, and epidemic forms. *Seminars Oncol* 1984; 11:47

Chapter 8.   Children with AIDS and the Public Risk

Ammann AJ. Is there an acquired immune deficiency syndrome in infants and children? *Pediatrics* 1983; 72:430

Centers for Disease Control. *Morb Mortal Wkly Rep* 1983; 32:358

_____. AIDS, United States. *Morb Mortal Wkly Rep* 1984; 32:688

_____. Apparent transmission of HTLV-III/LAV from a child to a mother providing health care. *Morb Mortal Wkly Rep* 1986; 35:75

Curran JW. AIDS—Two years later. *N Engl J Med* 1983; 309:609

Friedland GH, Saltzman BR, Rogers MF, et al. Lack of transmission of HTLV-III infection to household contacts of patients with AIDS or ARC with oral candidiasis. *N Engl J Med* 1986; 314:344

Gordon RS. *AIDS Memorandum* 1983; 1:11

Jaffe HW, Feorino PM, Darrow WW, et al. Persistent infection with HTLV-III/LAV in apparently healthy homosexual men. *Ann Intern Med* 1985; 102:627

Oleske J, Minneror A, Cooper R Jr, et al. Immune deficiency syndrome in children. *J Am Med Assoc* 1983; 249:2345

Rubinstein A. *Acquired Immunodeficiency Syndrome in Infants. Current Problems in Pediatrics.* Year Book Medical Publishers, Chicago, 1986

Rubinstein A, Sicklick M, Gupta A, et al. Acquired immunodeficiency with reversed T₄/T₈ ratios in infants born to promiscuous and drug addicted mothers. *J Am Med Assoc* 1983; 249:2350

Chapter 9.   AIDS and the Blood Supply

Centers for Disease Control. The safety of hepatitis B virus vaccine. *Morb Mortal Wkly Rep* 1983; 32, 134

_____. Transfusion malaria. *Morb Mortal Wkly Rep* 1983; 32:222

_____. Update: Acquired immunodeficiency syndrome (AIDS)—United States. *Morb Mortal Wkly Rep* 1984; 33:337

Curran JW, et al. Acquired immunodeficiency syndrome (AIDS) associated with transfusion. *N Engl J Med* 1984; 310:69

Feorino PM. Lymphadenopathy associated virus infection of a blood donor-recipient pair with acquired immunodeficiency syndrome. *Science* 1984; 225:69

Gallo RC, et al. Frequent detection and isolation of cytopathic retroviruses (HTLV-III) from patients with AIDS and at high risk for AIDS. *Science* 1984; 224:500

Klatzmann D et al. Selective tropism of lymphadenopathy associated virus (LAV) for helper-inducer T lymphocytes. *Science* 1984; 225:59

Kuritsky JN et al. Results of nationwide screening of blood and plasma for antibodies to human T-cell lymphotrophic virus, type III. *Blood* 1986; 26:205

National Hemophilia Foundation. AIDS Update. March 1985

Recommendations to Decrease the Risk of Transmitting Infectious Diseases from Blood Donors. Office of Biologics, National Center for Drugs and Biologics, Food and Drug Administration, Bethesda, MD, March 1983

Revised Definition of High Risk Groups with Respect to Acquired Immunodeficiency Syndrome (AIDS) Transmission. Office of Biologics Research and Review, National Center for Drugs and Biologics, Food and Drug Administration, Bethesda, MD, September 3, 1985

Schorr JB et al. Prevalence of HTLV-III antibody in American blood donors. *N Engl J Med* 1985; 313:384

Stevens C. Correspondence. *N Engl J Med* 1983; 308:1163

Chapter 10. The Haitian Link

Centers for Disease Control. Update on acquired immune deficiency syndrome (AIDS)—United States. *Morb Mortal Wkly Rep* 1982; 31:507–508

Clumeck N, Van de Perre P, Carael M, et al. Heterosexual promiscuity in African patients with AIDS. *N Engl J Med* 1985; 313:182

Frank E, Siegal FP, Siegal M, Vieira J, et al. T-cell subsets in Haitians with tuberculosis (TB): Predictive value for acquired immune deficiency syndrome (AIDS). (Abstract) *23rd Interscience Conference on antimicrobial Agents and Chemotherapy* 1983; 261

Harwood A, ed. *Ethnicity and Medical Care: Haitian Americans.* Harvard University Press, Cambridge, 1979

Leonides JR and Hyppolite N. Haiti and the acquired immunodeficiency syndrome. *Ann Intern Med* 1983; 98:1020–1021

Lundahl M. *Peasants and Poverty: A Study in Haiti.* Croom Helm, London, 1979

Macek C. Acquired immunodeficiency syndrome cause(s) still elusive. *J Am Med Assoc* 1982; 248:1423–1431

Metraux A. *La Voudou Haitien.* Gallimard, Paris, 1958; 150–157

Pape JW, Liautaud B, Thomas F, Mathurin JR, et al. Characteristics of the acquired immunodeficiency syndrome (AIDS) in Haiti. *N Engl J Med* 1983; 309:945–950

Pearce RB. Intestinal protozoal infections and AIDS (letter) *Lancet* 1983; 2:51

Piot P, Quinn TC, Taelman H, et al. Acquired immunodeficiency syndrome in a heterosexual population in Zaire. *Lancet* 1984; ii:65–69

Pitchenik AE, Fischl MA, Dickenson GM, Becker DM, et al. Opportunistic infections and Kaposi's sarcoma among Haitians: Evidence of a new acquired immunodeficiency state. *Ann Intern Med* 1983; 98:277–284

Van de Perre P, Rouvroy D, Lepage P, et al. Acquired immunodeficiency syndrome in Rwanda. *Lancet* 1984; ii:62–65

Vieira J, Frank E, Spira TJ, and Landesman SH. Acquired immune deficiency in Haitians: Opportunistic infections in previously healthy Haitian immigrants. *N Engl J Med* 1983; 308:125–129

Chapter 11.   AIDS in Prisons

Centers for Disease Control. Recommendation for assisting in the prevention of perinatal transmission of human T-lymphotropic virus type III/lymphadenopathy-associated virus and acquired immunodeficiency syndrome. 1985; 48:721–732

————. Update: Acquired immunodeficiency syndrome—United States. *Morb Mortal Wkly Rep* 1986; 35:17–21

————. Acquired immunodeficiency syndrome in correctional facilities. A report of the National Institute of Justice and the American Correctional Association. *Morb Mortal Wkly Rep* 1986; 35:195–199

Friedland GH, Saltzman BR, Rogers MF, et al. Lack of transmission of HTLV-III/LAV infection to household contacts of patients with AIDS and AIDS-related complex with oral candidiasis. *N Engl J Med* 1986; 314:344–348

Hammet TM. *AIDS in Correctional Facilities: Issues and Options*. U.S. Department of Justice, National Institute of Justice. Prepublication copy, January 1986

Hardy AM, Allen JR, Morgan M, et al. The incidence rate of acquired immune deficiency syndrome in selected population. *J Am Med Assoc* 1985; 253:17–22

Personal communications: Health administrators of State of New York Department of Corrections, Florida Department of Corrections, California State Department of Corrections, and Dr. M. Rooney, Medical Director, Department of Correction, New York City

Sande M. Transmission of AIDS: The case against casual contagion. *N Engl J Med* 1986; 314:380–381

Chapter 12.   Ethical Issues in AIDS

Bayer R, Levine C, and Murray TH. Guidelines for confidentiality in research on AIDS. *IRB: A Review on Human Subjects Research* 1984; 6(6):1–7

Centers for Disease Control. An evaluation of the acquired immunodeficiency syndrome (AIDS) reported in health care personnel—United States. *Morb Mortal Wkly Rep* 1983; 32:358–360

————. Status of acquired immunodeficiency syndrome (AIDS)—update United States. *Morb Mortal Wkly Rep* 1986; 35:78

Curran J. AIDS—Two years later. *N Engl J Med* 1983; 309:610

Dubos R. *The Mirage of Health*. Harper and Row, New York, 1959

Golubjatnikov R, Pfister J, and Tillotson T. Homosexual promiscuity and the fear of AIDS. *Lancet* 1983; 681

Healy C. AIDS and the professional ethic. *Austr Nurses J* Feb 14, 1985; 10

Jonsen A. Ethics and AIDS. *Bull Am Toll Surg* 1985; 70(6):16–18

Judson F. Fear of AIDS and gonorrhea rates in homosexual men. *Lancet* Sept 17, 1983; 159–160

Krieger L. AIDS reporting code aims to protect privacy. *Am Med News* 1983; 26(37):20

Lieberson J. Anatomy of an epidemic. *New York Review of Books*, August 18, 1983, pp. 17–22

Marwick C. Confidentiality issues may cloud epidemiologic studies of AIDS. *J Am Med Assoc* 1983; 250(15):1945

National Research Council. Committee for the Study of Inborn Errors of Metabolism. *Genetic Screening: Programs, Principles, and Research.* National Academy of Sciences, Washington, DC, 1975

Odyssey of AIDS victim ends in death. *Am Med News* Nov 1983, p. 3

Rechy J. An exchange on AIDS. *New York Review of Books*, October 13, 1983, pp. 43–44

Shipp ER. Quarantine for AIDS patients discussed by city council. *New York Times*, October 30, 1985, p. 16

Steinbrook R, Le B, Tarpack J, Dilley JW, and Volberding PA. Ethical dilemmas in caring for patients with acquired immunodeficiency syndrome. *Ann Intern Med* 1985; 103(5):787–790

Weiss K. AIDS turmoil in the medical profession. *The New Physician* 1983; 32(6):14, 16

Chapter 14. Economic Costs of AIDS

Arno PS. The non-profit sector's response to the AIDS epidemic: Community-based services in San Francisco. *Am J Public Health*, forthcoming

Arno PS. *The Contributions and Limitations of Voluntarism: Community-Based Services and the AIDS Epidemic.* Paper presented at AIDS: Public Policy Dimensions Conference, New York City, January 16–17, 1986

Arno PS and Hughes RG. *Local Responses to the AIDS Epidemic: New York and San Francisco.* Paper presented at the Annual Meetings of the American Public Health Association, Washington, DC, November 1985

Baxter RC and Ksell TE. *Needs Assessment, Acquired Immune Deficiency Syndrome.* New Jersey State Department of Health, Division of Epidemiology, Trenton, New Jersey, April 1985

Davis K and Rowland D. Uninsured and underserved: Inequities in health care in the United States. *Milbank Memorial Fund Quarterly/Health and Society* 1983; 61(2)

Groopman JE and Detsky A. Epidemic of the acquired immunodeficiency syndrome: A need for economic and social planning. *Ann Intern Med* 1983; 99(2):259–261

Hardy AM, Rauch K, Echenberg DF, Morgan WM, and Curran JW. The economic impact of the first 10,000 cases of AIDS in the United States. *J Am Med Assoc* 1986; 255:209–211

Intergovernmental Health Policy Project. *A Review of State and Local Government Initiatives Affecting AIDS.* George Washington University, November 1985

Landesman SH, Ginzburg HM, and Weiss SH. The AIDS epidemic. *N Engl J Med* 1985; 312(8):521–525

Lee PR and Arno PS. *AIDS and Health Policy.* Paper presented at AIDS: Public Policy Dimensions Conference, New York City, January 16–17, 1986

McHolland GF and Weller W. *Summary Report on California AIDS Victims: Quantitative Analysis.* California Department of Health Services, 1986

Monheit AM, Hagan M, Berk, and Wilensky G. *Unemployment, Health Insurance and Medical Care Utilization.* National Center for Health Services Research, Washington, DC, 1984

Newcomer RJ, Benjamin AE, and Sattler CE. Equity incentives in medicaid program eligibility. In *Long Term Care of the Elderly: Public Policy Issues,* Harrington C, Newcomer RJ, Estes CL, and Associates (eds). Sage, Beverly Hills, 1985

Rice DP. Estimating the cost of illness. *Health Economics Series No. 6.* Public Health Service Publication No. 947-6. U.S. Government Printing Office, Washington, DC, 1966

San Francisco Department of Public Health. *San Francisco's Response to AIDS: Status Up-Date,* October 8, 1985

Scitovsky AA, Cline M, and Lee PR. *Medical Care Costs of AIDS Patients Treated in San Francisco.* Paper presented at the Annual Meetings of the American Public Health Association, Washington, DC, November 19, 1985

Scitovsky AA, Rice DP, Showstack J, and Lee PR. *The Direct and Indirect Economic Costs of Acquired Immune Deficiency Syndrome, 1985, 1986 and 1990.* Final Report prepared for the Centers for Disease Control, Task Order 282-85-0061, #2, 1986

Sencer DJ and Botnick VE. *Report to the Mayor: New York City's Response to the AIDS Crisis.* The City of New York, Office of the Mayor, December, 1985

Swartz K. Statement before the U.S. Senate Subcommittee on Health of the Committee on Finance, April 27, 1984

U.S. Conference of Mayors. *Local Responses to Acquired Immune Deficiency Syndrome (AIDS): A Report of 55 Cities,* Washington, DC, 1984

West Bay Hospital Conference. *Monthly AIDS Hospital Utilization Report,*
San Mateo, California, October 25, 1985
————. *Quarterly AIDS Utilization Report.* San Mateo, California, March
5, 1986

**Chapter 15. Public Health and the Gay Perspective: Creating a
Basis for Trust**

1. Testimony of Katy Taylor, Human Rights Specialist, New York City
Commission on Human Rights, House Subcommittee on Intergovernmental Relations and Human Resources, September 13, 1985; "Anti-gay
Violence and Victimization in 1985," A Report by the Violence Project of
the National Gay and Lesbian Task Force, April 1986.
2. Then Secretary of Health and Human Services Margaret Heckler drew
angry criticism from the gay community when, during her speech at the
first International Conference on AIDS in Atlanta in April 1985, she said,
"We must conquer [AIDS] before it infects the heterosexual population
and threatens the health of the general population."
3. Office of Technology Assessment, *Review of the Public Health Service's
Response to AIDS,* February 1985.
4. Appropriate models are the Assurance of Confidentiality granted by the
Centers for Disease Control for its AIDS surveillance work and the
Certificate of Confidentiality granted the National Institutes of Health
large study of the natural history of AIDS among homosexual men, both
of which make identifying information subpoena-proof.
5. At some point it may still be necessary to take measures against an
occasional recalcitrant individual. But health officials already have such
authority without having to invoke special quarantine powers, and such
steps should be taken only when all other remedies are exhausted and with
full respect for the individual's due-process rights.
6. It should be noted that public health officials may claim a correlation
between knowledge of antibody status and changed behavior, but this has
yet to be proven. Nonetheless, they are willing to base major education
programs on the test, despite serious risks to the individual.
7. Under pressure from the White House, the U.S. Centers for Disease
Control (CDC), in December 1985, imposed strict limitations on explicit-
ness in any CDC-funded AIDS education program. In some communities,
where federal dollars are the only source of education money, this will
severely limit the potential success of education efforts.

Chapter 17.   Prospects for AIDS Therapy and Vaccine

Anand R, Moore JL, Skinivasun M, et al. Ansamycin inhibits replication and infectivity of HTLV-III/LAV (Abstract). In *The International Conference of the Acquired Immunodeficiency Syndrome: Abstracts*. The American College of Physicians, Philadelphia, 1985

De Clerco E. Suramin: A potent inhibitor of the reverse transcriptase of RNA tumor viruses. *Cancer Lett* 1979; 8:9–22

Dormont D, Spire B, Barre-Sinoussi FC, et al. Inhibition of RNA dependent DNA polymerases of two primate retroviruses (LAV and AIDS virus) by ammonium-21-tungsto-9-antimoniate (HPA-23). *Ann Inst Pasteur/Virol* 1985; 136E:75–83

Francis DP and Petricciani JC. The prospects for and pathways toward a vaccine for AIDS. *N Engl J Med* 1985; 313(25):1586–1590

Grieco MH, Reddy MM, Manvar D, et al. In vivo immunomodulation of isoprinosine in patients with the acquired immunodeficiency syndrome and related complexes. *Ann Intern Med* 1984; 101(2):206–207

Groopman JE, Gottlieb MS, Goodman J, et al. Recombinant alpha-2 interferon therapy for Kaposi's sarcoma associated with the acquired immunodeficiency syndrome. *Ann Intern Med* 1984; 100:671–676

Hirsch MS and Kaplan JC. Prospects of therapy for infections with human T-lymphotropic virus type III. *Ann Intern Med* 1985; 103:750–755

Ho DD, Hartshorn KL, Rota TR, et al. Recombinant human interferon alpha-2 suppresses HTLV-III replication in vitro. *Lancet* 1985; 1:602–604

Klatzmann E and Montagnier L. Approaches to AIDS therapy. *Nature* 1986; 319:10–11

Krown SE, Real FX, Cunningham-Rundles S, et al. Preliminary observations on the effect of recombinant leukocyte A interferon in homosexual men with Kaposi's sarcoma. *N Engl J Med* 1983; 308:1071–1076

Lane HC et al. Use of interleukin-2 in patients with acquired immunodeficiency syndrome. *J Biol Resp Mod* 1984; 3:512–516

Marwin C. Task Force formed to coordinate study testing of AIDS therapies. *J Am Med Assoc* 1986; 225(10):1233–1242

Marx JL. The slow insidious natures of the HTLV's. *Science* 1986; 231:450–451

McCormick JB, Getchell JP, Mitchell SW, and Hicks DR. Ribavirin suppresses replication of lymphadenopathy-associated virus in cultures of human adult T lymphocytes. *Lancet* 1984; 2:1367–1369

Mitsuya H, Popovic M, Yarchoan R, Matsushita S, Gallo RC, and Broder S. Suramin protection of T cells in vitro against infectivity and cytopathic effect of HTLV-III. *Science* 1984; 226:172–174

Pitha P, Bilello JA, and Riggin CH. Effect of interferon on retrovirus replication. *Tex Rep Biol Med* 1981; 2(41):603–609

Pompidoiu A et al. In vitro inhibition of HTLV-III/LAV infected lymphocytes by dithiocait and Nosine Pranobex. *Lancet* 1985; 1:1423

Rozenbaum W, Dormont D, Spire B, et al. Antimoniotungstate (HPA-23) treatment of three patients with AIDS and one with prodrome (letter). *Lancet* 1985; 1:450–451

Sandstrom EG, Kaplan JC, Byington RE, and Hirsch MS. Inhibition of human T cell lymphotrophic virus type III in vitro by phosphonoformate. *Lancet* 1985; 1:1480–1482

Siegel JN et al. T-cell suppression and contrasuppression induced by histamine H-2 and H-1 receptor agonists, respectively. *Proc Natl Acad Sci* 1982; 79:5052

Trainin, A et al. Attempted treatment of acquired immunodeficiency syndrome with thymic humoral factor. *J Med Sci* 1984; 20:1195–1196

Tsang P et al. Modulation of T and B lymphocyte functions by isoprinosine in homosexual subjects with prodromata and in patients with acquired immune deficiency syndrome (AIDS). *J Clin Immunol* 1984; 4(6):469

Chapter 19.   Preventing AIDS

Centers for Disease Control. Acquired immune deficiency syndrome (AIDS): Precautions for clinical and laboratory staffs. *Morb Mortal Wkly Rep* 1982; 31:577

————. Prevention of acquired immune deficiency syndrome (AIDS): Report of interagency recommendations. *Morb Mortal Wkly Rep* 1983; 32:101

————. Provisional Public Health Service interagency recommendations for screening donated blood and plasma for antibody to the virus causing acquired immunodeficiency syndrome. *Morb Mortal Wkly Rep* 1985; 34:5–7

————. Update: Public Health Service Workshop on human T-lymphotropic virus type III antibody testing—United States. *Morb Mortal Wkly Rep* 1985; 34:477–478

————. Heterosexual transmission of human T-lymphotropic virus type III/lymphadenopathy-associated virus. *Morb Mortal Wkly Rep* 1985; 34:561–563

————. Update: Evaluation of human T-lymphotropic virus type III/lymphadenopathy-associated virus infection in health-care personnel—United States. *Morb Mortal Wkly Rep* 1985; 34:575–578

————. Recommendations for preventing transmission of infection with human T-lymphotropic virus type III/lymphadenopathy-associated virus in the workplace. *Morb Mortal Wkly Rep* 1985; 34:681–695

————. Additional recommendations to reduce sexual and drug abuse-related transmission of human T-lymphotropic virus type III/lymphadenopathy-associated virus. *Morb Mortal Wkly Rep* 1986; 35:152–155

————. Recommendations for preventing transmission of infection with human T-lymphotropic virus type III/lymphadenopathy-associated virus during invasive procedures. *Morb Mortal Wkly Rep* 1986; 35:221–223

Conant MA, Spicer DW, and Smith CD. Herpes simplex virus transmission: Condom studies. *Sex Transm Dis* 1984; 11:94–95

Judson FN, Bodin GF, Levin MJ, Ehret JM, and Masters HB. In vitro tests demonstrate condoms provide an effective barrier against chlamydia trachomatis and herpes simplex virus. Abstract in Program of the International Society for STD Research, Seattle, Washington, August 1-3, 1983:176

Mason JO. Public Health Service plan for the prevention and control of acquired immune deficiency syndrome. *Public Health Reports* 1985; 100:453–455

Weiss SH, Saxinger C, Rechtman D, Grieco MH, Nadler J, et al. HTLV-III infection among health care workers: Association with needle-stick injuries. *J Am Med Assoc* 1985; 254:2089–2093

Chapter 20. Psychological and Social Issues of AIDS and Strategies for Survival

Allison H, Gripton J, and Rodway M. Social work services as a component of palliative care with terminal cancer patients. *Social Work in Health Care* 1983; 8(4):30

Dunkel J and Hatfield S. Counter-transference issues in working with persons with AIDS. *Social Work* 1986; 31(2):114–117

Kastenbaum R. Death and development through the life span. In *New Meanings of Death,* ed. Feigel H. McGraw-Hill, New York, 1977, p. 42

Kubler-Ross E. *On Death and Dying.* Macmillan, New York, 1968, p. 5

Lopez D and Getzel G. Helping gay AIDS patients in crisis. *Social Casework* Sept. 1984, pp. 387–394

Sande M. Transmission of AIDS: A case against casual contagion. *N Engl J Med* 1986; 314(6):380–382

Chapter 21. AIDS and Mental Health

Beck AT and Emery G. *Anxiety Disorders and Phobias*. Basic Books, New York, 1985

Dilley JW, Ochitill HN, Perl M, and Volberding PA. Findings in psychiatric consultations with patients with AIDS. *Am J Psych* 1985; 142:82–85

Goldblum PG and Delaney M: *Gay Health Workbook: An AIDS Survival Manual* (in press)

Holland JC and Tross S. The psychosocial and neuropsychiatric sequelae of the acquired immunodeficiency syndrome and related disorders. *Ann Int Med* 1985; 103:760–764

Horowitz MJ. *Stress Response Syndrome*. Jason Aronson, New York, 1976

Longman Dictionary of Psychology and Psychiatry. Longman, New York, 1984

May R. *Psychology and the Human Dilemma*. Van Nostrand, Princeton, 1967

Perry SW and Tross S. Psychiatric problems of AIDS inpatients at the New York Hospital: Preliminary report. *Public Health Reports* 1984; 99:200–205

Index

Index 373

ARC. *See* AIDS-related complex
(ARC)
asialo GM₁, 46
atypical tuberculosis, 73–74. *See
also* tuberculosis
Auerbach, David, 20
autoimmune disease, 13, 41–42
autopsy, 128
azidothymide, 211

bacterial infections, 99; *Listeria,*
75–76; *Nocardia,* 75;
salmonellosis, 74–75;
tuberculosis, 72–73
bargaining, 296
bathhouses, 163–164
B cells, 39, 41; AIDS defects of,
76; EBV and, 58
bereavement, 298–301
biologic response modification,
205–208
bisexuals. *See* homosexuals
blacks, 253
bladder control, 224, 228
bleeding, 52. *See also* symptoms
blood: disorders, 88, 118–119;
donors, 113–115, 241, 313;
products and usage of, 105–108;
screening, 8–10, 21, 24, 95,
105, 109–113, 149 152,
164–165, 241, 254 (*see also*
human T-lymphotropic virus
type III/lymphadenopathy-
associated virus [HTLV-III/
LAV]); and the transmission of
AIDS, 235–236. *See also* blood
transfusions
blood transfusions: autologous,
113; and CMV infections, 28;
from a dedicated donor,
113–114; and the epidemiology

of AIDS, 19–21, 22; and
hepatitis, 60–61, 106; and risk
of AIDS, 94–95; and
transmission of AIDS, 6, 64,
104, 106, 122, 241, 313
body fluids: analyzing, 45; HTLV-
III/LAV presence in, 5, 24; and
the immune system, 39–40; and
transmission of AIDS, 100–101,
227. *See also* specific fluids
body temperature, 49
bone marrow transplantation, 204.
See also organ transplantation
bowel control, 224, 228
brain infections, 52–53, 68, 75,
99. *See also* neurological
symptoms
Brandt, Edward N., 144
Bridges, Fabian, 147–148
Broder, Samuel, 210
bronchoscopy, 66, 95
bruising, 52. *See also* symptoms
Buchanan, Patrick, 144
Burkitt's lymphoma, 58, 82, 86
butyl nitrites (poppers), 16–17,
26–27

California, 165; antidiscrimination
legislation, 195; and financing of
patient care, 173–174, 177–178.
See also San Francisco
cancer, 259; and AIDS, 80–88,
EBV and, 58; herpes simplex
virus and, 59; and the immune
system, 43, 86; lymphomas, 58,
85–87. *See also* Kaposi's
sarcoma (KS)
Candida infections, 50–51;
Candida albicans, 78, 118; and
the immunology of AIDS, 44;
and Kaposi's sarcoma, 83; SCID
and, 41

Contributors

Victor Gong, MD. Editor. In private practice, Internal Medicine, Baltimore, Maryland.

Norman Rudnick, MS. Editor. Science editor and writer, physicist, with background in biomedical science.

Peter S. Arno, PhD. Department of Health Care Administration, Baruch College, Mt. Sinai School of Medicine, City University of New York.

Gretchen M. Aumann, BSN. PhD candidate in Medical Ethics, Institute for the Medical Humanities, University of Texas Medical Branch, Galveston.

Leonard H. Calabrese, DO, FACP. Head, Section on Clinical Immunology, Department of Rheumatic and Immunologic Disease, Cleveland Clinic Foundation, Ohio.

Keewhan Choi, PhD. Formerly Assistant Director, Division of Surveillance and Epidemiological Studies, Centers for Disease Control, Atlanta, Georgia.

James W. Dilley, MD. Project Director, University of California, San Francisco, AIDS Health Project.

The Rev. William A. Doubleday, MDiv. Professor Doubleday is Director of Field Education, The General Theological Seminary, New York City. Chair of Episcopal Bishop of New York's Committee on AIDS Ministries. Formerly, Pastoral Care Coordinator for Patients with AIDS, St. Luke's-Roosevelt Hospital Center.

Nirmal K. Fernando, MD. Assistant Professor of Infectious Disease, University of Medicine and Dentistry of New Jersey-Rutgers Medical School.

Peter B. Goldblum, PhD, MPH. Educational Developmental Specialist; University of California, San Francisco, AIDS Health Project.

Benjamin Greer, MD. In private practice in San Francisco, East Bay, California.

Helen L. Grierson, PhD. Assistant Professor of Pathology and Laboratory Medicine, University of Nebraska Medical Center, Omaha.

Isabel C. Guerrero, MD. Medical Director, Mid-state Correctional Facility Hospital, New Jersey; private practice in infectious diseases and internal medicine. Former Medical Epidemiologist, Centers for Disease Control, Atlanta, Georgia.

Robert L. Hirsch, MD. Former Medical Director, Greater New York Blood Program, New York Blood Center, now retired.

Peter Ho, MD. Until his untimely death from lymphoma, Dr. Ho was with the Department of Infectious Disease, St. Michael's Medical Center, Newark, New Jersey.

Edward S. Johnson, MD. Assistant Director of Infectious Disease, Director of AIDS Clinic and AIDS Hotline, St. Michael's Medical Center, Newark, New Jersey.

Alan C. Koenigsfest, BS in Criminal Justice. Administrative Analyst I, New Jersey Department of Corrections, Central Office.

Philip R. Lee, MD. Professor of Social Medicine, Director, Institute for Health Policy Studies, University of California, San Francisco.

Virginia Lehman, MSW, ACSW. Department of Social Work, Bellevue Hospital Center, New York, affiliated with New York University School of Medicine.

Jeffrey Levi. Executive Director, National Gay and Lesbian Task Force, Washington, DC.

Thomas H. Murray, PhD. Professor, Ethics and Public Policy, Institute for the Medical Humanities, University of Texas Medical Branch, Galveston.

Mary Cuff Plante, RN, MA, CS. Clinical Instructor of Medicine, New York University Medical Center, New York City.

Abby R. Rubenfeld, Esq. Legal Director, Lambda Legal Defense and Education Fund, New York City.

Arye Rubinstein, MD. Professor of Pediatrics, Microbiology, and Immunology; Director, NIH AIDS Research Project, Albert Einstein College of Medicine, New York City.

Noreen Russell, MSW, ACSW. New York University School of Medicine; clinical social worker in private practice in New York City.

Leonard Scarpinato, DO, MACP. In private practice, internal medicine, Long Beach CA; Assistant Director of Medical Education, Pacific Hospital, Long Beach; Assistant Professor of Internal Medicine, College of Osteopathic Medicine of the Pacific; Los Angeles County AIDS Forum; Long Beach AD HOC AIDS Committee.

Michael Scoppetuolo, MD. Associate attending at Clara Maas Medical Center, Belleville, New Jersey; Adjunct attending Solid Tumor Service at Memorial-Sloan Kettering Hospital, New York City.

John W. Sensakovic, PhD, MD. Director of Nosocomial Disease Laboratory, Director Medical Education, St. Michael's Medical Center, Newark, New Jersey.

Daniel Shindler, MD. Assistant Professor of Medicine, University of Medicine and Dentistry of New Jersey-Rutgers Medical School.

Mervyn F. Silverman, MD, MPH. President, American Foundation for AIDS Research; Director, The Robert Wood Johnson Foundation, AIDS Health Services Program.

Jeffrey Vieira, MD. Chief, Infectious Diseases Service, The Brooklyn Hospital-The Caledonian Hospital, Brooklyn, NY.